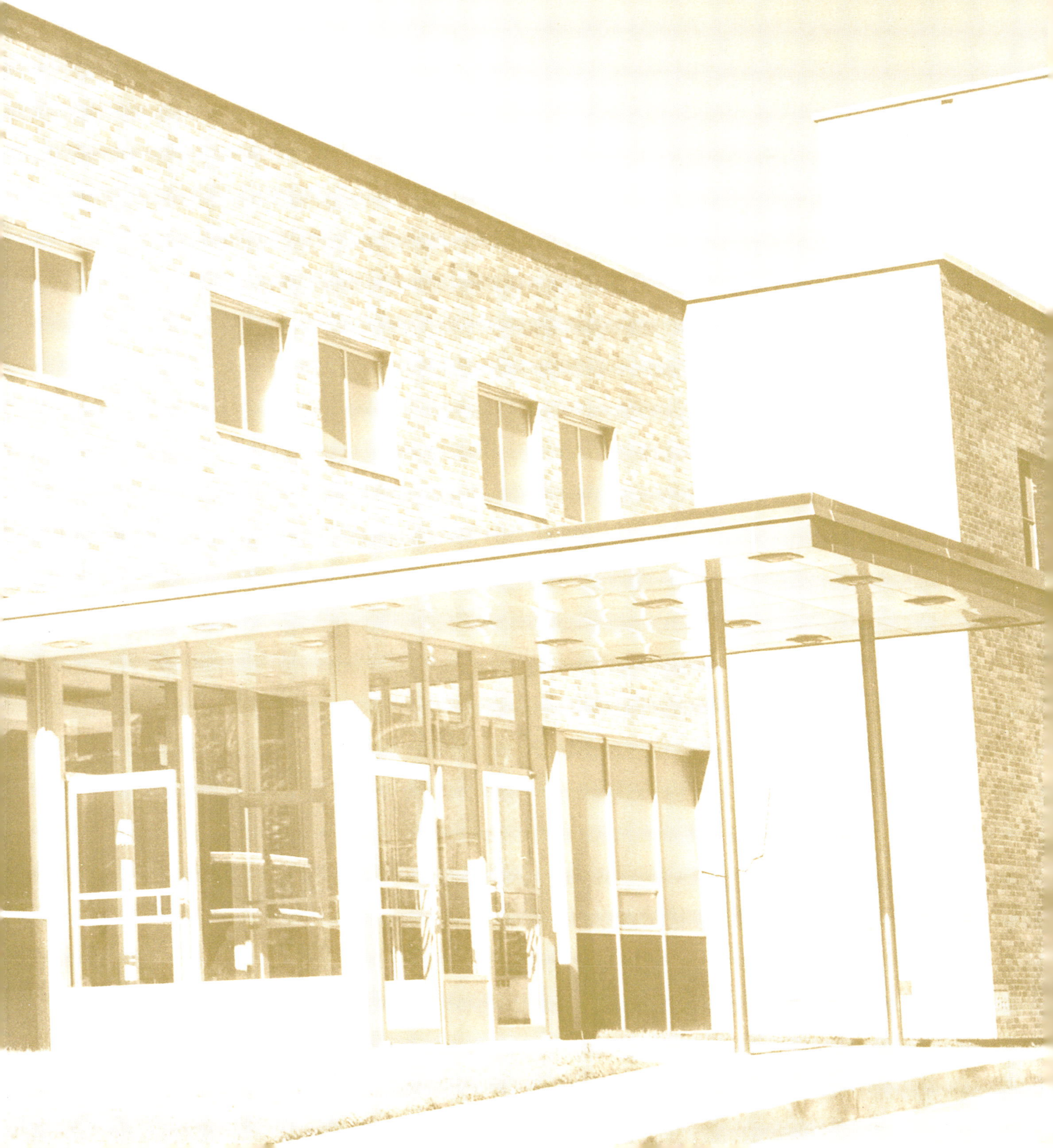

INDIANA
1914 — 2014
REGIONAL MEDICAL CENTER

Honoring our past — 100th Anniversary — Embracing our Future

BY PATRICIA SWINGER

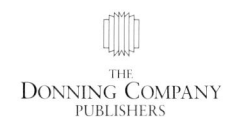

THE
DONNING COMPANY
PUBLISHERS

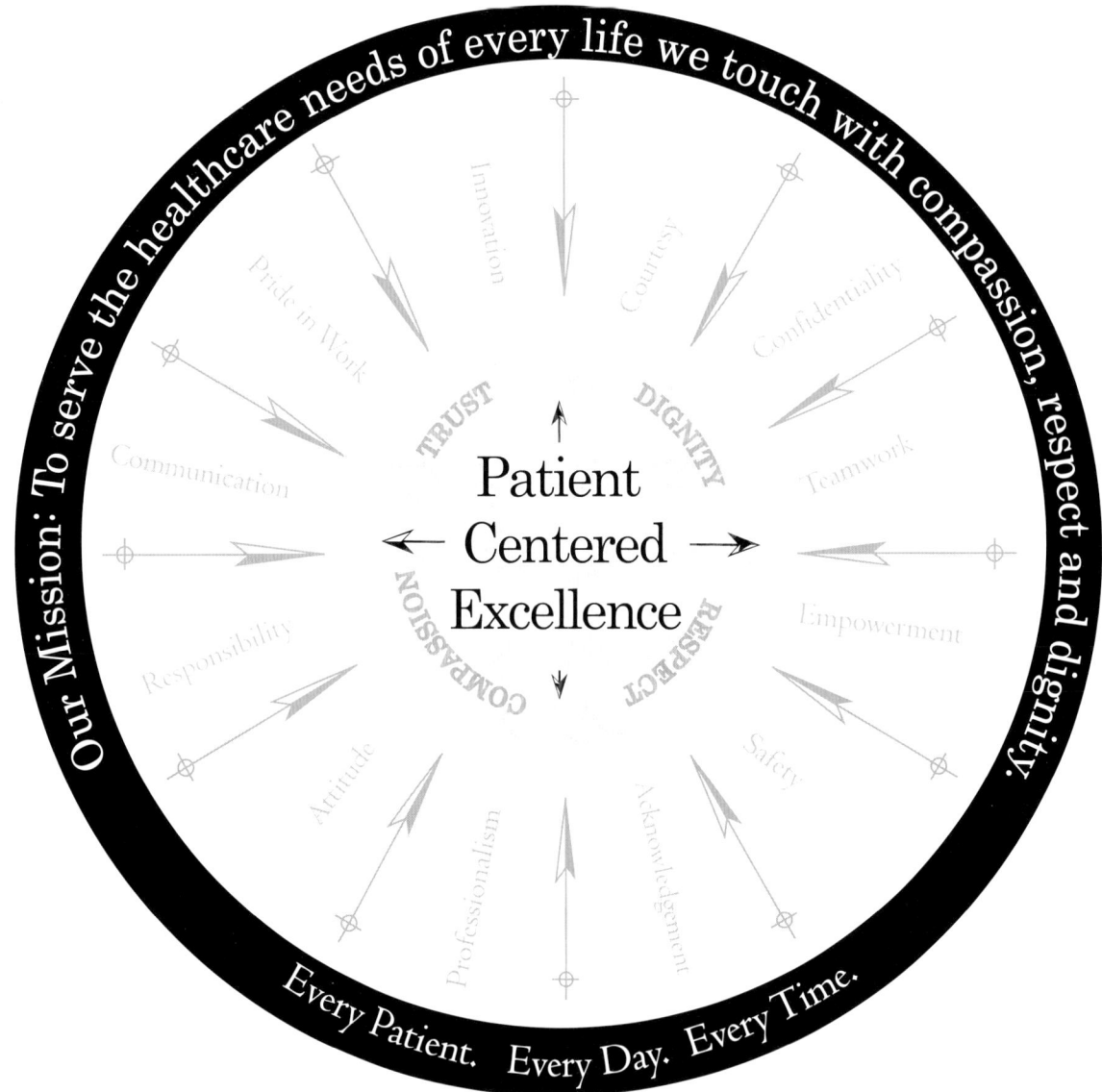

Mission, Vision & Values

Mission
To serve the healthcare needs of every life we touch with compassion, respect and dignity

Vision
To be the best community Hospital in the country

Values
Patient-Centered Excellence, Respect, Compassion, Dignity and Trust

Honoring Our Past

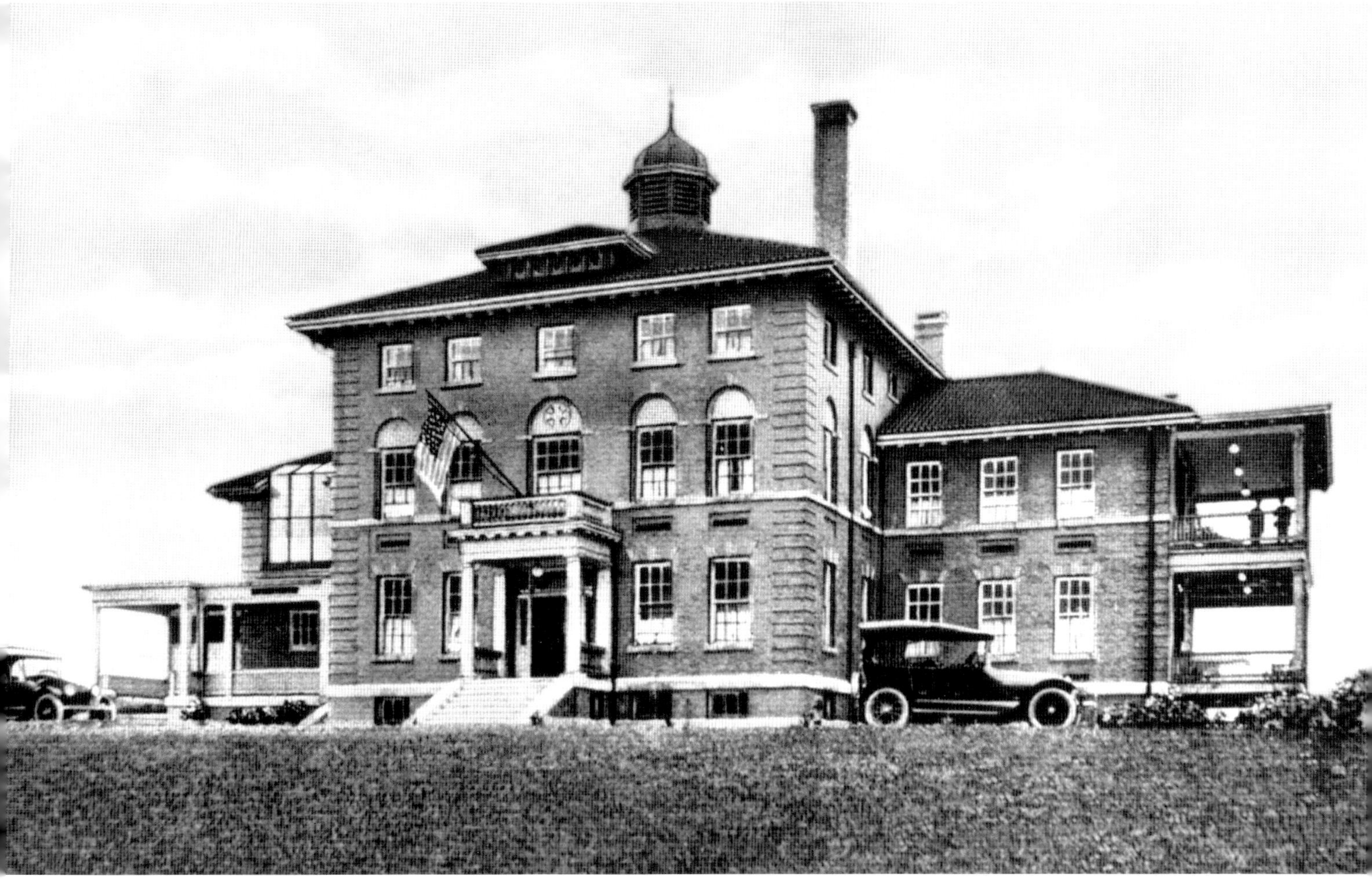

Embracing Our Future

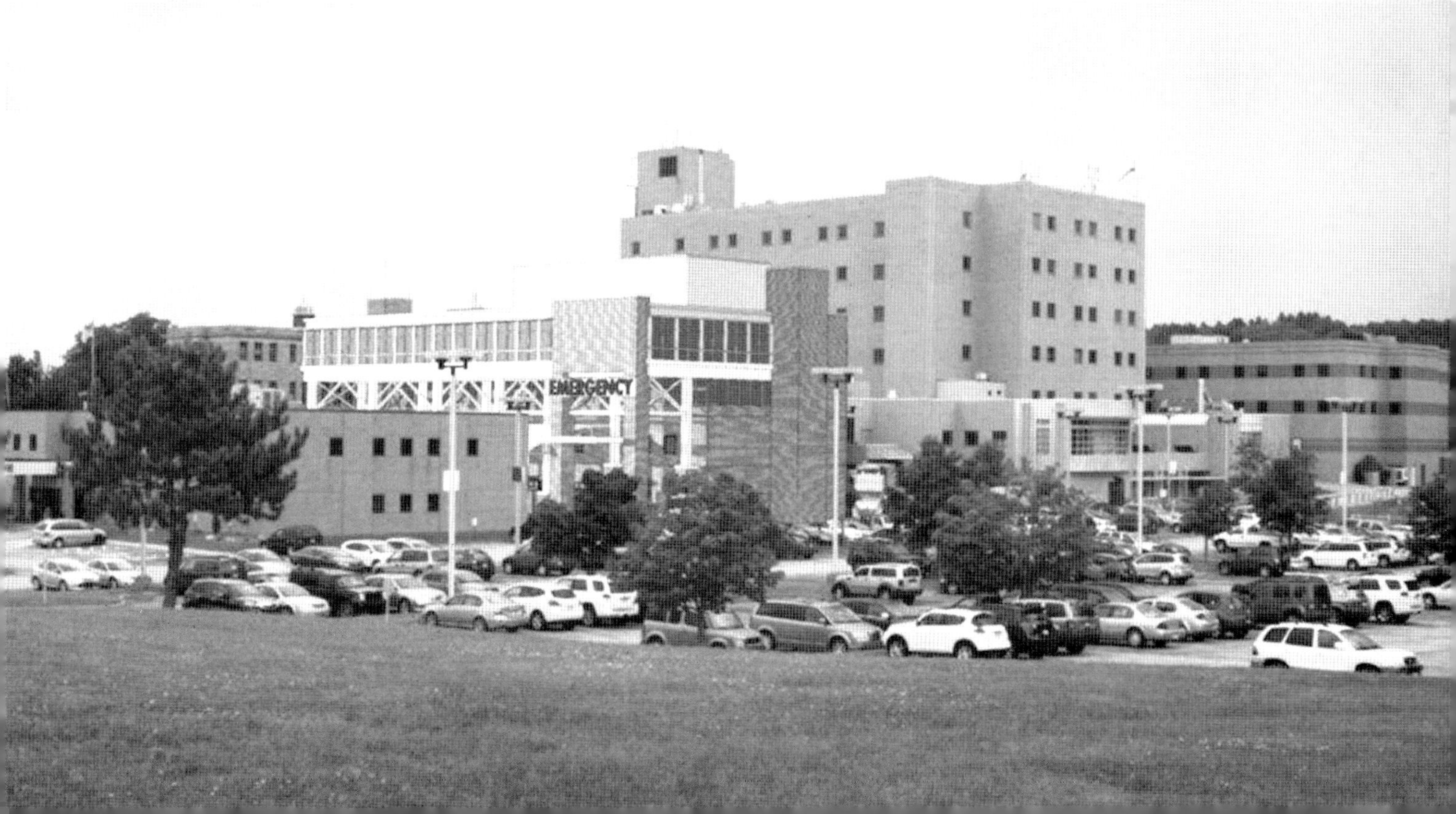

Copyright © 2014 by Indiana Regional Medical Center

All rights reserved, including the right to reproduce this work in any form whatsoever without permission in writing from the publisher, except for brief passages in connection with a review. For information, please write:

The Donning Company Publishers
184 Business Park Drive, Suite 206
Virginia Beach, VA 23462

Steve Mull, General Manager
Barbara Buchanan, Office Manager
Pamela Koch, Senior Editor
Brett Oliver, Graphic Designer
Kathy Adams, Imaging Artist
Nathan Stufflebean, Research and Marketing Supervisor
Susan Adams, Project Research Coordinator

Mary Miller, Project Director

Library of Congress Cataloging-in-Publication Data

Swinger, Patricia, 1951– author.
  Indiana Regional Medical Center 1914–2014 : honoring our past, embracing our future / by Patricia Swinger.
    p. ; cm.
  Includes bibliographical references.
  ISBN 978-1-57864-859-7 (hard cover : alk. paper)
  I. Title.
  [DNLM: 1. Indiana Regional Medical Center (Indiana, Pa.) 2. Indiana Hospital (Indiana, Pa.) 3. Hospitals, Community—history—Pennsylvania. 4. History, 20th Century—Pennsylvania. WX 28 AP4]
  RA981.P4
  362.1109748'89—dc23
                    2013029122

Printed in the United States of America at Walsworth Publishing Company

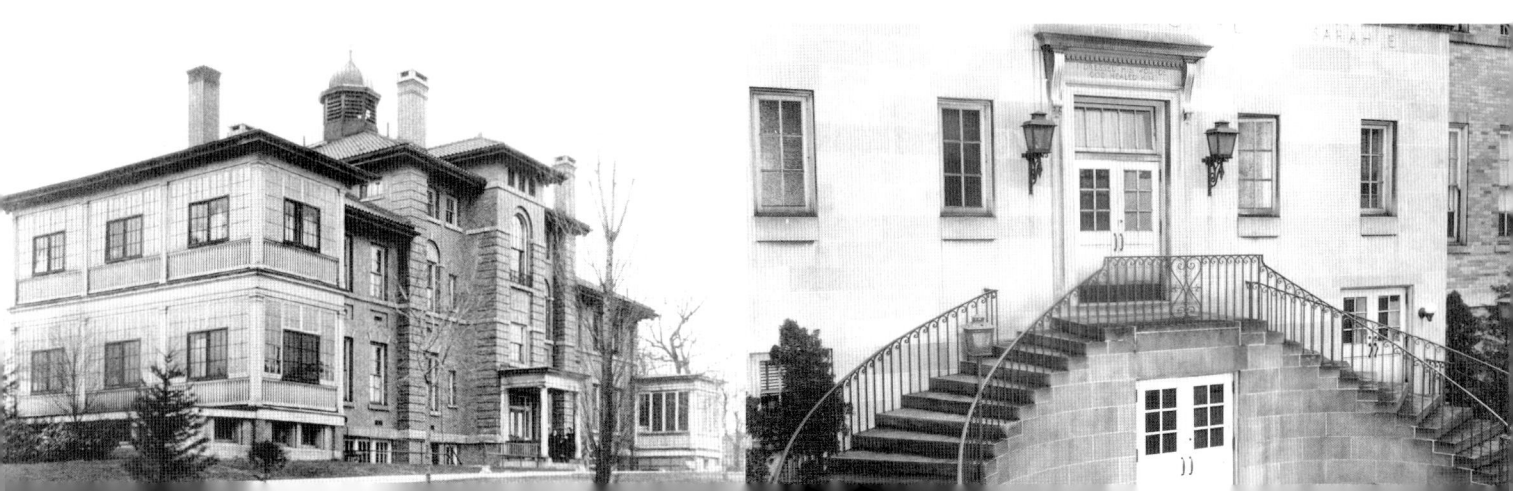

CONTENTS

Foreword
—6—

Acknowledgments
—7—

Chapter 1: The Origins of Indiana Hospital
—8—

Chapter 2: The Women of Indiana Hospital
—20—

Chapter 3: A Sense of Civic Duty
—28—

Chapter 4: The "Hospital on the Hill" Matures
—36—

Chapter 5: Turbulence, Tradition, and the Tower
—52—

Chapter 6: The Preferred Regional Health Services Provider
—70—

Chapter 7: A New Era, A New Commitment, A New Identity
—90—

Chapter 8: Honoring Our Past, Embracing Our Future
—114—

IRMC Family Album
—130—

Selected References
—142—

About the Author
—144—

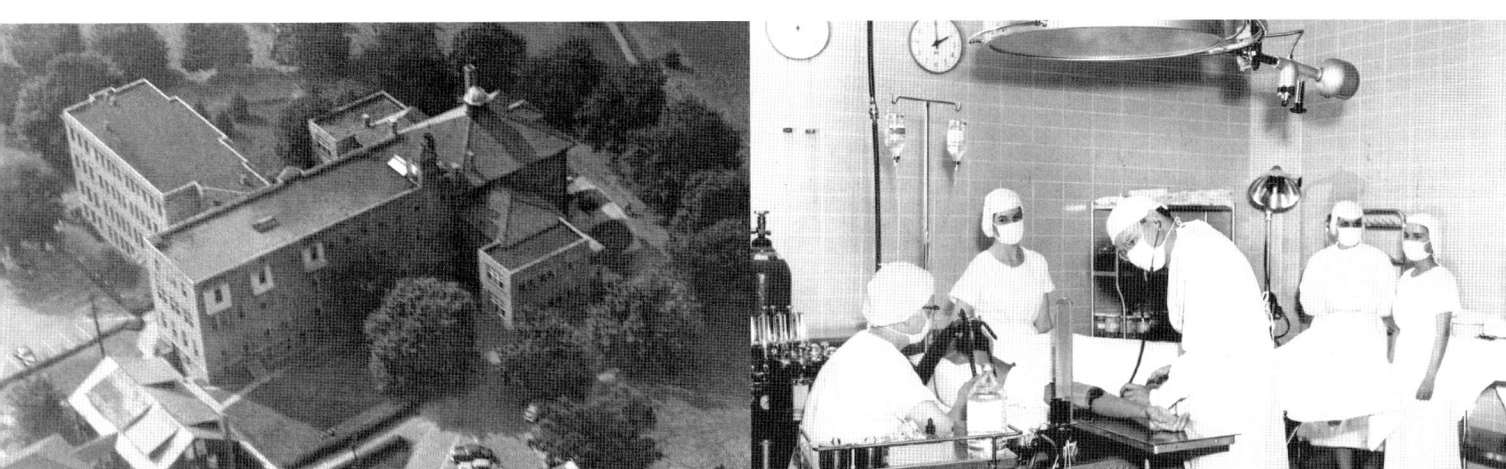

FOREWORD

Dr. Charles Rink, an Indiana Hospital physician, offered the following resolution on the death of Dr. Benjamin Coe:

Medical practice in all of its branches is both science and art. One who practices the science alone becomes the machine of Medicine. One who practices the art alone becomes the quack and charlatan of Medicine. One who practices both the science and art and adds to these, devotion to his profession, a sincerity of purpose, and loyalty to his patients has a combination of qualities that makes his professional life outstanding in any community.

Written in the board of directors minutes
—dated December 1938

We have been blessed over one hundred years to have outstanding physicians who are selfless and committed to the cause of providing the very best health care to the communities we serve. They have always been and will be in the forefront of our thoughts, actions, and decisions. We vow to work with them to perfect the art and science of medicine and its delivery to the communities we serve.

Over our one hundred years, it would be immeasurable to calculate that difference that this hospital—which became a regional medical center in 2002—has made in the quality of life of the citizens of Indiana County and beyond. We have been caretakers for their health and well-being, and business stewards for the economic impact it has had on the region. It is nothing to be taken for granted, and as we move forward, the number of community hospitals is going to dwindle. We believe we are in a very unique position to try to maintain that community ownership here, but it is going to become very rare. It is a blessing to the community.

We are also very blessed to have a robust business community and the tradition of partnering we have within it. Indiana is an incredible community. We are so fortunate to

Administrators

September 23, 1914
Dr. F. F. Moore of Lucerne selected as physician in charge of the hospital for the first six months.

October 15, 1914–December 3, 1917
Miss Sara Mogart of Johnstown
First Superintendent of the hospital
Resigned for Red Cross Duty—WWI

December 3, 1917–September 1, 1918
Miss Eliza Dill elected Acting Superintendent
Resigned for Red Cross Duty—WWI

September 8, 1918–August 1920
Miss Bess F. Dale elected Acting Superintendent
Elected as the Superintendent in November 1919

July 26, 1920–June 1922
Miss Lenore Byers, Superintendent

May 23, 1922–May 1929
Mrs. E. F. Allison, Superintendent

July 7, 1929–March 1, 1944
Miss Lillian A. Hollohan, Superintendent
Granted a 3-month leave of absence due to ill health
Miss Adeline Hauxhurst appointed Acting Superintendent
Miss Hollohan returned on December 15, 1943, and Miss Hauxhurst became Assistant Administrator

March 15, 1944–May 1, 1965
Miss Adeline W. Hauxhurst, Superintendent

May 1, 1965–June 1, 1966
Mr. William Peters, Administrator

June 1, 1966–April 14, 1967
Miss Adeline W. Hauxhurst, Interim Administrator

April 17, 1967–May 1, 1970
Mr. George Ferrey, Administrator

June 10, 1970–September 28, 1981
Mr. Donald Smith, Administrator

September 28, 1981–February 22, 1982
Dr. Henry Mitchell, Interim Administrator

February 22, 1982–September 30, 1983
Mr. Donald Valentine, Chief Executive Officer

September 30, 1983–December 28, 1984
Administrative Committee
Larry Marshall, Dr. Larry Kachik, Mrs. Leona Shank, and Mr. Jeryl Gates

December 28, 1984–May 7, 1998
Mr. Donald Sandoval, President and Chief Executive Officer

May 7, 1998–February 11, 1999
Dr. Robert Parker, Acting President and Chief Executive Officer

February 11, 1999–Present
Mr. Stephen A. Wolfe, President and Chief Executive Officer

live in an area where it is so beautiful. It is not an urban setting, but it has a nice blend of people and business. As a former Chamber president, I had the opportunity to interact with all the great businesses that are out there, providing jobs and growing our county. We believe the hospital is a very important part of that economic development as well. If you do not have a first-class acute care hospital, it is going to be very difficult to recruit and retain future business—especially if you are not delivering babies, taking care of children, and providing care to all segments of our population.

In our unique case, it is not about shareholders. This hospital is owned and run by the community.

So many generations have sacrificed and worked hard so we could have what we have today to try to make the most of those assets. For generations, many worked for hardly anything at all; it was really a mission, a ministry. I am just honored to be a small part of where we are now and where we are headed.

On behalf of Indiana Regional Medical Center, I would like to thank everyone who has played a role in our evolution. As the title explains, we will continue to honor our humble past, and embrace our exciting future.

Stephen A. Wolfe, President & CEO

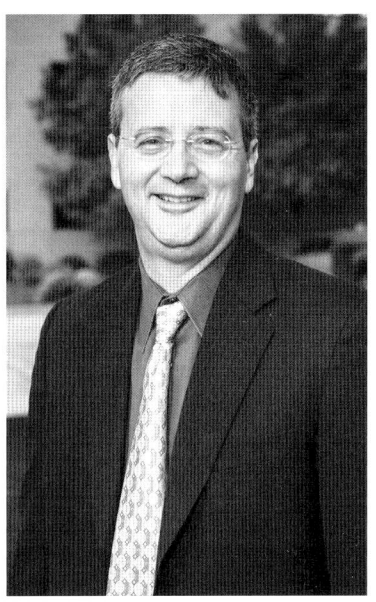

ACKNOWLEDGMENTS

Indiana Regional Medical Center would like to thank the members of the 100th Anniversary Committee who have given so much of their time to prepare a memorable commemoration of this historic moment in the hospital's history. We want to extend a special thanks to Laura Jeffrey, who spent untold hours searching for photos, scouring through records to check facts, and working with the author to complete the manuscript.

Robert Parker, MD, Chair	Heather Reed
James Garrettson, MD	Mark Richards
Louise Hildebrand	Marge Scheeren
Laura Jeffrey	Larry Sedlemeyer
Stephen Margita	Nancy Smith
Jim Miller	Cindy Virgil
Diane Petras	Dawn Zoldak

In addition, we would like to thank those who were also willing to give of their time to be interviewed for the book in order to tell this worthwhile story.

Ralph Brown, MD
John Busovicki, historian
Alex Juhasz, MD
Bernice Leslie, RN
Edward McDowell, MD
Dominic Paccapaniccia
Danny Sacco
James Wakefield, Mack descendant
Dr. and Mrs. Ralph Waldo
Eileen Watchko
Dr. and Mrs. Melvin Williams
Stephen A. Wolfe

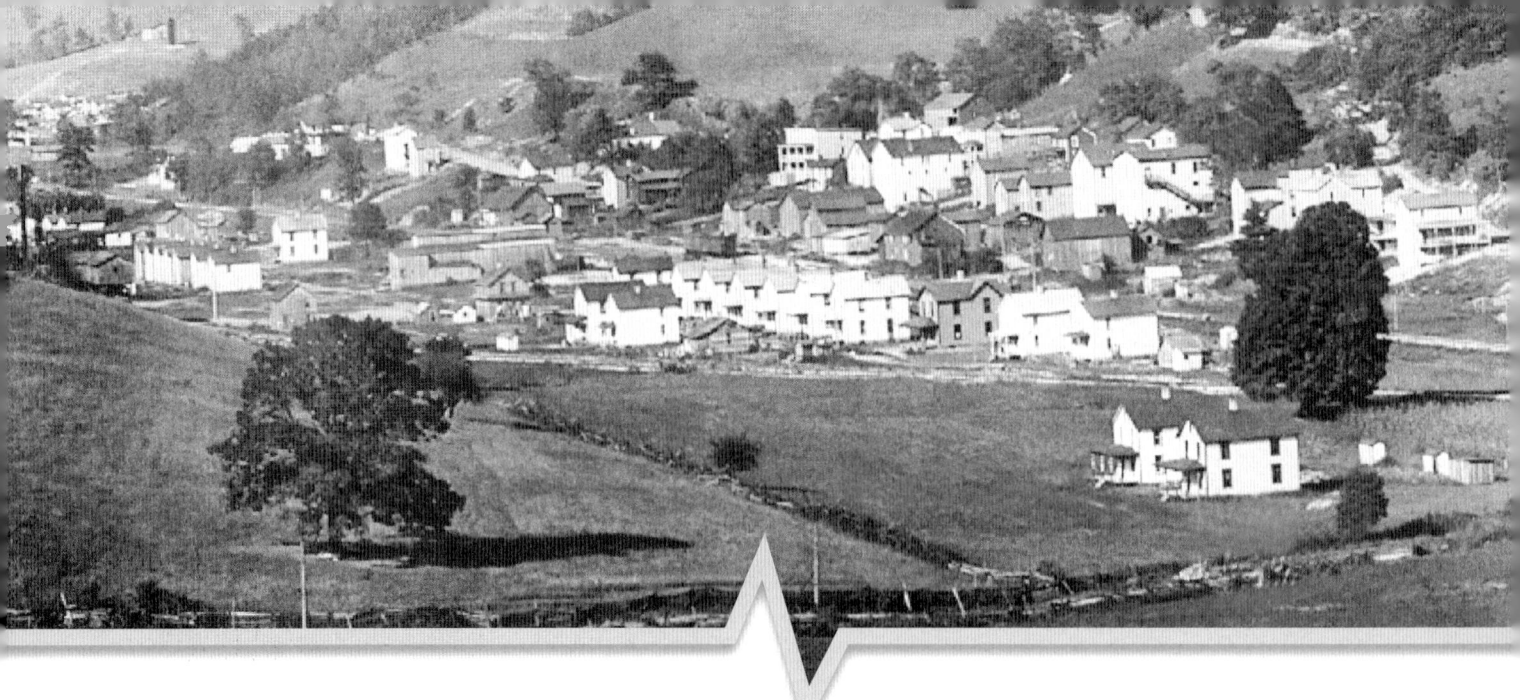

CHAPTER 1

The Origins of Indiana Hospital

*"How many desolate creatures on the earth
have learnt the simple dues of fellowship
and social comfort, in a hospital."*
—Elizabeth Barrett Browning

In the early 1800s, and for nearly another century to come, most Americans gave birth and endured illness and even surgery at home. And so it was in Indiana County at the time. Many of the early hospitals emerged from institutions—notably almshouses—that provided care and custody for the ailing poor. Rooted in this tradition of charity, numerous hospitals can trace their ancestry to community efforts to shelter and care for the chronically ill, deprived, and disabled. Other hospitals resulted from efforts to provide essential civilian disaster relief, such as in neighboring Cambria County when Clara Barton and the Red Cross assisted with the 1889 Johnstown Flood.

Religious orders began caring for the ill, the insane, and the indigent in the early 1800s. Some of the hospitals started by the St. Vincent de Paul Sisters of Charity remain in operation to this day, and the Protestant nursing movement, which began in Germany, came to Pennsylvania in 1850. That trend, the belief that we all have both a moral and spiritual obligation to care for those less fortunate than ourselves, remains a vital component of medical care to this day. When Indiana Hospital was first organized, its seal consisted of a "circular device depicting the Good Samaritan assisting the wounded traveler." And when John S. Mack's donation made Indiana Hospital's first major expansion possible, engraved in the stone over the new wing's entrance was the phrase, "I dressed his wounds; God healed him."

Life in rural early America, though hard and fraught with challenges, was at least free of the plagues and infirmities brought on by the crowded and impoverished

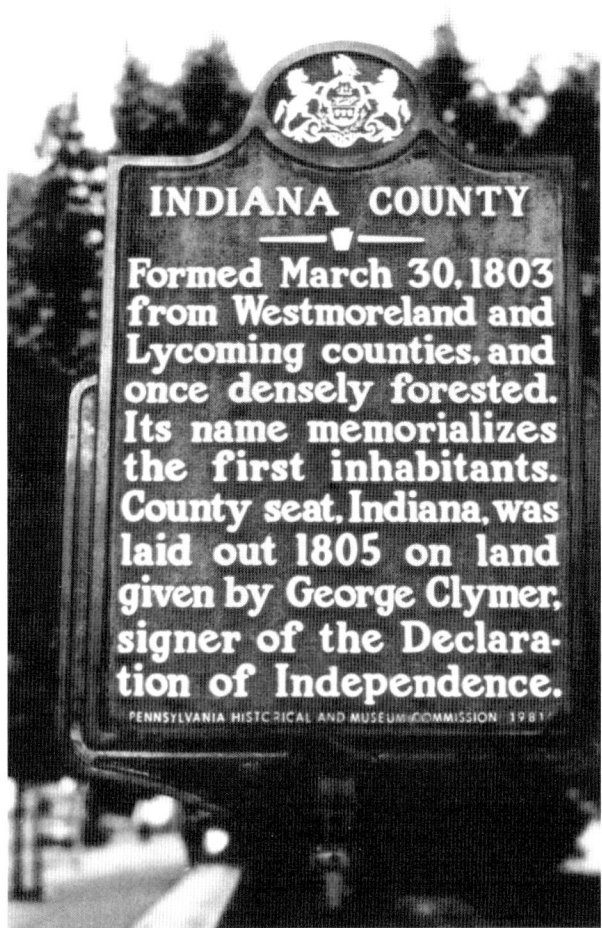

The people of Indiana County treasure their proud history, which includes its earliest Native Americans, the colonists who played an integral part in the Revolutionary War, and the many immigrants who came here seeking a better life.

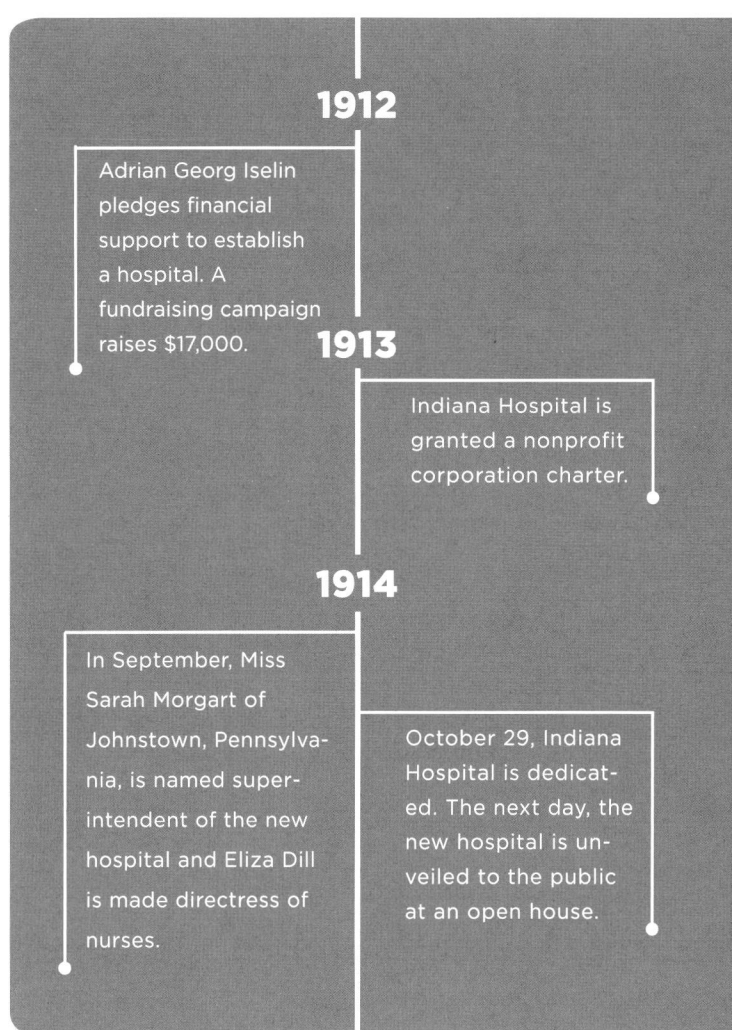

1912
Adrian Georg Iselin pledges financial support to establish a hospital. A fundraising campaign raises $17,000.

1913
Indiana Hospital is granted a nonprofit corporation charter.

1914
In September, Miss Sarah Morgart of Johnstown, Pennsylvania, is named superintendent of the new hospital and Eliza Dill is made directress of nurses.

October 29, Indiana Hospital is dedicated. The next day, the new hospital is unveiled to the public at an open house.

conditions of America's early industrial and urban areas. While life expectancies in 1850 hovered around forty, that statistic is misleading, distorted by the fact that work-related injuries on the farm and elsewhere were often fatal. For women, childbirth posed a major threat. One in eight births resulted in loss of the mother's life. Like most things, health care was a do-it-yourself proposition. With few physicians available and most of them minimally trained, common illnesses were treated with home remedies handed down from generation to generation.

The American hospital as we know it today emerged over the course of about sixty years, beginning around the time of the Civil War. Physician-staffed hospitals with professional nursing and specialized departments and services were products of urbanization and economic expansion during the Second Industrial Revolution. About 1880, asepsis (sterilizing) opened broad new horizons for medicine, and as health care providers looked to the future with a new sense of hope, hospitals became symbolic of their new optimism and authority.

Of all the institutions in U.S. society, the hospital evolved to become the most appreciated, most aligned, and often least understood. Besides serving as havens of healing for the sick and injured, hospitals also became a "business," branching into research and education, and often becoming one of the largest employers in the community. Given all that they have become—and will yet transform into—hospitals will always indelibly be identified with the communities they serve.

The first physician recorded as having actually located in Indiana was Dr. Jonathan French. A native of New Hampshire, Dr. French received his medical education in Vermont. He practiced first in York, Pennsylvania, and then in nearby Kittanning, before moving to Indiana in 1807 where he practiced until his death in August 1814.

Indiana County itself had only been organized since 1803. George Clymer, signer of the Declaration of Independence and a substantial contributor to George Washington and his troops, donated 250 acres of his own land to form the center of the county seat. Indiana County's first major town was Saltsburg where, between 1813 and 1860, roughly one-third of all the salt in the United States was produced. In 1818, Blairsville was founded and played an important role as a port city along the Connemaugh River.

Indiana County's earliest industry, besides agriculture, was lumber. By 1820 seventeen sawmills were busy cutting oak, pine, hickory, and hemlock. Towns sprang up when loggers and lumberjacks brought their families with them to camp. By 1840 the number of sawmills had grown to seventy-four. The logging industry in Indiana County kept pace with another vital industry—coal. Used to boil the saltwater from which the salt was extracted, nearly 20,000 tons of coal were being produced annually by 1840.

Indiana County's early industries, and the injuries and illnesses that resulted from them, were the primary impetus for the development of the county's various hospitals. Twelve years passed from the time the idea of Indiana Hospital was conceived to the day it welcomed its first patients. In the interim, a number of small hospitals opened, most of them extensions of a physician's private practice, while a community of people learned how to work together for a common purpose.

The timing was just right. During the early 1900s, a number of factors contributed to the growth and refinement of hospitals across the country. For one, science was advancing and expanding the medical profession's knowledge. The industrial age provided the technology needed to create the tools for diagnosing and curing illnesses—surgical tools, diagnostic equipment, and pharmaceuticals. The Progressive Movement, itself a response to the excesses and hazards of the industrial age, swept the country from 1890 to 1920. The emerging middle class, also created by America's industrialization, was now advocating for social and political reforms. Finally, at the most basic level, the industrial age brought work-related hazards like never before.

By 1914 when Indiana Hospital was organized, most of the people in Indiana County either worked on a farm or in the coal mines. The majority of the county's more than 66,000 residents were immigrants. Seeking freedom and opportunity, they came from Poland, Eastern Europe, and Italy. Immigrants from Ireland, Scotland, and Wales dominated the mines. Safety warnings posted around the mines were written in seven different languages. Despite the warnings, the accidents and illnesses that arose created the need for hospitals and the medical care they provided.

1883 THE BLAIRSVILLE INFIRMARY

By all accounts, the "Blairsville Infirmary" as it was known was the first hospital in Indiana County though no information remains to tell us how large it was. Founded in 1883 by Dr. Israel P. Klingensmith, an eminent physician and surgeon, it was located on West Market Street near Liberty Street in Blairsville. When Dr. Klingensmith died on September 28, 1904, his widow Mary and his as-

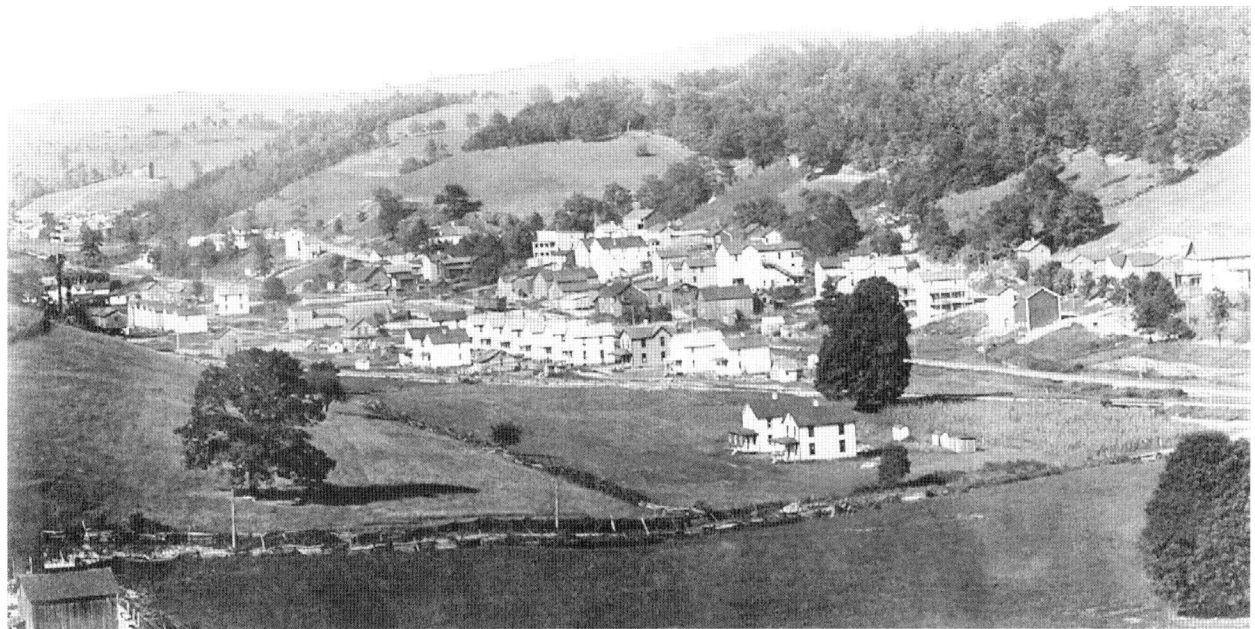
Dixonville, Pennsylvania, 1905. The large house on the far right is the Dixonville Hospital. Photo courtesy of John Busovicki.

sociate, Dr. Homer M. Wellman, continued the hospital. Facing bankruptcy, the hospital closed in 1909.

1902 INDIANA HOSPITAL

The twelve-year saga toward the organization of Indiana Hospital began in 1902 when a Grand Jury recommended that "a well-equipped hospital for the reception and treatment of diseased persons and surgical operations should be established; that the county officials should give the project aid and, if possible, assist with a substantial contribution."

A hospital association was organized, and on August 21, 1903, Mrs. Sue Williard, the association's president, conducted a mass meeting in the courthouse. A week later they reported that a local resident named A. S. Cunningham offered to donate three acres at the edge of Indiana's city limits, and that the B.R. & P. Railroad had promised at least $3,000 a year for the support of a hospital. For the next few years, nothing of note occurred toward the creation of Indiana Hospital. In the interim, two other hospitals opened: one in Dixonville and the other near Heilwood.

1905 DIXONVILLE HOSPITAL

Dr. Benjamin Coe started the Dixonville Hospital in his residence in 1905, the one most often given the distinction of being the first hospital in Indiana County. A few years later, Dr. Coe moved his family and the hospital to Clymer. According to one source, "the brick building was constructed by R. L. Ferrier of Clymer and had seventeen rooms plus an operating room and basement." Other sources tell of the addition of "a wing of two rooms plus an operating room" to the hospital. Among the papers handed down to descendants of John Mack, who would later play a very important role in the hospital's future, was a note handwritten by Mrs. Maude McDevitt, RN, though the nature of her association with Dr. Coe and the hospital remains unknown. "It can be truly said that the Dixonville Hospital and Dr. Coe were pioneers in medicine and surgery in Indiana County in 'The Horse and Buggy Days,'" she wrote. "There was no eight-hour duty in those days; every one connected with the hospital worked hard and late until the last task was finished. It was not unusual to operate in the middle of the night on a patient driven cross-country in a covered hack, sometimes an operating wagon. Many medical students just out of college were given from two to five years of training under the competent instruction and guidance of Dr. Coe, many entering the field of surgery in which every one has been very successful." The physicians working under Dr. Coe's expert tutelage included Dr. B. F. Bowers, who was the hospital's resident physician.

The other hospital was one started by a Dr. R. F. McHenry in a humble three-room miner's shanty in Heilwood. Over the next few years, Dr. McHenry moved his hospital first to a small house, which was later used as a garage, and then to a seven-room house where it remained until 1909. Apparently, the hospital was supported, at least in part, by the Penn-Mary Coal Company and is the first recorded instance of a coal company's participation in the provision of health care. The company began assessing its employees five cents per month in 1905, and the following year, mine superintendent H. P. Dowler raised it to twenty cents per month. The assessment, and the care it provided, covered only injured miners.

1907 INDIANA HOSPITAL

In early 1907, the New Century Club, a local civic organization, formed a committee "to devise plans by which a hospital could be secured." The committee members included Mrs. Williard, Mrs. G. P. McCartney, and Mrs. M. C. Watson. On March 20 a public meeting was again held, this time in Cunningham's Hall with John M. Leech serving as chairman. The committee proposed the chartering of the Indiana County Hospital Association using funds raised through subscriptions to build and furnish a hospital. Thirty directors—fifteen men and fifteen women—were elected, and Mrs. Williard was made president.

While rumors began circulating in July 1907 that a judge by the name of Harry White might donate land for the hospital, three acres on the north edge of Indiana was donated by a group of landowners. Pleased with the location, the committee announced, "The land is the very spot [they] had in view to purchase if it could not be secured as a gift."

Other donations soon followed. In August 1907, the will of T. J. Robinson, a local resident, bequeathed $1,000 to the Indiana County Hospital Association "for the purpose of endowing a bed or room to be known as the Thomas J. Robinson room or bed: said room or bed shall be for the free use of any poor American citizen of West Wheatfield Township." The will included a provision to revoke the bequest at the end of five years if the hospital failed to come to fruition.

In September 1908, the Hospital Association entered into a $10 per month, five-year lease with the County Commissioner's Office for the Elmer Campbell house, presumably to be used for the Association's office and an interim site for the hospital. Shortly thereafter, the Association applied to the State Board of Charities for a $20,000 grant, but in January 1909, the headlines read "State Refused to Help the Hospital." Apparently, no one from Indiana went to Pittsburgh for the hearings with the board officials. As Mrs. Williard herself admitted, "As all other hospitals usually have a half-dozen persons pleading for an increase, it can be seen that general apathy has more to do with the failure of the appropriation than the State Board of Charities."

1908 SIMPSON-NEAL HOSPITAL

Rumors once again began swirling throughout the community in early 1908 that Dr. George E. Simpson had plans to build a new hospital in Indiana. By that September, a headline appeared that read "Simpson Building a Modern Structure." The following February, headlines again teased the residents of Indiana

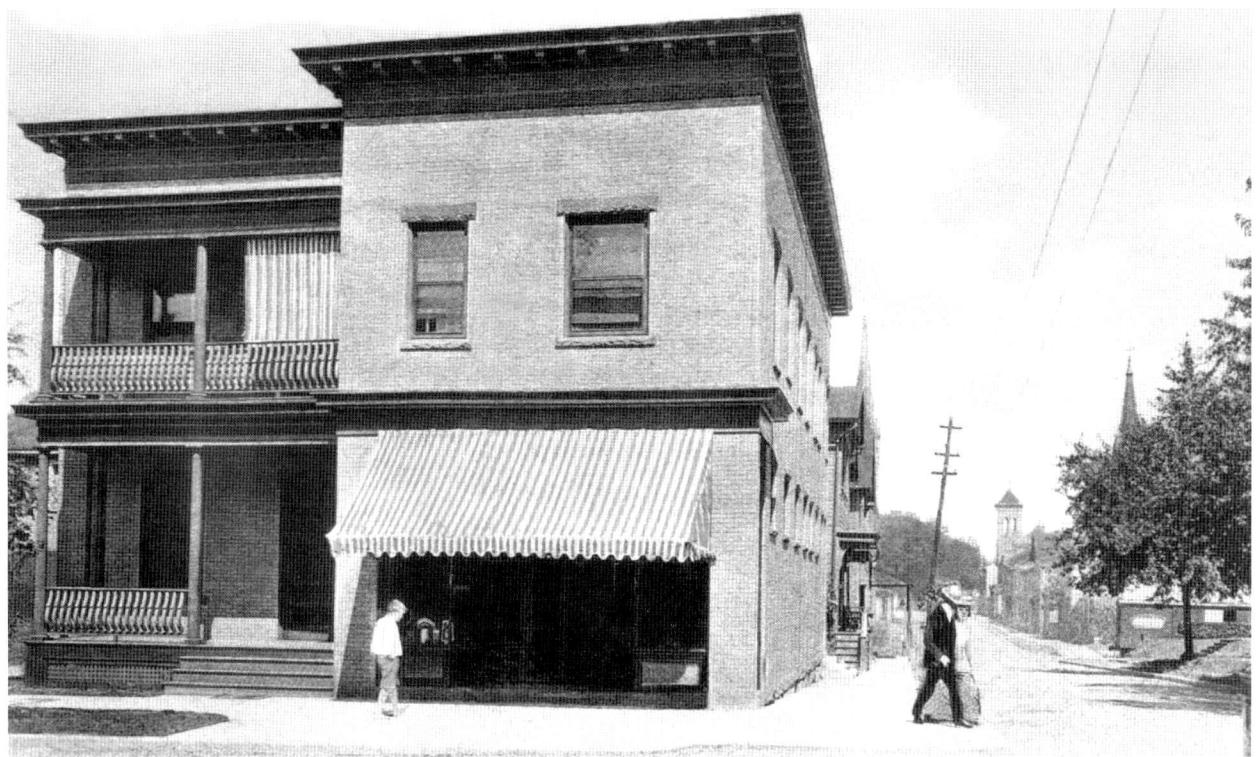

The Simpson-Neal Hospital at Church and Ninth Streets in Indiana. Photo courtesy of John Busovicki.

County announcing that Dr. Simpson and Dr. Harry B. Neal "Will Open a Hospital for Use of the Public" in "the near future." Two eager citizens, Mary Palmer and Fannie W. Nixon, who had donated equipment for two rooms in the proposed Indiana County Hospital, transferred their gift to the Simpson-Neal Hospital.

The formal opening of the hospital at the corner of Church and Ninth Streets on April 3, 1909, attracted over five hundred visitors. When the hospital opened for patients on Monday, April 5, four beds were already occupied. The entire second floor of the building was dedicated to the hospital, which had ten beds and room for five more, an operating room, a recovery room, a waiting room, and a large roomy porch. The facilities were open to all of Indiana County's approximately seventy practicing physicians. Head nurse Anna Pollock and her assistant, Miss Kelley, had apartments within the hospital.

It is this hospital that is credited with performing the first Caesarean section in an Indiana County hospital. Injured miners received first aid there and were frequently then sent by train to Punxsutawney if further treatment was required.

1908 SALTSBURG

In November 1908, Dr. E. B. Earhart purchased the Rumbaugh homestead in Saltsburg from Mrs. Eliza-

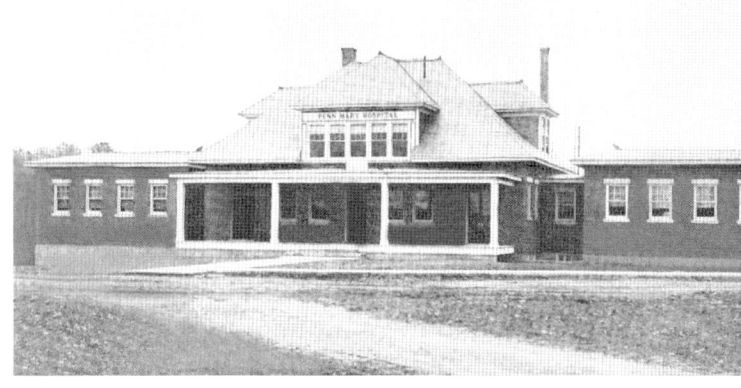

The Penn-Mary Hospital in Heilwood, 1909. Photo courtesy of John Busovicki.

beth R. Martin for $3,200. The headlines read, "Saltsburg now in line for Hospital." Though the twenty-bed hospital was expected to open in June 1, 1909, its opening was delayed until August 15, 1909.

1909 PENN-MARY

In October 1909, the Penn-Mary Coal Company expanded the little hospital first organized by Dr. McHenry by building a thoroughly modern brick hospital in Heilwood at a cost of $25,000. It had two wards, four private rooms, and an operating room furnished by funds assessed from the miners since 1905. A local citizen, Raymond Malengo, chronicled the hospital's new location as "one of the most beautiful spots in Indiana County," and noted, "The corners were all rounded—not a right-angled corner in the building," he said. The first building erected solely for hospital purposes in Indiana County, it remained under the charge of Dr. McHenry.

The June 7, 1916, edition of the *Indiana Progress* described the hospital in glowing detail.

> At the front entrance is a large waiting room for American people and a nurses' office. The physicians' rooms, nurses' office, dining room and a living room are fitted out with plain oak. The balance of the building is furnished with sanitary steel enameled furniture. All doors are four feet wide and made of sanitary enameled oak. All fixtures are brass or nickel, perfectly plain.

> The building has modern equipment of electric lights, which are detachable and transferable, the light being furnished from the power plant at the works of the coal company. The heat is the most modern hot water system obtainable. Sterilizers for the operating rooms and typhoid sterilizers are equipped with fifteen horsepower high steam pressure boiler, which also supplies the high pressure steam to the laundry which is arranged for the immediate sterilization of soiled linens, or other materials.

> Off the operating room is an etherizing room, which is perfectly plain. In this room all anesthetics are started, thus avoiding all shock to the patient from sight of instruments or by preparation in the operating room.

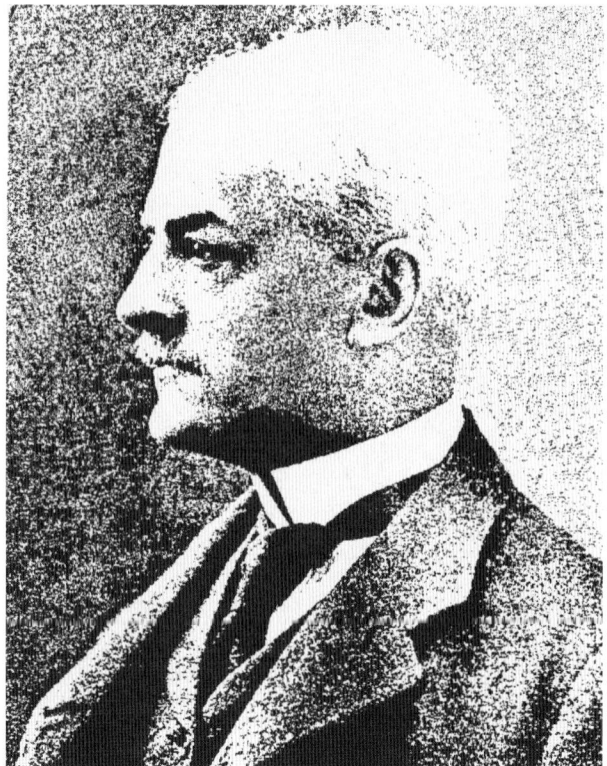

Adrian Georg Iselin Jr., 1846-1935, was a prime benefactor to Indiana Hospital.

Up until now, the predecessors to the Penn-Mary Hospital had been only for the treatment of injured miners. But with the new hospital, the assessment was increased to forty cents per month and covered both accidental injuries and illnesses of all Penn-Mary Coal Company employees and their families. According to one article written by Bill Graff of the *Indiana Gazette*, others were charged one dollar a day for ward services and fifteen dollars per week for private rooms. Twenty-four patients could be cared for in the wards.

The Iselin Family Connection

Adrian Iselin Jr. was born in 1846, the first son in a family of Swiss investment bankers who lived in New York City. His father, Adrian Sr., was the chief investor in the Rochester and Pittsburgh Coal and Iron Company, whose first mines were located in Jefferson County, Pennsylvania, in an area known as the Saw Mill Run Valley. By 1890, the company had acquired over five thousand acres of coal lands. The company had also purchased several small railroads, which they consolidated into one large railway company, the Buffalo, Rochester and Pittsburgh Railroad.

When Adrian Jr. took the helm following his father's death in 1905, he expanded the company into Indiana County, Pennsylvania. Following in his father's footsteps, Adrian Jr. was an ardent philanthropist. Before Indiana Hospital, the family was also responsible for building the Adrian Hospital in Punxsutawney.

1912 INDIANA HOSPITAL

After another three-year lull, Mrs. Williard called another meeting of the Indiana County Hospital Association in 1912. John A. Scott received a letter from Adrian Iselin Jr. of New York City, whose wealth from both the railroad and coal industries was substantial. In his letter, Mr. Iselin offered to contribute at least $40,000 toward a hospital building provided that local citizens could find a suitable site, prepare it for construction, and then take charge of the hospital once built. A committee of seven consisting of John Scott as chairman, T. E. Hildebrand, Rev. N. P. McNelis, J. R. Richards, Joseph W. Clements, P. McGovern, and Elder Peelor was appointed to take on the task. They raised $17,000 and purchased a fifty-four-acre tract just south of the fairgrounds from the George C. Dickey estate and Edward and Joseph P. Mack for $16,500.

Judge S. J. Telford granted the hospital's charter in January 1913, and a board of directors was chosen consisting of John P. Elkin, president; John Fisher, vice president; J. Wood Clark, secretary; T. E. Hildebrand,

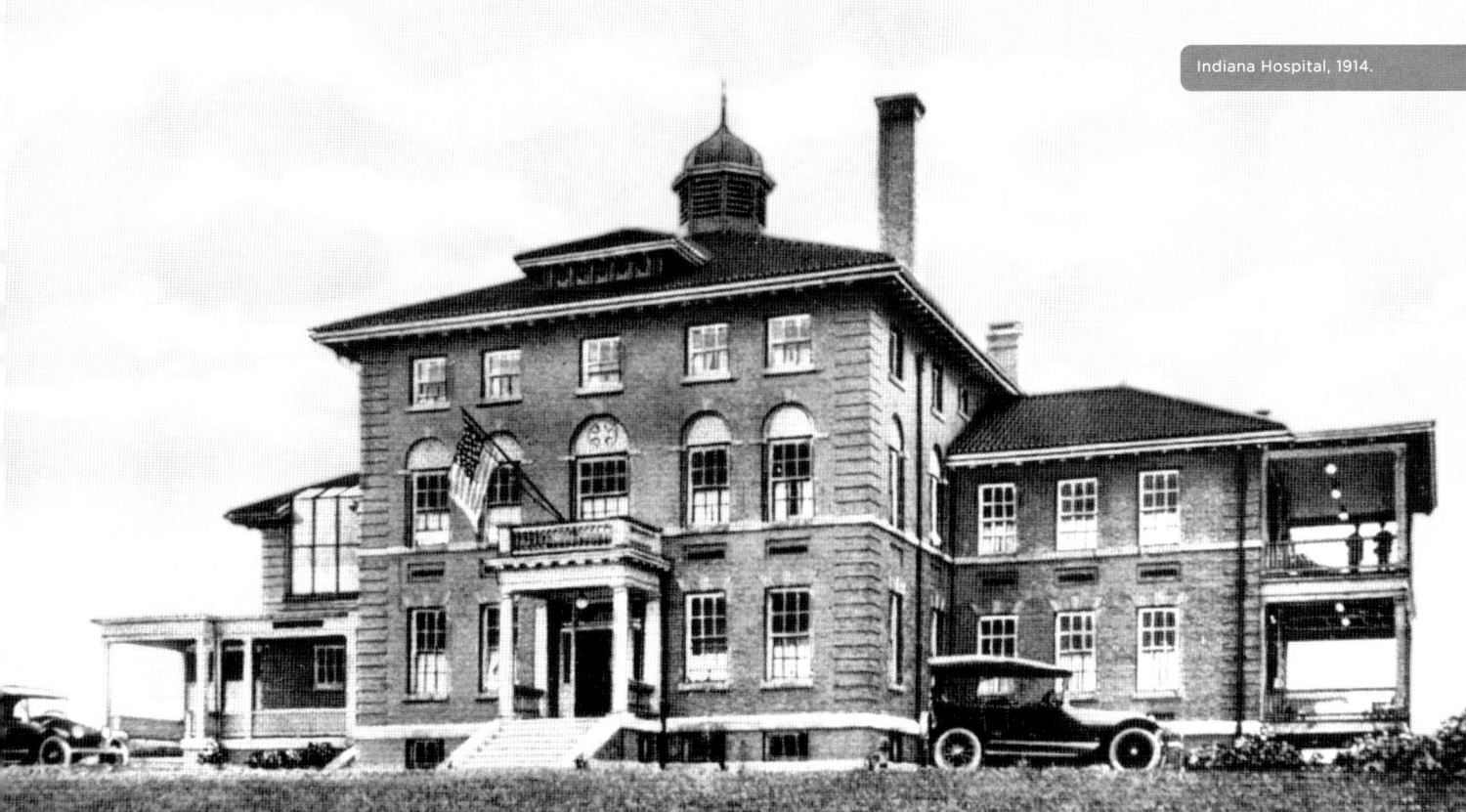

Indiana Hospital, 1914.

treasurer; and L. W. Robinson, Harry W. Wilson, Mrs. Williard, Miss Mary McKnight, Joseph W. Clements, A. W. Calloway, A. S. Cunningham, Henry Hall, A. W. Mabon, Rev. N. P. McNelis, John A. Scott, and D. B. Taylor. On April 5, a subcommittee from the House Committee on Appropriations visited Indiana for the purpose of looking over the site for the proposed new hospital, which was seeking state aid. The subcommittee "let it be known that a favorable report would be returned to the general committee."

In addition to the funds raised to purchase the land, the Board of Directors spent $9,000 to grade the site, install sewers and electric lines, and build a 1,500-foot-long concrete roadway, unusual in those days, leading to the hospital. The building was erected by Hyde-Murphy Company, Rochester and Pittsburgh Coal Company's trust firm of contractors, at a cost of $125,000, which Adrian Iselin Jr. donated in memory of his wife, Louise. With a footprint of 80´ x 140´, it consisted of three stories plus a basement. With accommodations for forty-five beds, the hospital had thirteen private rooms, most of them on the third floor and three of which were to be used by the superintendent and nurses. Miss Georgine Iselin, sister of Adrian Iselin, donated $16,000 worth of equipment and furniture. Eight physicians and surgeons were elected to serve Indiana Hospital for one year without compensation. They included physicians Dr. W. A. Simpson, Dr. H. B. Buterbaugh, Dr. William F. Weitzel, all of Indiana, and Dr. A. W. Clark of Ernest. The surgeons were Dr. G. E. Simpson and Dr. William D. Gates of Indiana, Dr. Berry F. Coe of Clymer and Dr. R. F. McHenry of Heilwood.

The Iselin family entourage arrived at the hospital's dedication by train on October 29, 1914, greeted by local dignitaries amid a great deal of fanfare. The Honorable John P. Elkin, associate justice of the Pennsyl-

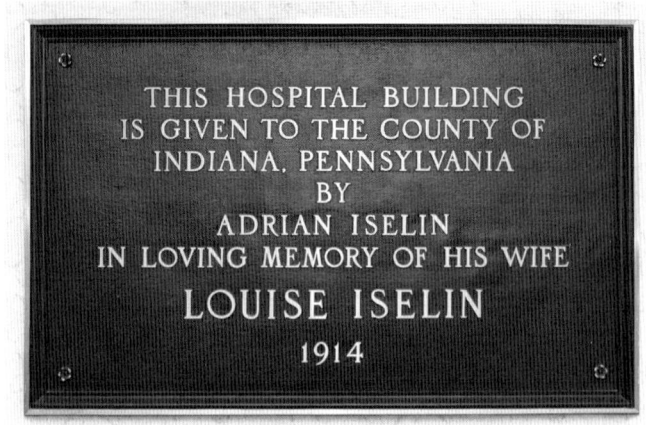

This original plaque dedicating the hospital to Adrian Iselin's wife Louise remains a visible part of Indiana Hospital's history.

vania Supreme Court, addressed the crowd gathered on the grounds around the entrance. The *Indiana Evening Gazette* gave the following account of the ceremony in the romantic language of the day, marveling at the wonders of this new hospital:

The skies were dull and overcast, but inside the new Indiana County General Hospital this afternoon, all was brightness and light, when the most modern institution of its kind in this part of the state was formally turned over to the Indiana directorate by the donors, Adrian Iselin Jr. and his sister, Miss Georgine Iselin.

From one until two o'clock there was a steady stream of automobiles on their way to the new institution, carrying those persons who had contributed to the general fund, and who, with Mr. Iselin and his party from New York City, were the honored guests of the directors at the dedication.

The ceremonies, although formal in a sense, were nevertheless highly interesting and on Sabbath, when the doors of the institution are, for the first time, thrown open for the reception of patients, the Hospital will come into its own, and the directors

Indiana, Pa., Oct. 26, 1914

The Board of Directors of the Indiana Hospital met upon notice by the Secretary at the office of the Secretary at 7:30 P.M. Present: Messrs. Cunningham, Hall, McNelis, Scott, Fisher, Miss McKnight, Mrs. Williard, and Clark, Mr. Clements arriving later.

On motion of Mr. Scott, seconded by Father McNelis, Mr. Adrian Iselin, Jr. and Miss Georgine Iselin, of New York City, were elected honorary members of the Board of the Indiana Hospital for life, and the Secretary was instructed to notify them of this action.

The following Resolutions were then presented by Mr. Scott and unanimously adopted upon his motion, seconded by Mr. Clements, and direction given to the Secretary that a copy be sent to the parties named therein.

1. "Resolved. That we, the Board of Directors of the Indiana Hospital, do hereby tender our sincere and hearty thanks to Adrian Iselin, Jr. of the City of New York, for his magnificent generosity in tendering to the people of the County of Indiana, Pennsylvania, a splendid hospital building, with permanent equipments, for the use of the entire people who are residents of Indiana County, irrespective of nationality or religious belief."

2. "Resolved that we, the Board of Directors of the Indiana Hospital do hereby tender our most appreciative feelings toward Miss Georgine Iselin, of New Rochelle, New York, who so generously and lavishly equipped the hospital building at Indiana, Pennsylvania, and which was presented to the County of Indiana by her brother, Adrian Iselin, Jr."

The October 26, 1914, minutes of the Board of Directors' meeting expresses their gratitude to both Adrian Iselin and his sister Georgine for their generosity.

Indiana Evening Gazette.

TELEPHONE- Local 138-x
OFFICE S. Carpenter Ave.

READ- "Evening Gazette Classified Ads, on the Second Page They Bring Results

VOLUME 11 –No. 30.   INDIANA, PA., THURSDAY, OCTOBER 29, 1914   TWO CENTS

Get Ready For The Big Hallowe'en Celebration On Friday

THREE INJURED IN AUTO COLLISION

Two Cars Met Head-on at the Corner of Grant Street and Wayne Avenue Today.

ALL ARE IN THE HOSPITAL.

Three persons were seriously in-

New Indiana County General Hospital Is Formally Dedicated This Afternnon

Invitations For Pennsylvania Day

Interesting Event To Be Held at State College on Friday.

Simple Ceremonies Marked the Presentation of $165,000 Institution to the Residents of Indiana County.

READY FOR PATIENTS SABBATH

Photo Drama Not Shown At The Pit

Picture of the Creation Will Not

THE LINE OF MARCH HALLOWE'EN PARADE

Chief Marshal D. W. Simpson Issues Officials Orders for Tomorrow's Celebration

WEATHER PROMISED FAIR.

The October 29, 1914, edition of the *Indiana Evening Gazette* reported the details of the hospital and its dedication ceremony.

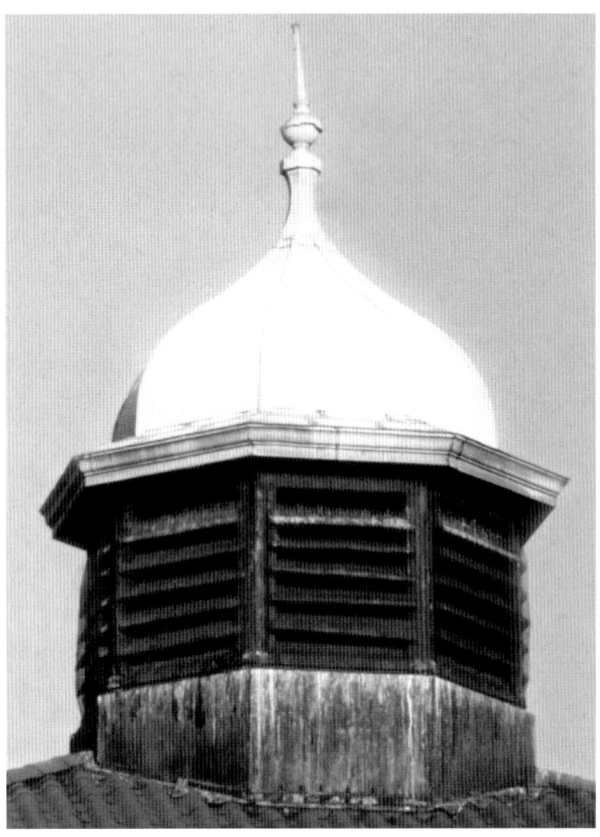

Since the hospital's first days, the cupola has served as a symbol of hope and healing for the people of Indiana County.

and all those who were in any way responsible for the building of it, will see a most successful culmination of their efforts.

Speaking for Mr. Iselin and his sister, Lucius W. Robinson, general manager of the Buffalo, Rochester & Pittsburgh Railway, in a brief though concise address, turned over the new institution to Indiana County. In behalf of the Board of Directors and subscribers to the fund, Justice John P. Elkin, President of the Board of Directors, made the acceptance. During the course of the afternoon, Prof. Cogswell of the Indiana Normal School and his student musicians rendered a beautiful program. Following the ceremonies, the guests were taken for a complete inspection of the hospital and many were the exclamations of delight and pleasure heard from them.

The new structure is of brick, three stories and a basement. It is absolutely fireproof, built according to the latest approved methods for hospital constructions. It is sanitary in every detail, even the doorknobs being of the easily cleaned, germproof glass design.

The system of reflex ceiling lights is used, which does away with the annoyance of glaring lights affecting the patients. With the exception of the telephone bell, there is not a bell or noise-making device in the building. Entrance is gained to the hospital by pressing a button, which lights an

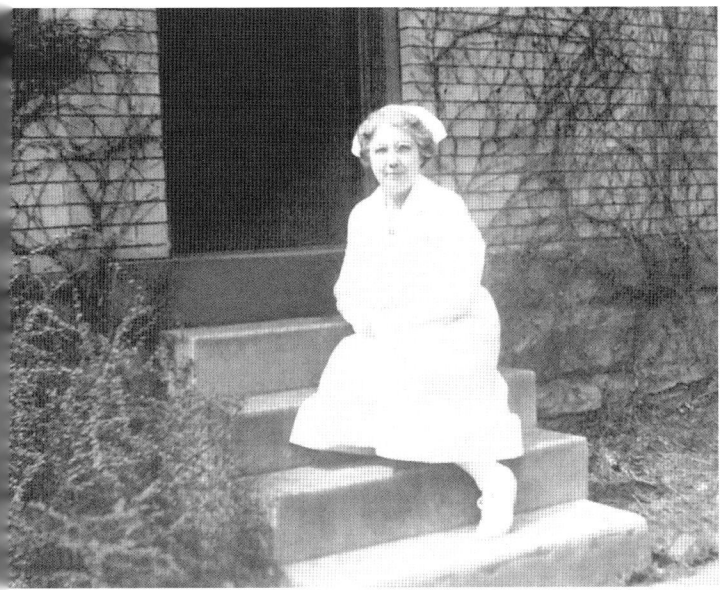
Floy Shaffer Campbell, pictured here in April 1946, was in the first group of nurses to graduate from Indiana Hospital School of Nursing in 1918.

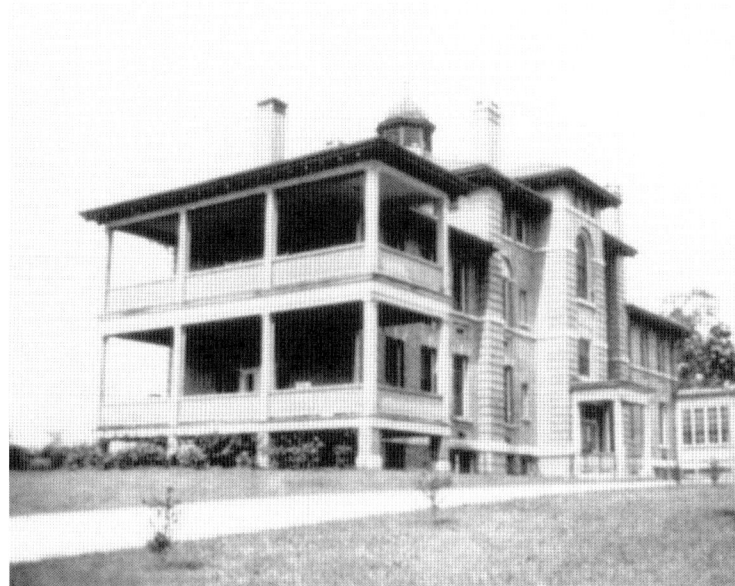
Indiana Hospital's open-air porches, seen clearly from the side view, had their own therapeutic purposes for treating respiratory illnesses.

electric bulb instead of ringing a bell. If a patient wants a nurse, he presses a button. A red light shows in a plate at the head of his cot and a similar one in the nurse's room. The light at the patient's cot cannot be extinguished until the nurse answers the call and presses another button.

Instead of the ordinary noisy elevator there is one of the automatic design. You step into it, push a button, indicating the floor at which you wish to stop, and the machine does the rest.

There are so many marvelous things about the arrangement and equipment of the building that one wonders how they were conceived and made to work together in harmony.

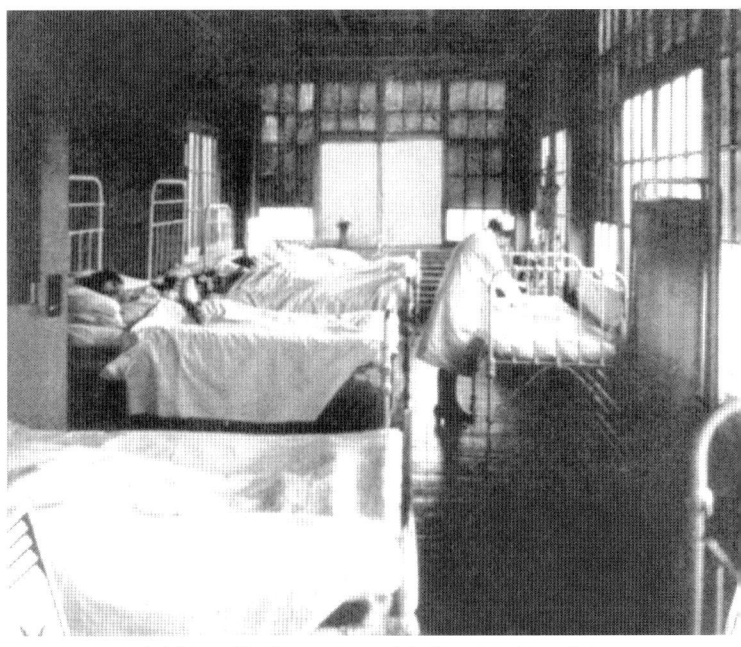
Men, women, and children all had separate wards in the original hospital.

Ironically, the glorious dedication day was marred only by a few unexpected early admissions to the hospital. Floy S. Campbell, a member of the first graduating class of nurses at Indiana Hospital, recalled an accident at the corner of Wayne Avenue and Grant Street in which Mrs. Sue McCormick suffered a compound fracture of her leg while on her way to attend the open house. She was taken to the Simpson-Neal Hospital and following surgery was brought by ambulance to the new hospital. Mrs. Boden, injured in the same accident, was also admitted, as was Mr. Harry Earhart, a pneumonia patient. Quite appropriately, the hospital's seal consisted of a "circular device depicting the Good Samaritan assisting the wounded traveler." The citizens of Indiana County finally had their hospital.

Chapter 1: The Origins of Indiana Hospital — 19

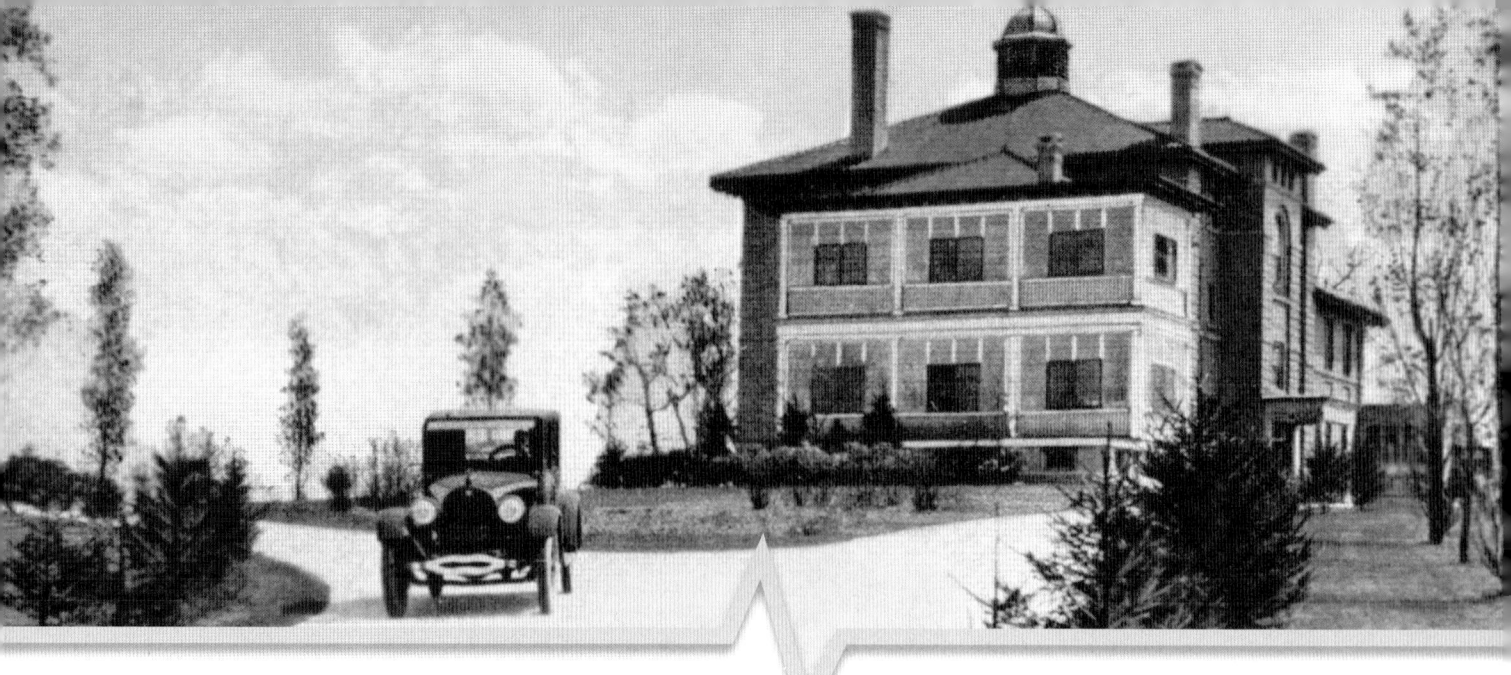

CHAPTER 2
The Women of Indiana Hospital

When the hospital's doors officially opened, Miss Sara M. Morgart (Mrs. Charles Leventry) was Superintendent of Hospital, and Miss Eliza B. Dill was Directress of Nurses. Miss Lulu Lee, the first night superintendent, Miss Lulu Moorhead, and Miss Ivay Huey assisted in preparing the hospital to receive its patients. Miss Morgart's few years of experience at Memorial Hospital in Johnstown qualified her for her salary of $480 per month for which she had "exclusive charge of the hospital with the exception of the medical and surgical departments." At the committee's recommendation, Dr. F. F. Moore of Lucerne was appointed as physician-in-charge for a six-month period at a fee of $50 per month.

During its first year of operation, Indiana Hospital admitted 632 patients: 235 of them private patients, 213 were subscription cases, and 184 charity cases. Income from the State of Pennsylvania amounted to $9,013.25 and from patients, $9,486.60. Donations of $7,698.15 brought the total to $26,198 against expenses of $28,181.11. Three hundred operations were performed, thirty-seven deaths occurred, and, since most women gave birth at home in those days, only fifteen births took place.

The Iselin family's contributions continued. Eleanora Iselin Kane, another sister of Mr. Iselin, presented the hospital with a "modern motor ambulance," with all the necessary equipment in March 1915, and Columbus O. Iselin, a brother, donated a modern x-ray unit costing $1,600.

With Indiana Hospital now in full operation, some of the smaller hospitals that sprang up before it now fell by the wayside. By 1913 the Saltsburg Hospital had accommodations for thirty-five patients but closed shortly after Dr. Earhart's death in January 1914. The Simpson-Neal Hospital merged with the newly chartered Indiana Hospital in 1913 and continued operating until October 1914 when the new Indiana Hospital opened. When the last of its patients was discharged

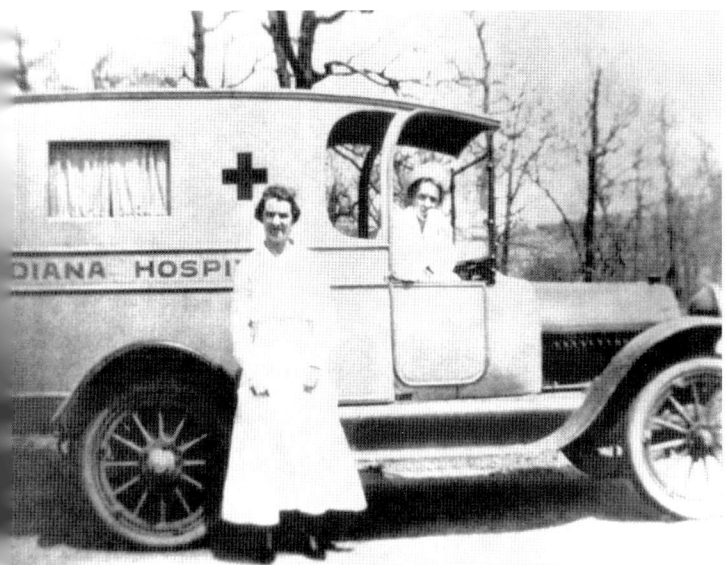

Adrian Iselin's other sister, Eleanora Iseline Kane, donated a "modern motor ambulance" to the hospital.

Opposite page: Visitors to Indiana Hospital were amazed to find that the road leading up to the hospital was not cobblestone or gravel, but cement.

in early 1915, the Simpson-Neal Hospital closed its doors. The Penn-Mary Hospital continued operations until the late 1920s.

Years later, Bertha Manner of the School of Nursing's Class of 1924 recalled fondly Dr. Benjamin Coe, who joined Indiana Hospital's staff upon the closing of the Dixonville Hospital. "You could hear his big booming voice a mile away, and when he stomped through a ward—and I do mean he stomped (he had an artificial leg, you know)—he cheerfully called out 'Hello Mama Mio' to everyone he passed. Everyone felt better just because he was around."

The Indiana Hospital Auxiliary was organized on January 21, 1916. To encourage community involvement in the hospital, the Board of Directors solicited one representative from each church to serve on the Auxiliary board. The first president, Mrs. D. B. Taylor, presided over meetings held monthly in the Municipal Building except for July and August. One hundred and sixty-three members strong, they supplied all the hospital's linens, sewed patient gowns, and hemmed diapers.

1915
- Fourteen students enroll in the first nursing class.
- The hospital receives a "modern motor ambulance," accompanying equipment, and an x-ray machine from the Iselin family.

1916
- The Indiana Hospital Auxiliary is organized.
- The nurses' home is constructed at a cost of $8,000.

1917
- The hospital's large porches are enclosed, increasing bed capacity to sixty.

1918
- Twelve nurses completing the three-year course receive diplomas.

1925
- Mrs. Eva Allison Farnsworth is made supervisor of nurses.

1926
- Indiana Hospital joins the American Hospital Association.

1929
- $276,000 is raised, $100,000 from the Rochester and Pittsburgh Coal Company, for additions and renovations to the hospital.

Chapter 2: The Women of Indiana Hospital

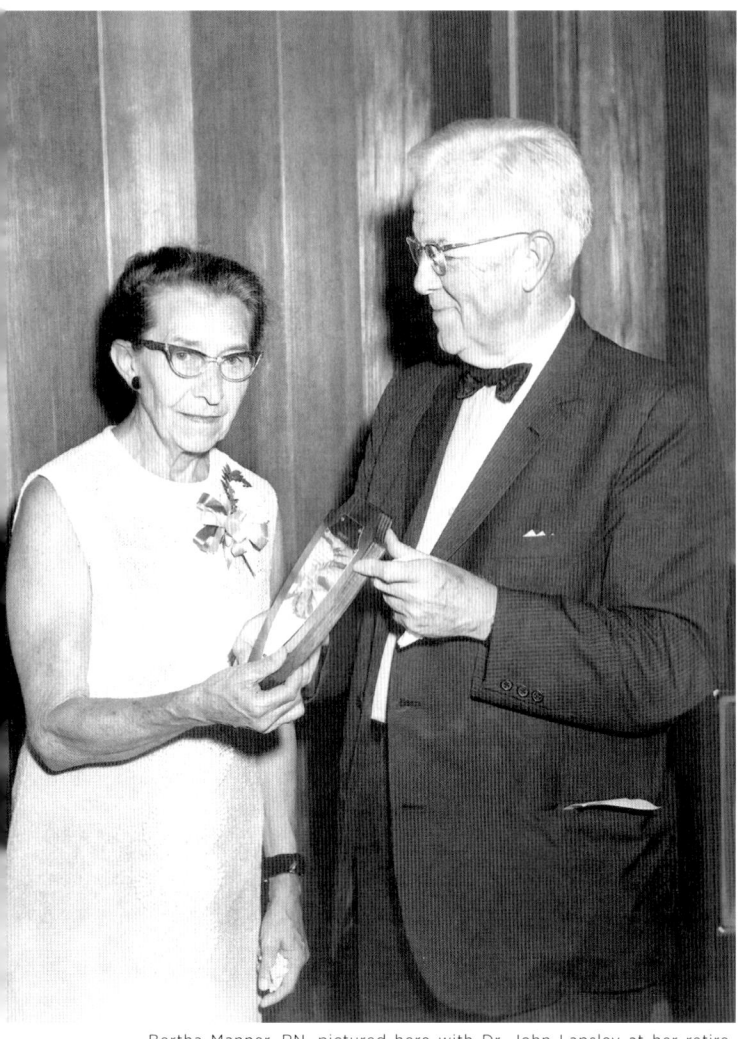

Bertha Manner, RN, pictured here with Dr. John Lapsley at her retirement, recalled many of the hospital's earliest physicians. Photo courtesy of *Indiana Gazette*.

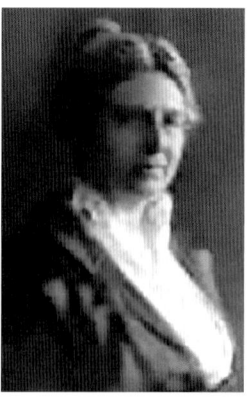

Mrs. D. B. Taylor was the first president of Indiana Hospital Auxiliary.

THE NURSES OF INDIANA HOSPITAL

The first class of fourteen student nurses started on January 1, 1915. At first, students were housed on the third floor of the hospital building; the overflow of students were placed in private homes and transported back and forth with the hospital's car. Only a high school diploma was required for entrance, and no entrance exam was given, but the students were on academic probation for their first three months. Opal Wetzel of the Class of 1922 once reminisced that, after the 10:30 p.m. lights-out inspection, they sometimes huddled in lockers in order to study after hours without being detected.

During the three-month probation period, the student nurse's uniform was a blue dress with a starched white collar and cuffs. Once past their probation period, they wore a blue striped uniform with a white bib, apron, long sleeves, and cuffs. Their caps, given to them at the end of their probation period, were made of muslin and starched to an unnatural level of stiffness that made them so brittle the drawstrings that gathered the back of the cap sometimes snapped like dry twigs. Discipline was very strict, and the punishment the nurses dreaded the most, besides losing a free half-day or even being "campused," was the loss of their cap—a visible sign to everyone that they'd done something wrong.

Students were not charged tuition and were given a stipend of six dollars a month the first year, eight dollars the second, and ten dollars a month during their final year. However, they constituted the overwhelming majority of the hospital's workforce. In crisply starched uniforms, caps, stockings, and shoes, the student nurses put in grueling twelve-hour days from 7 a.m. to 7 p.m. with "time off" for two hours of classroom instruction plus one-half day per week. However, when the work on the floor was heavy, classes were cancelled. Most of their time was devoted to patient care, though they were also expected to do the cleaning and prepare food for the patients. Nurses were assigned to night duty for three-month rotations and were expected to attend their regular daily classes for the duration. When that rotation was completed, the nurse was given one full day off.

The first teachers were hospital administrator Sara M. Morgart and directress of nurses Mrs. Eliza Dill Wineman. Staff doctors, including Drs. G. E. Simpson, W. D. Gates, F. F. Moore, H. B. Neal Sr., C. E. Rink, W. A. Simpson, Fred S. Clair, F. B. Stevenson, W. F. Weitzel, H. B. Buterbaugh, B. F. Coe, and A. H. Stewart, occasionally lectured to the classes. During their three-year course of study, the student nurses participated in a three-month program in obstetrics at Elizabeth Steel Magee Hospital in Pittsburgh. Except for the years 1918 to 1923 when wartime conditions at Magee forced the hospital to develop another affiliation with St. Francis Hospital in Pittsburgh, the affiliation with Magee continued until 1932 when obstetrical training was moved to Children's Hospital in Pittsburgh.

In 1916, a frame building was erected to house the nursing students. Built by contractor John Klingensmith at a cost of $8,000 the 37′ x 61′ building was three stories high and included a lecture hall, dining room, and bathrooms. At the same time, a 40′ x 40′ garage was built along with an addition to the hospital for the laundry. The rooms were large, dormitory-style rooms with four to six students sharing one room, one clothes closet, one toilet, and two lavatories.

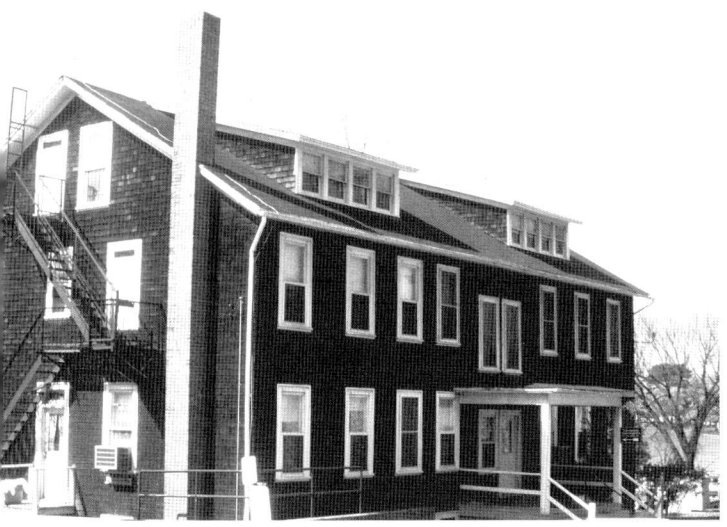
The three-story nurses' home was built in 1916.

In 1917, the hospital's capacity was expanded for the first time with the enclosure of the porches, increasing the hospital's capacity to sixty beds. The carpenter's union donated the labor, various local businesses donated lumber and supplies, and Pittsburgh Plate Glass Company donated the glass for the windows.

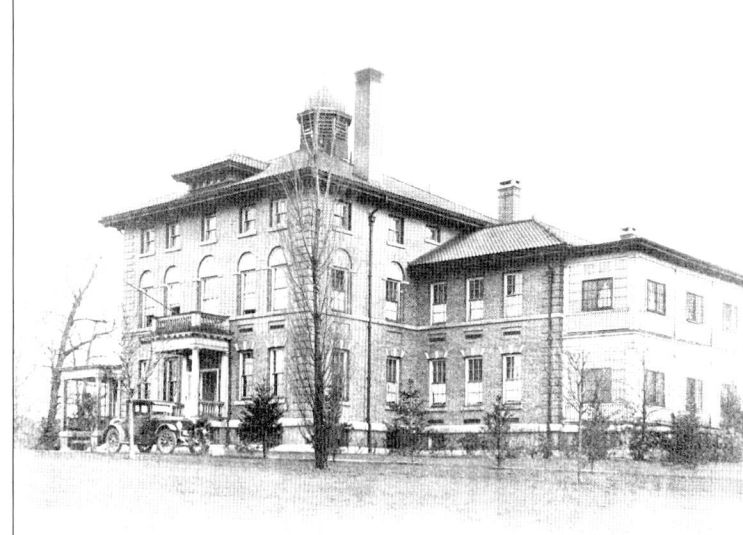

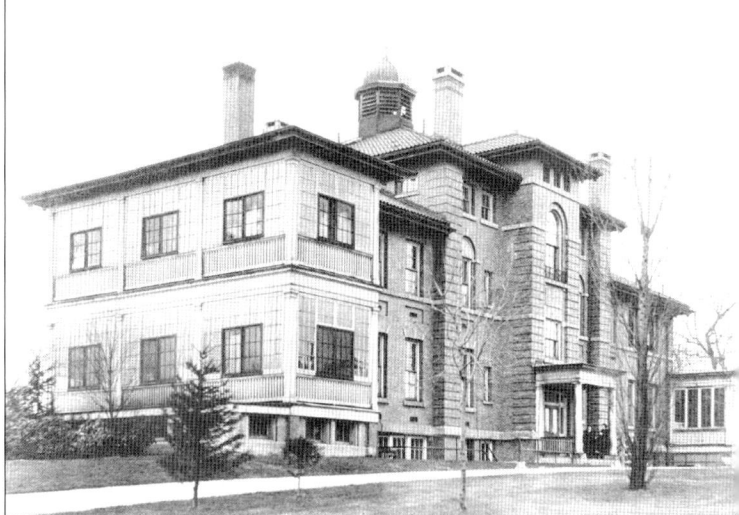
The hospital's porches were enclosed in 1917 to make room for more patients. Photos courtesy of *Indiana Gazette*.

WORLD WAR I

When World War I erupted in 1914, President Woodrow Wilson vowed to maintain the United States' neutrality. However, Germany's continued aggression on the seas led to increased public outcry. After repeated incidents

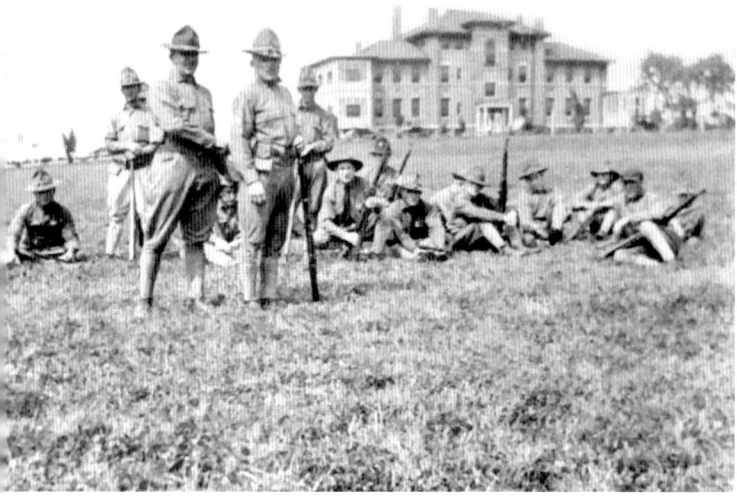

World War I soldiers used the grounds of Indiana Hospital for training.

and Germany's announced intention to continue unrestricted warfare in war-zone waters in 1917, the United States broke diplomatic relations with Germany. As America began steeling itself for war, Germany sunk four US merchant ships, prompting President Wilson to call for a formal declaration of war against Germany on April 2, 1917.

The United States' role in World War I was short-lived but vital, and Americans rushed to do their part to aid the war effort. The grounds of Indiana Hospital were filled with soldiers who were given permission to train there. Toward the end of 1917, Miss Sara Morgart, superintendent of Indiana Hospital, joined the Red Cross nursing service and got her orders to leave for France the next month.

On January 3, 1918, twelve of the initial fourteen students—Irene McKinstry, Olive McCrea, Nele Maher, Mary Gaster, Esther Griffith, Sara Sheilds, Vera Keagle, Mary Kelly, Stella Rickard, Nancy Bracken, Margaret Steving, and Floy Shaffer—completed the three-year training. A baccalaureate service was held in the Lutheran Church in

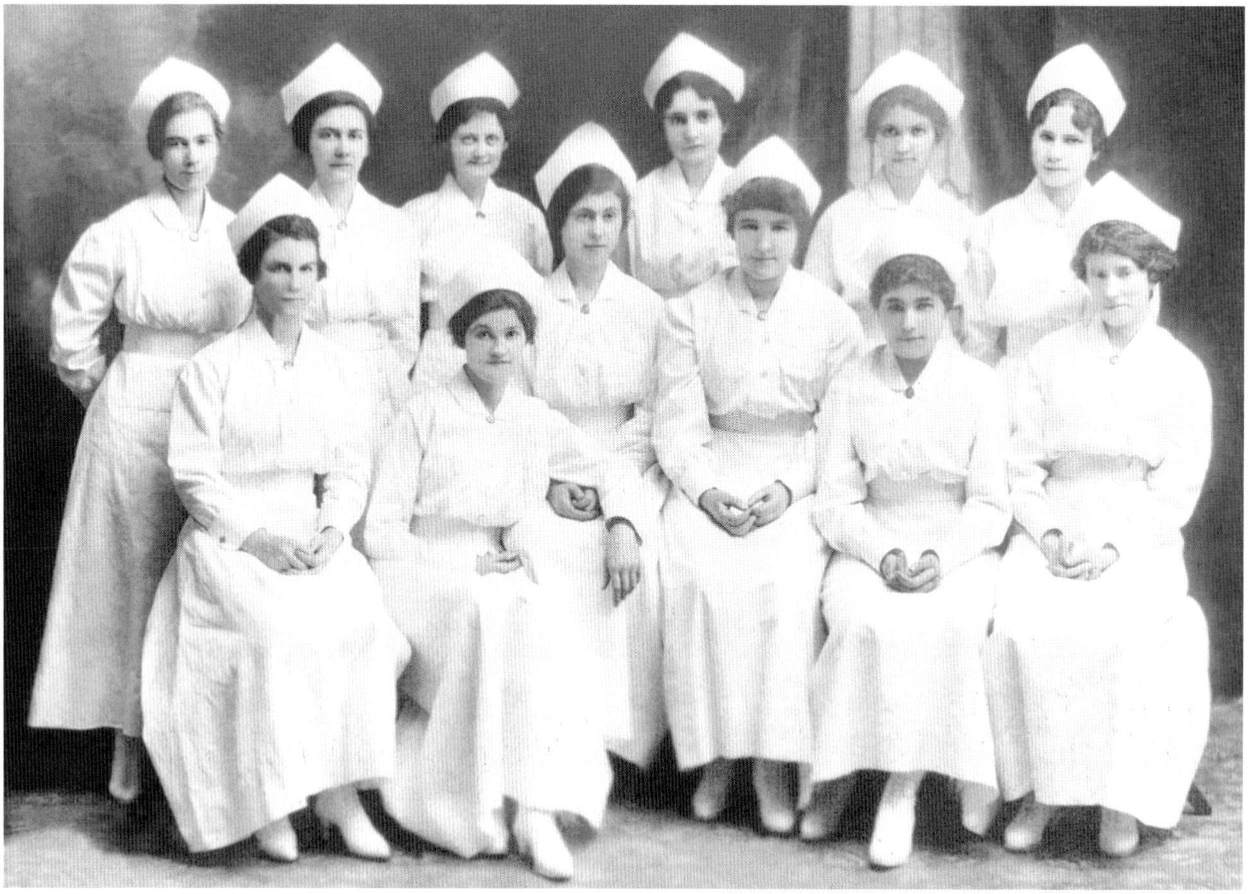

The first graduating class of Indiana Hospital School of Nursing, 1918.

Indiana Regional Medical Center

Indiana on December 20, 1917, and the graduates received their diplomas at commencement exercises held in the First Presbyterian Church in Indiana on January 3, 1918.

Shortly thereafter Sara Morgart left to fulfill her patriotic duty in France. Eliza Dill took over as hospital superintendent until the following October when Miss Dill also left for Army service at Camp Lee, Virginia, and Miss Bessie I. Dale became superintendent.

In fact, Miss Dill was among a group of seven nurses from the Indiana Hospital Army Nurses Unit who went to Camp Lee for preparatory training. Besides Eliza Dill the group included Mary Gaster, Floy Shaffer (later Mrs. Harry Campbell), Myrtle I. McKinstry (later Mrs. Joseph Jackson), Teresa Jones, Myrtle Gray, and Mary Jane Swan (later Mrs. Earl Gray). After training they were assigned to the Walter Reed Medical Center where for over a year they worked with wounded and crippled officers.

The Indiana Hospital Auxiliary opted to suspend all parties and other events for the duration of the war, and what funds they did raise were used to help furnish the nurses' home. But once the armistice was signed during November 1918, they were ready to resume their fundraising efforts for the hospital. On July 5, 1920, they held a countywide picnic. More than 6,000 people came out for the event, paying twenty-five cents per person admission or fifty cents per automobile. Everyone enjoyed the music of brass bands and the speeches made by local dignitaries. The men rolled up their sleeves and competed in boxing bouts and contests of all kinds. The ladies dressed their little ones in their finest for the baby show. The event raised $1,878.73, the equivalent of over $20,000 in today's dollars.

Whether or not Miss Morgart resumed her position as hospital superintendent following her military service

The Influenza Pandemic of 1918

Soldiers returning to the United States following duty in Europe during World War I brought with them the particularly virulent strain of influenza that was nicknamed "Spanish flu." The disease reached Indiana County around the end of September 1918. By early October nearly 600 people in Coal Run and McIntyre fell victim and nine people died. Coal operations all but ceased; schools and movie theaters closed. Funerals were held privately with only the immediate family, the minister, and funeral director present. Guards were posted to prevent people from entering or leaving the town. The State Department of Health set up a twenty-five-cot hospital in an army tent. The quarantine was ineffective, and within a week the situation at Ernest became critical. The number of deaths was estimated at nearly forty. All public gatherings were prohibited. An appeal was made for volunteer Red Cross flu workers, and an emergency seventy-five-bed hospital was set up in Ernest. By October 16 there were many more deaths, undertakers were extremely busy, the stock of caskets was depleted, and there was a shortage of gravediggers. By the time the disease ran its course the following year, more than 21.6 million people died from it worldwide.

is uncertain. Mrs. Allison took the position on May 23, 1922, followed by Miss Lillian Hollohan, who became the hospital's new superintendent on July 10, 1929.

As Indiana Hospital's nursing school enrollment continued to increase, more living space became necessary. The contract for a new nurses' dormitory was given to Longwill Brothers of Indiana in September 1922. The frame structure costing $6,000 was ready for its occupants in January 1923.

In 1926 Indiana Hospital became a member of the American Hospital Association. Under the auspices of the Indiana Rotary Club and other civic organizations, the first crippled children's diagnostic clinic was held October 19, 1926, and the first operative clinic in March 1927. Over the coming year, a total of twelve such clinics were held in which 236 children were examined and fifty operations performed. Of those, 168 of the children were orthopedic cases.

In 1929 the hospital announced its plans to expand with a new three-story wing in addition to making a number of interior improvements, including an elevator.

Elder Peelor, chairman of the fund drive, launched the campaign to raise $250,000 in May. The following month, Rochester and Pittsburgh Coal Company pledged $100,000 toward the project, contingent upon the county's ability to raise the remaining $150,000. Clearfield Bituminous Coal Corporation donated $25,000 toward the project and M. Bennett & Sons another $12,000. Two area Boy Scout troops helped with the fund drive by placing bumper stickers on automobiles that read "Open Your Heart for Humanity's Sake." By July the fund drive was oversubscribed at $276,000.

Monies from the capital campaign were also used to expand living space for the growing School of Nurs-

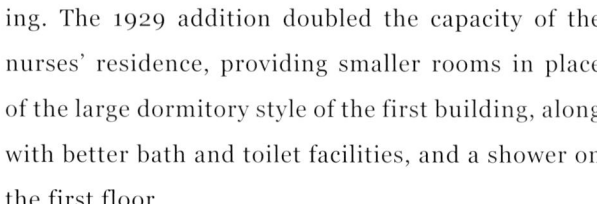

1923
The only year during which the Indiana Hospital School of Nursing did not graduate students was 1923.

ing. The 1929 addition doubled the capacity of the nurses' residence, providing smaller rooms in place of the large dormitory style of the first building, along with better bath and toilet facilities, and a shower on the first floor.

THE COAL CONNECTION

In the early 1900s, Pennsylvania had more coal company towns than any other state in the nation. By 1920, the Rochester and Pittsburgh Coal and Iron Company had fifteen mines operating in Indiana County alone, the largest of which was in Ernest where they employed one thousand men. Miners and their families lived in the company towns or "patch towns," as they were known. They lived in company-built row houses and attended company-built churches and schools. Most were paid subsistence wages in company currency, which the miners used to purchase goods at the company store.

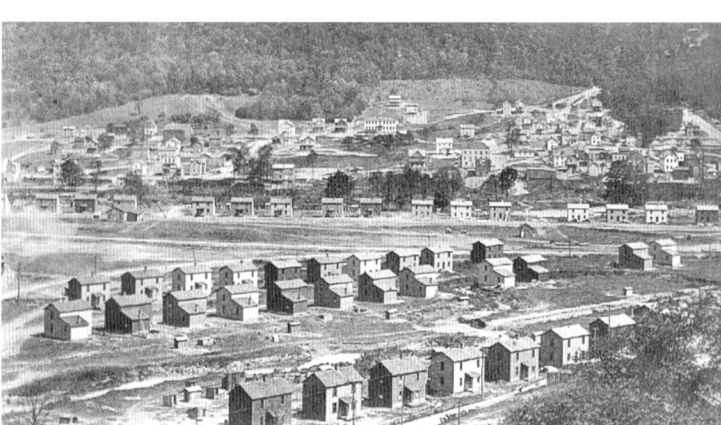

Ernest, Pennsylvania, was founded in 1903 by the Rochester and Pittsburgh Coal Company. The large building in the center was the company store. Photo courtesy of John Busovicki.

Clymer, Pennsylvania, in 1908 with its rows of company houses. Photo courtesy of John Busovicki.

Far from being magnanimous, the company towns actually served to control the mineworkers, virtually imprisoning them in a state of poverty. But, at least their basic needs were provided, including health care. Indiana County native Raymond Malengo set down his recollections of his hometown of Alverda, Pennsylvania, in a short missive he titled *In Memory of a Little Town*.

> Around 1920 the local coal company hired Dr. William Heiser from Georgia to take care of the miners and their families. Dr. Heiser moved his wife Josephine and daughter Sadie to Alverda and established an office which, years later, was moved to the company store. Dr. Heiser was known to everyone as simply "Doc." Dr. James O'Conner was the next company doctor in Alverda and the last one the town had.

Besides the coal company doctors, private hospitals continued springing up in the area during the decade known as "The Roaring Twenties." The first specialized hospital to open in Indiana County was Stevenson Hospital on South Ninth Street in Indiana. Dr. S. B. Stevenson founded the hospital, which opened in 1921 especially for eye, ear, nose, and throat patients. It had private rooms, an office, an x-ray room, and operating rooms. Dr. Stevenson also organized the Western Pennsylvania Eye, Ear, Nose, and Throat Society and served as the group's first president.

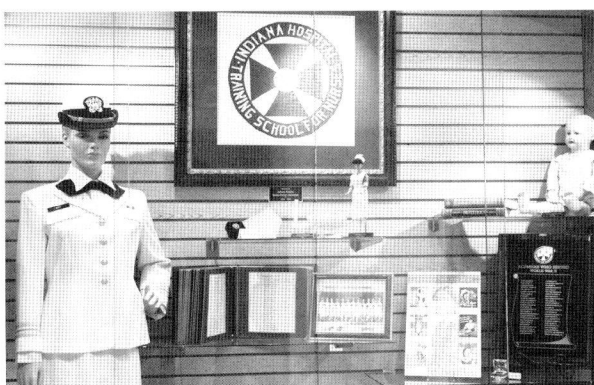
So important have the nurses been to the hospital that their starched caps, capes, Bunsen burners, and syringes remain displayed to remind everyone of Indiana Hospital's history.

In 1929, Dr. W. D. Gates built the Gates Hospital as an annex to his residence on Philadelphia Street in Indiana. It consisted of private rooms, a nursery, an operating room, and offices. Dr. J. W. Campbell joined Dr. Gates and, after his death in 1935, continued operating the hospital into the early 1950s.

Year End 1927

The following statistics provide a snapshot of Indiana Hospital for the year ending September 30, 1927:

Patients admitted: 1,514
Charity patients: 196

Total receipts were $69,405.95. Of that:

Fees received from patients: $29,745.39
Proceeds from the boarding of
  special nurses: $2,247.25
Delivery room fees received: $270.00
Nursery fees received: $301.50
Operating room fees: $3,075.00
Anesthesia fees: $1,797.95
Laboratory fees: $2,806.00
X-ray fees: $2,157.50
State appropriations: $8,900.00

Total costs were $67,227.08 consisting of:

Administration: $6,027.36
Household: $25,133.15
Plant operation: $10,693.15
Maintenance: $1,150.32
Insurance: $2,366.57
Professional care: $21,856.53

A hospital farm brought in receipts of $1,077.81 against an outlay of $768.32.

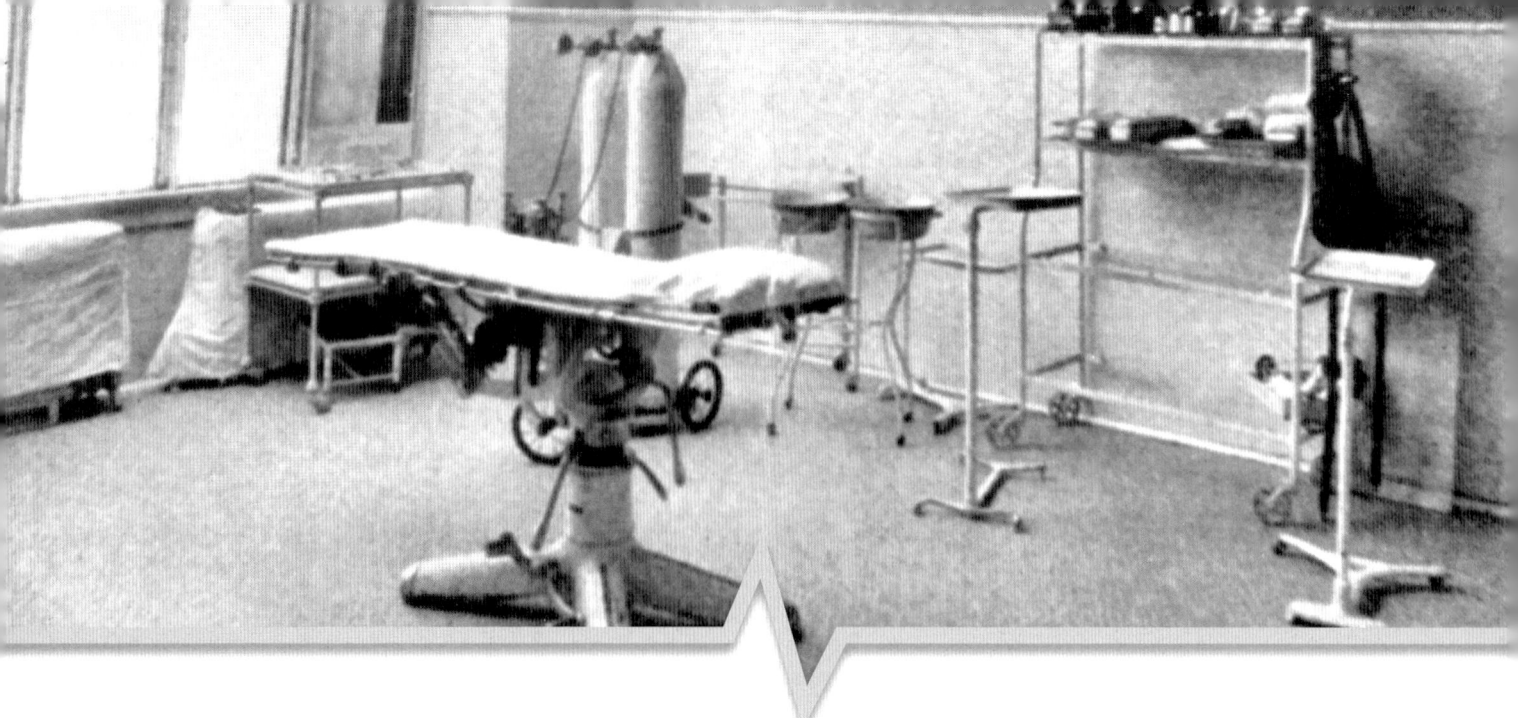

CHAPTER 3
A Sense of Civic Duty

From the very beginning, Indiana Hospital was the result of a community of people committed to each other's care. Local businesses contributed generously, and the residents volunteered in droves. On January 22, 1930, the Indiana Hospital Auxiliary expanded that community involvement by inviting the area's young people to participate in the care of patients. The Junior Auxiliary was organized to help care for the babies and children in the hospital, and Dr. Charles Rink addressed their first meeting at the Legion Hall on February 14. In March, the members began their first project of sewing "bathrobes and bloomers for the small girls." The Auxiliary itself issued its first cookbook that year and sold chances on a brand new Maytag washing machine. At ten cents per chance, they raised $189.90 and by October donated $500 to purchase three cribs and three children's beds along with mattresses.

Indiana Hospital's new three-story wing was completed in November 1930 and officially opened on May 12, 1931, increasing the hospital's capacity to 154 beds. John G. McCrory, president of McCrory stores, a chain of five-and-dime stores based in York, Pennsylvania, donated funds for an elevator.

At the same time the new wing was opening, Indiana Hospital received a small windfall associated with the closing of Dixonville Hospital. Since its inception, more than $40,000 had been spent for new equipment including a modern laundry, an x-ray, and an ambulance. The hospital's capacity was now twenty beds, and a nurses' home had been erected in 1925 at a cost of $10,000. When the hospital closed during the spring of 1931, all the equipment was donated to Indiana Hospital.

In 1934, Indiana Hospital became a member of the Hospital Association of Pennsylvania and acquired its first electrocardiograph machine.

In the early to mid-1930s, prepaid hospitalization and group hospital insurance became more common. As

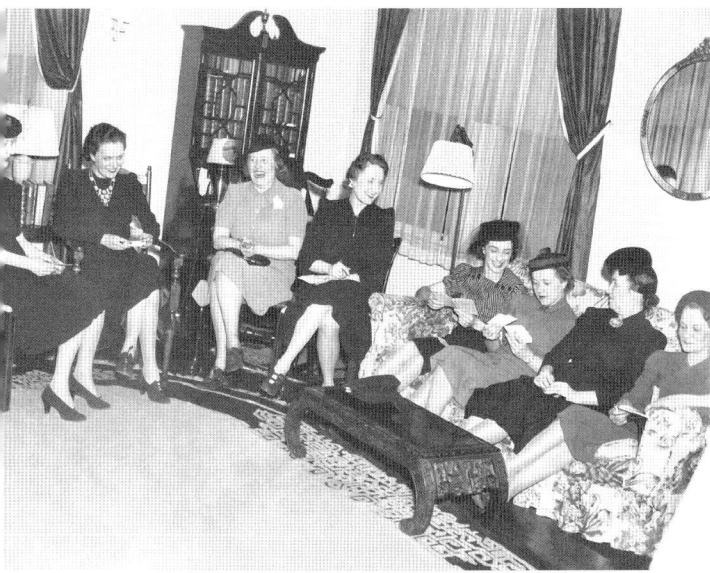

Indiana Hospital Auxiliary's Charity Ball Committee, 1937. Left to right: Mrs. Effie Johnson, Judy Meisser, Mrs. Betty Coulter, Patty Lewis, Lorraine Miller, Mary Kredel, Jean Whitmyre, Edith McCarthy.

Opposite page: An operating room in Indiana Hospital, circa 1930.

the public learned the value of such plans and more people took advantage of prepaid hospital care, the number of hospital admissions increased. Not long after the first major expansion was completed, the need arose once again. This time, the hospital that Adrian Iselin Jr. helped start, John S. Mack would now take to the next level.

Up to that point, Indiana Hospital was too small to be recognized by the state as a complete training school for nurses or to qualify to apply for interns. Mr. Mack was serving on the hospital's board of directors as plans were being devised to once again expand the hospital's capacity. One option was to build a central heating plant, thus freeing up space in the main hospital building. It was a good plan. Having all the power facilities located in a separate building would reduce the hazards of fire and keep smoke and dirt caused by the production of heat away from the hospital. The central plant was to be a one-story brick building with a 230-foot-long pedestrian tunnel connecting the heating plant to the main hospital building and carrying all steam lines to the hospital as well

1930

On January 22, the Junior Auxiliary is organized for the care of babies and children in the hospital.

In November, the first big addition to the hospital is completed bringing bed capacity to 154.

1934

1935

The hospital joins the Hospital Association of Pennsylvania and acquires an electrocardiograph machine.

John Sephus Mack of McKeesport, Pennsylvania, volunteers to build an additional fifty-bed wing on the main hospital building as a memorial to his parents, John M. and Sarah E. Mack.

John Mack also donates 1,500 shares of G. C. Murphy stock to Indiana Hospital.

1936

1937

The Junior Auxiliary raises $375 to purchase an oxygen tent.

On National Hospital Day, a new brick residence for nurses and personnel is completed.

1938

A central heating plant is completed at a cost of $21,000.

The Mack Wing is erected, bringing the hospital's bed capacity to 200.

1939

A pedestrian tunnel, 230 feet long, is built to connect the heating plant to the main hospital buildings. The tunnel carries all steam lines to the hospital and nurses' quarters.

The Mack Maternity Wing is opened and dedicated on September 21.

Chapter 3: A Sense of Civic Duty — 29

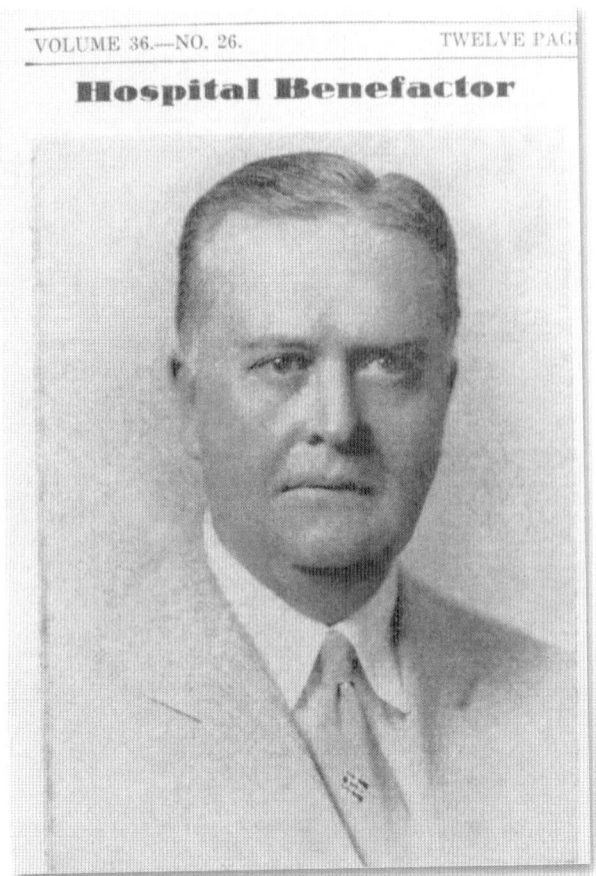

John S. Mack, successful businessman and generous philanthropist.

McCrorey with an "e"

Two cousins from Indiana County started two of the biggest five-and-dime chains of stores in the country, McCrory's and G. C. Murphy Company. J. G. McCrory opened his first store in Scottdale, Pennsylvania, in 1882. Born with his last name spelled "McCrorey," the owner of the chain of five-and-dime stores changed it, dropping the "e," to save money on his store signs.

as to the nurses' quarters. Despite the merits of this plan, Mr. Mack realized it was not enough to create the additional bed space the hospital needed, so he volunteered to build an additional wing of fifty beds onto the main building.

John Sephus Mack was born in Brush Valley, Pennsylvania, on March 9, 1880, the only son among John McCrory Mack and Sarah E. Mack's six children. He received a public school education, took a business course at Johnstown, Pennsylvania, in 1899, and immediately took a job working in the stockroom of a J. G. McCrory Company five-and-dime store where he earned $5.00 per week. By 1908, at the age of twenty-eight, he became general manager of the entire chain of stores. When George C. Murphy, who had himself gotten his start as manager of a McCrory store, died in 1909 after starting his own chain, John S. Mack, along with Walter Shaw, purchased the G. C. Murphy chain of twelve stores and quickly expanded it.

On October 1, 1935, Mr. Mack, now president of G. C. Murphy Company, created the J. S. Mack Trust Fund, transferring 1,500 shares of G. C. Murphy Company stock to the hospital as a memorial to his parents, John M. and Sarah E. Mack. The net income of the stock, then valued at $202,500, was to be used to provide hospitalization, medication, and nursing for needy patients, with preference being given to Brush Valley Township residents and maternity cases.

The new wing of Indiana Hospital would not be realized for several years, and the man who, despite his success, preferred to think of himself as "a dirt farmer" apparently did not want to wait to help the folks of Brush Valley. The J. S. Mack Foundation sponsored the Brush Valley Maternity Hospital, which opened in June 1937. Located in the old Truby Mansion, the hospital was endowed with $200,000 through the Foundation. It included a delivery room, nursery, utility room, x-ray, and a patient ward. The staff members were Dr. T. H. Roney and nurses Dean K. Tyger and Esther Stewart.

The Indiana Hospital Auxiliary

1933: The Auxiliary held its first benefit dance on February 17 in the Armory, netting $50.25.

1934: Three more beds, six bedside tables, and a piano were purchased for the children's ward.

1936: The Junior Auxiliary raised $375 to purchase an oxygen tent.

1937: The Auxiliary held its first charity ball at the Country Club. Admission was $1.50 per couple.

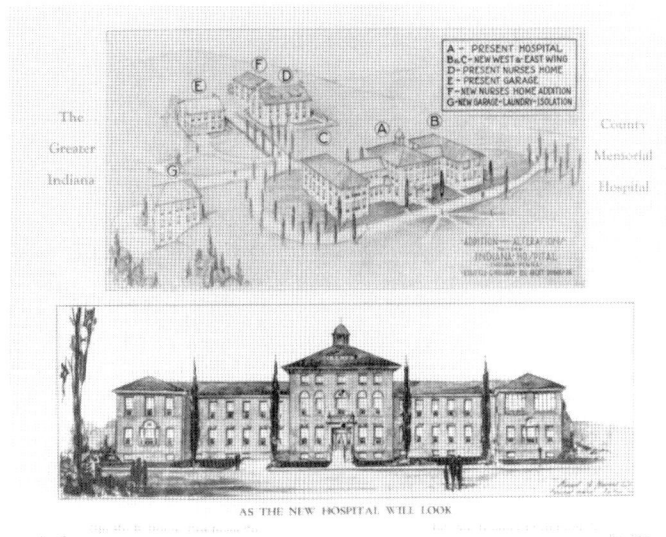

Sketches of the hospital show expansions to the nurses' housing, garages, and laundry facilities.

Not only did Indiana Hospital need room for more patients, it also needed more room for its nurses. The hospital already had two nurses' homes on the grounds; one a frame building and the other, built with a portion of the $280,000 pledged in the 1929 capital campaign, was a combination stone and shingle structure. This time, no capital campaign was necessary, and in 1937 a new nurses' home was built at a cost of $35,000. The new brick building was opened for inspection on National Hospital Day on May 12, 1937. The new nurses' home contained, in addition to the dormitories and classrooms for nurses in training, a fully equipped kitchen where students were taught to prepare practical dietetics.

Finally, the August 10, 1938, edition of the *Indiana Evening Gazette* announced that the Board of Trustees of Indiana Hospital awarded contracts for the construction of the new maternity wing and power plant to the Westmoreland Construction Company. The construction was to be completed within a seven-month period at a cost of $109,000 for the new wing and $20,000 for the power plant.

Robert E. Tomb, a prominent local architect, designed the new wing to Indiana Hospital. The four-story brick addition measuring forty-by-eighty-six feet in area was to be connected to the main building by ramps, announced Blair Sutton, chairman of the building committee. The basement of the new wing was to be constructed as a receiving floor.

Ultimately, the Mack Wing, as it came to be known, cost $115,000 to build and was furnished and equipped

Homer City

A hospital to be built by the Works Progress Administration, a Depression-era program designed to provide jobs on public works projects, was proposed for Homer City in May 1937. At a "mass meeting" on July 22, James M. Higgins, a WPA engineer, assured a crowd that $34,000 in federal funds was already approved. The local community, however, had to raise $30,000 for materials and supplies. The effort failed.

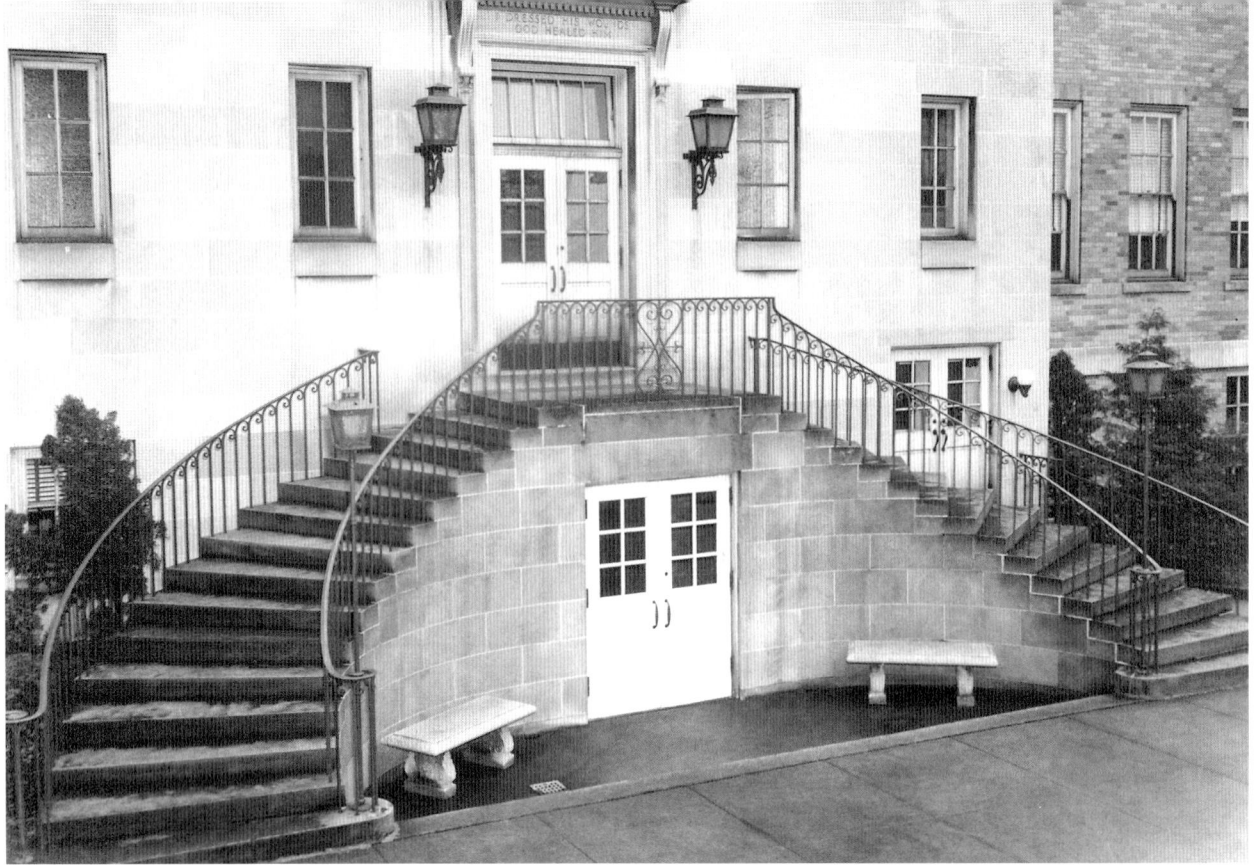

The portico of the new J. S. Mack Memorial Wing became the new entrance to the hospital.

by the hospital's board of directors. Dedicated to the care of maternity patients, the new fifty-bed wing brought the hospital's total capacity up to two hundred beds, five times the size of the original hospital.

More than five hundred people gathered around the main entrance to the new wing on September 21, 1939, to hear John Mack give the address dedicating the wing in memory of his parents, John and Sarah Mack. Seated on the portico along with Mr. and Mrs. Mack were hospital superintendent Lillian Hollahan and Dr. Charles Rink, who gratefully accepted the keys to the new wing from Mr. Mack. The Indiana High School Band entertained the crowd, and after the ceremony, guests were invited to tour the new wing as well as the power plant while tea was served in the nurses' home.

Everything about the new wing was designed with care, compassion, and sensitivity to the maternity patients for whom it was built. On the ground floor was an emergency room complete with operating room, medical examination rooms, and a prenatal maternity clinic. Expectant

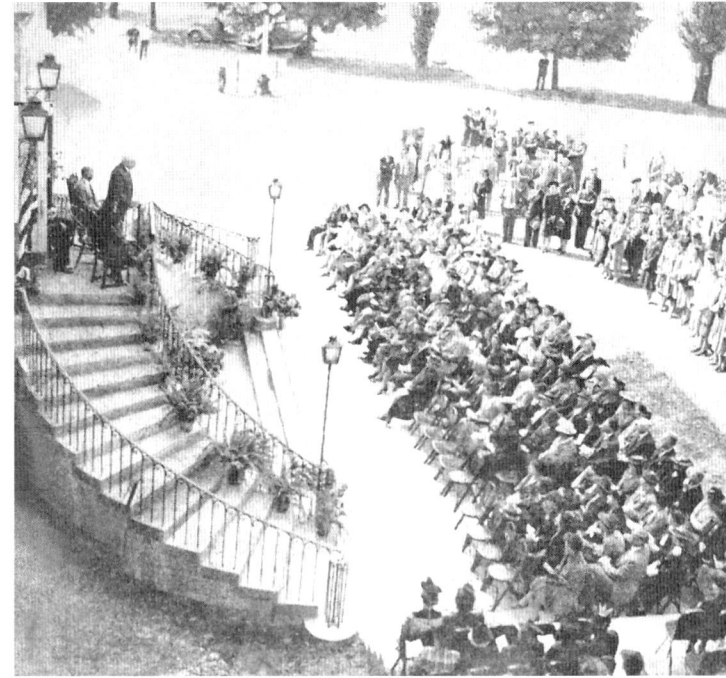

Hundreds of townspeople, business owners, and supporters showed up for the dedication of the J. S. Mack Memorial Wing on September 21, 1939.

mothers entered the clinic through a separate entrance and waiting room to shelter them from the sight of accident patients arriving at the emergency room. The x-ray division and clinical laboratories were also located on the ground floor in the wing erected in 1930.

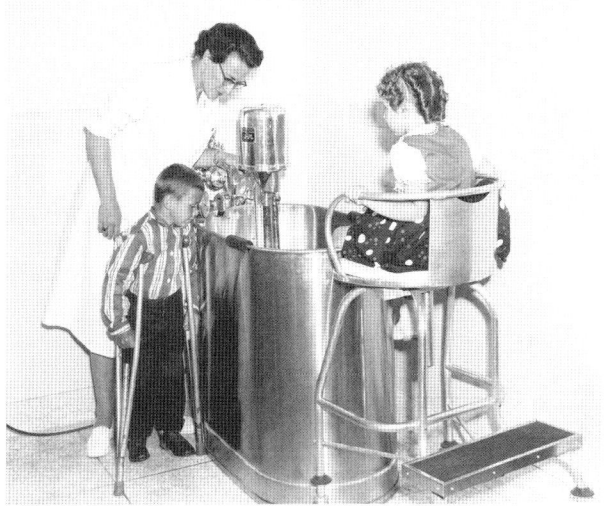
Indiana Hospital began holding clinics for crippled children as early as 1926. During the 1950s, as seen here, the major health threat to children was polio.

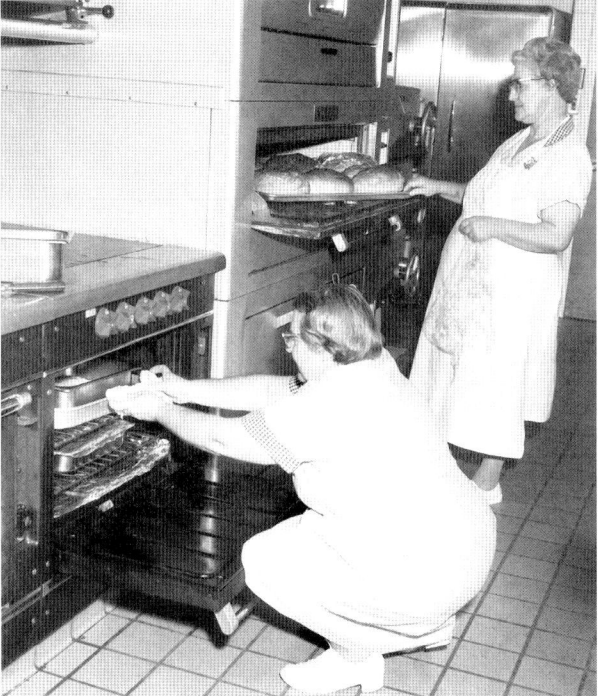
The cooks prepare fresh food to help with the patients' recovery. Photo courtesy of *Indiana Gazette*.

graduated nine students, leaving an enrollment of forty-two young ladies with another twenty-eight new students waiting to be admitted for the fall term. Besides being able to award its own diplomas, there was another change for the nursing school—the no-tuition/paid stipend policy had to be discontinued.

Since opening its doors in 1914, Indiana Hospital had admitted a total of 49,216 patients. The total number of patients admitted during the year ending September 1, 1939, was 3,830; 1,569 of them were admitted as free patients.

When the J. S. Mack Wing was dedicated in 1939, Indiana Hospital's staff and leadership consisted of the following:

THE BOARD OF DIRECTORS
A. J. Musser, President, Coal Operator
W. W. Taylor, Merchant
Dr. Charles E. Rink, Physician
J. Anthony Grapp, Banker
Mrs. Gertrude Blaxter
George J. Feit, Lawyer
James Stewart, Miner and Teacher
J. Blair Sutton, County Employee
John M. Miller, Auto Dealer
John McEwen, Coal Miner
C. Gilbert Wolfenden, State Senator
Ellsworth Campbell, Coal and Ice Dealer
L. W. Householder, Coal Operator
J. S. Mack, Merchant
W. C. Bennett, Retired
Joseph Luxenberg, Merchant
Robert Fisher, Lawyer

ADMINISTRATIVE STAFF AND RESIDENT PHYSICIANS
Miss Lillian A. Hollohan, Administrator
Miss Adeline Hawxhurst, Manager Business Office
Miss Lillie Mae Haupt, Director of Nurses
Dr. S. V. Algin, Pathologist
Dr. Wilson Dougherty, Physician
Dr. B. L. Silverblatt, Physician
Dr. B. Franklin Lear, Physician

THE MEDICAL STAFF
Dr. H. B. Neal, President, Physician
Dr. C. E. Simpson, Surgeon
Dr. F. J. Kellam, Surgeon
Dr. C. P. Reed, Surgeon
Dr. J. C. Lee, Surgeon
Dr. W. L. Whitten, Surgeon
Dr. T. W. Kredel, Surgeon
Dr. W. A. Simpson, Physician
Dr. George Martin, Surgeon
Dr. C. H. Bee, Physician
Dr. C. E. Rink, Physician
Dr. H. B. Buterbaugh, Specialist
Dr. T. J. McNelis, Specialist
Dr. F. B. Stevenson, Specialist
Dr. W. F. Weitzel, Specialist
Dr. Wilbur Gibson, Dentist
Dr. R. J. Hobaugh, Dentist

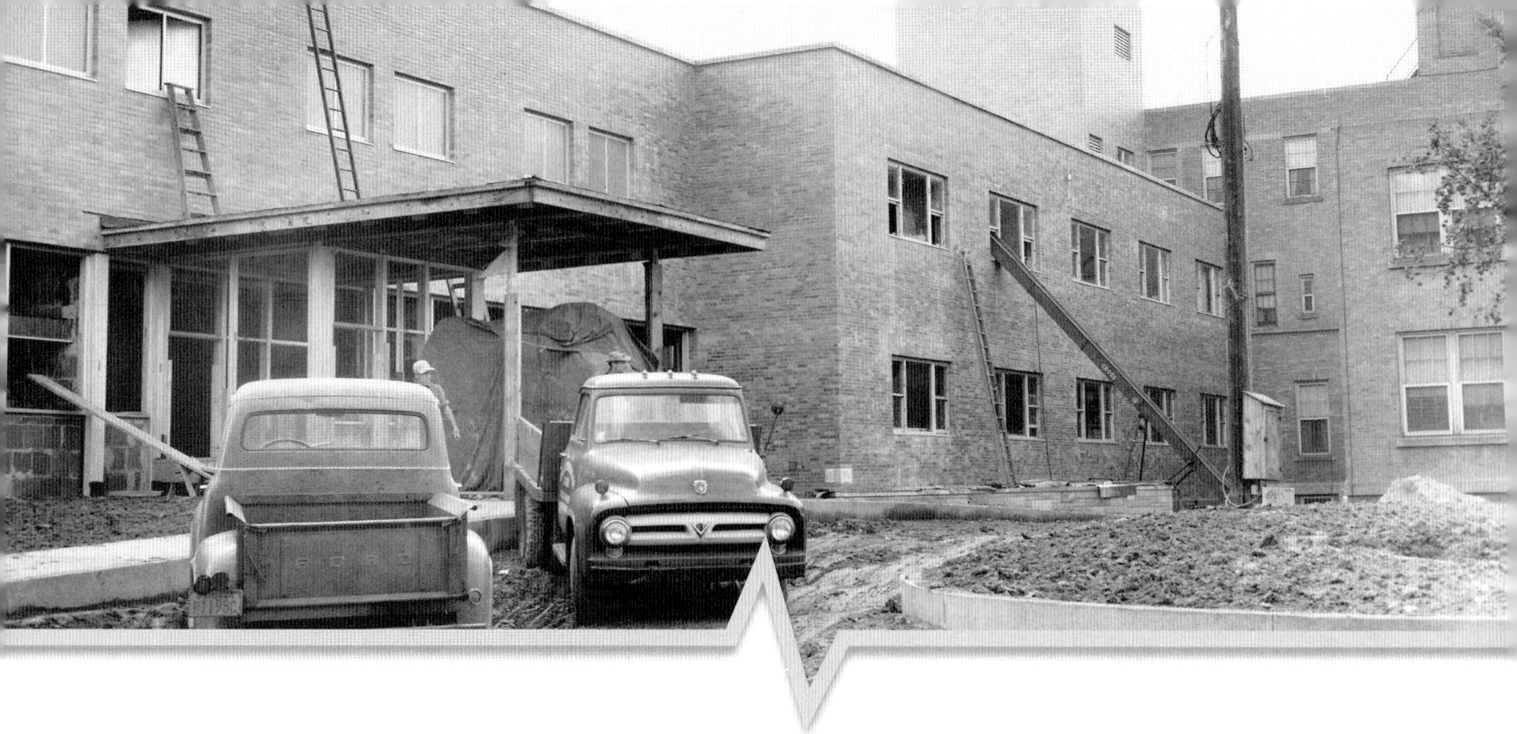

CHAPTER 4
The "Hospital on the Hill" Matures

Excitement over Indiana Hospital's new wing was marred only by the passing of John S. Mack, who died on September 27, 1940, one year and six days following the dedication of the wing he built in honor of his parents, John and Sarah Mack. The trust John S. Mack established back in 1935 was substantial enough to keep the Mack name alive, however. After January 1, 1941, the fund generated enough income to provide care for needy residents of Brush Valley Township, in addition to providing for the maintenance and repair of the Mack Memorial Wing.

In the meantime, the winds of war were once again blowing through Europe. Historians generally agree that World War II began on September 1, 1939, with Germany's invasion of Poland. As with the first "war to end all wars," the United States under President Franklin Roosevelt attempted to maintain a policy of nonintervention. That sentiment quickly changed, however, when the Japanese, having joined Germany and other Axis nations, attacked Pearl Harbor on December 7, 1941. With a horrified nation's full-throated support, the United States declared war on Japan the very next day, followed by declarations of war against Germany and Italy on December 12.

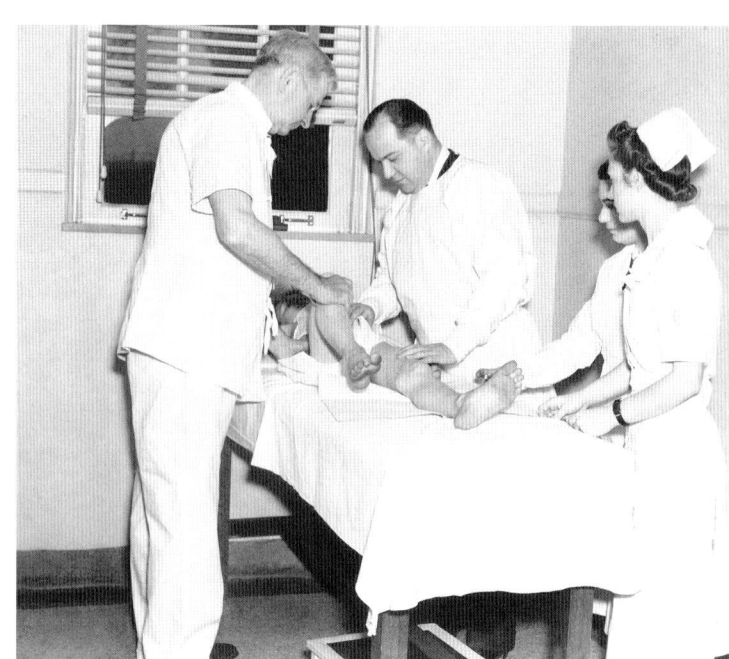

Surgeons examine a young patient while nurses look on.

Top: Construction gets underway on the 1958 wing.

36 —⎯⎯⎯ Indiana Regional Medical Center

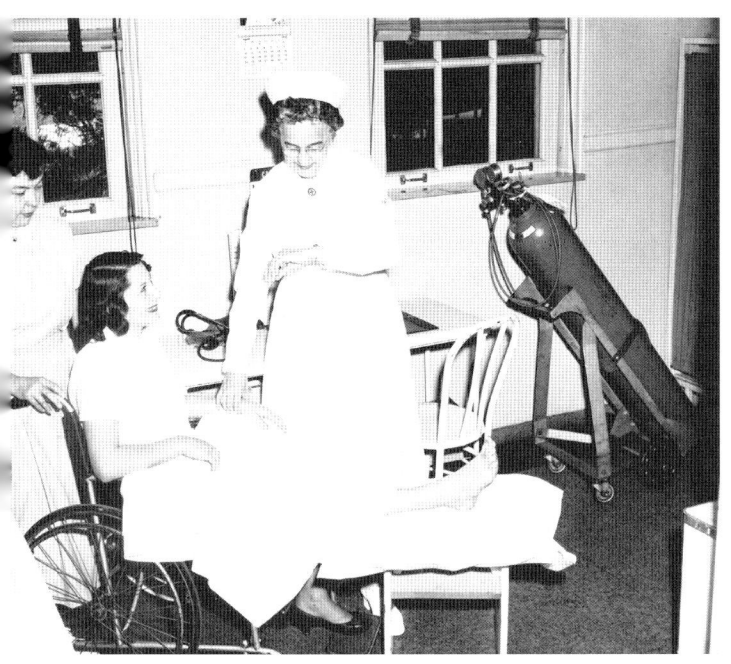

A nurse, starched white uniform and smiling face, tends to a patient brought in by a candy striper, 1955.

diana Hospital again turned its attention to the quality of its facilities, recognizing the need for a more modern educational facility for the School of Nursing. The Board of Directors launched a capital campaign, appealing to the community to help erect a large addition to the 1937 building to house more students. The new nurses' home and educational unit, which opened in October 1947, included dormitory space, classrooms, a kitchen for teaching dietetics, and an auditorium. Among donations from the County Medical Society and others, movie star and Indiana native Jimmy Stewart generously donated several thousand dollars to the school, enough to purchase educational equipment, a sound projector and screen for the recitation room, furnishings for the lounge and auditorium, and equipment for the nursing arts laboratory. Another generous donation made possible the Jean R. McElhaney Memorial Library, which made the latest books and publications on nursing available to the student nurses and faculty. The Indiana Hospital School of Nursing received the full approval of the Pennsylvania State Board of Nurse Examiners.

TWO FORMIDABLE WOMEN

Long before women entered the mainstream workforce, women frequently oversaw the day-to-day operations of hospitals, perhaps because the preponderance of patient care fell to the nurses. But in the mid-to-late 1940s, two women rose to leadership

Indiana's Famous Native Son

As actor Jimmy Stewart was rising to movie star fame, his father, Alex Stewart, had his own brand of fame in his hometown of Indiana. A man who Dr. Ralph Waldo described as "the town character," he was famous for arriving late to church in his familiar but slightly shabby tweed jacket. "He would toddle down the church aisle to about the third row," Jo Waldo recalled, making a conspicuous entrance. Alex was also famous for his lack of driving skills. The family lived in a nice house on top of Vinegar Hill and the road down beneath had a concrete retaining wall. "Everyone called it Alex Stewart's wall," said Dr. Waldo, "because of all the marks he left on it."

Understandably proud of their son's achievements, the family's hardware store window was always filled with memorabilia from Jimmy's movies. Hoping to cash in on that fame, one day Alex Stewart came to the emergency room on his horse's behalf. Dr. Waldo was called down to the emergency room. "My son bought this hospital a new x-ray machine, and my horse has a bad leg," Alex told him. Dr. Waldo then called Dr. Jacobson, the radiologist, who agreed to x-ray the horse's leg. The portable x-ray machine was brought to the emergency room, Alex brought his horse up from the fairgrounds where he kept him, and Dr. Jacobson x-rayed the horse's leg, only to determine that he was quite all right. Alex Stewart left entirely satisfied.

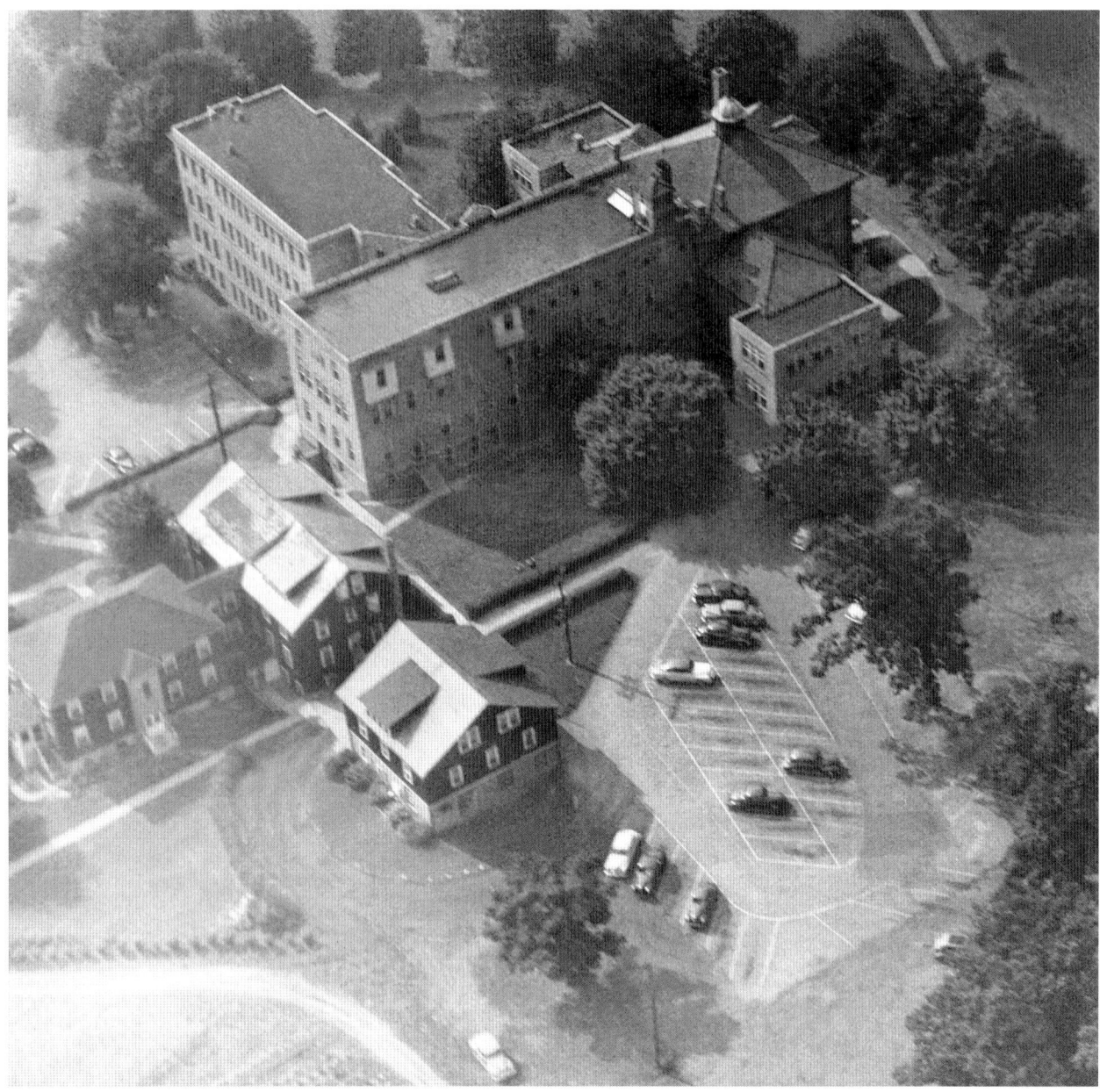

An aerial view of the hospital in the early 1950s.

positions and, through the full force of their dedication, made an indelible mark on the history of Indiana Hospital.

Hospital Superintendent Lillian Hollohan resigned her post in March 1944. She was succeeded by a woman who, for the next twenty years, inspired both fear and admiration in the hearts and minds of everyone associated with Indiana Hospital.

Adeline Hawxhurst began her career at the hospital on August 26, 1915, working as a bookkeeper. She received her education at the Model School, known later as Keith School, followed by two years at Indiana State Normal School. In early 1929 she was made office manager, with two employees working under her supervision. From 1939 to 1943, Miss Hawxhurst was the assistant administrator, and when Miss Hollohan resigned, she was asked to take the position of administrator. To meet the challenges of her new responsibilities, Adeline took a special course in hospital administration at the University of Chicago in 1948 and was admitted to the American College of Hospital Administrators in 1954.

Dr. Ralph Waldo, who first started working at Indiana Hospital in 1949 before being called to military duty, approached the pragmatic Miss Hawxhurst with an offer she was delighted to accept on behalf of the physicians who were trying to wean their patients away from house calls in favor of the hospital's emergency room. "I came to Indiana Hospital and asked Miss Hawxhurst if she'd hire me," Dr. Waldo recalled. "I told her I would run the emergency room and take care of all the free patients. Miss Hawxhurst was very happy, and the physicians were happy, too, because I was going to do that work for them. So I took all the histories and did the examinations on the free patients, and if a doctor didn't get there in time, I delivered the babies." His wife, Jo Waldo, remembers Miss Hawxhurst as an imposing figure, entirely dedicated to her work. "If ever an administrator had only one thing on their mind—the hospital—that was her. She had no other life . . . she was passionate and unswerving."

The possibility exists, of course, that members of the hospital's board of directors influenced Miss Hawxhurst, and not everyone embraced the concept of a woman in charge. Nonetheless, if she did not inspire affection from some of the physicians, certainly an atmosphere of mutual respect existed between them. Dr. Melvin Williams, who did not join the staff until 1967, summed it up: "She was tough," he said. "We got along very well but she was the boss . . . no doubt about that."

The other notable woman who made her mark on Indiana Hospital was Miss Nettie Bealer, a woman who Jo Waldo described as "another formidable soul." She was hired as Director of Nursing in 1948, a post she held until her retirement in 1965. Upon her arrival, the nursing school affiliated with the Indiana University of Pennsylvania where nursing students could take classes in biological and physical sciences.

Nettie Bealer demanded precision from the nurses who worked under her supervision. At a time when physicians wore suits and ties to the hospital, Miss Bealer and her nurses were in impossibly starched, blindingly white uniforms. Careful not to interfere with the physician's orders or instructions, she was quick to go to bat in defense of her nurses when a problem arose. She ran an efficient operation but, despite her stern demeanor, was a compassionate caregiver. Beverly Capriani, a nurse from those days, told Jo Waldo that where Miss Bealer was concerned, "the patients always came first—at any cost."

During Miss Nettie Bealer's tenure as Director of Nursing, Indiana Hospital nursing students became members of the local, district, state, and national Student Nurses Association.

THE MINER'S FUND

How well the coal companies took care of employees could probably be debated long and hard, but they did, at least, help provide medical care for the miners and their families. For three dollars per month, deducted from their pay, the physician took care of the entire family, making house calls and providing medicines. Dr. Ralph Brown, whose fledgling practice in Homer City was not quite keeping him busy, got a call from "one of the bigwigs" at the Rochester and Pittsburgh Coal Company asking him to become a company doctor. After talking with some other doctors, he decided it was a good way to get started but sometimes found it a daunting job, providing all their needs. "I had cold pills, nerve pills, sleeping pills, blood pressure pills. If they had seven kids, I took care of them."

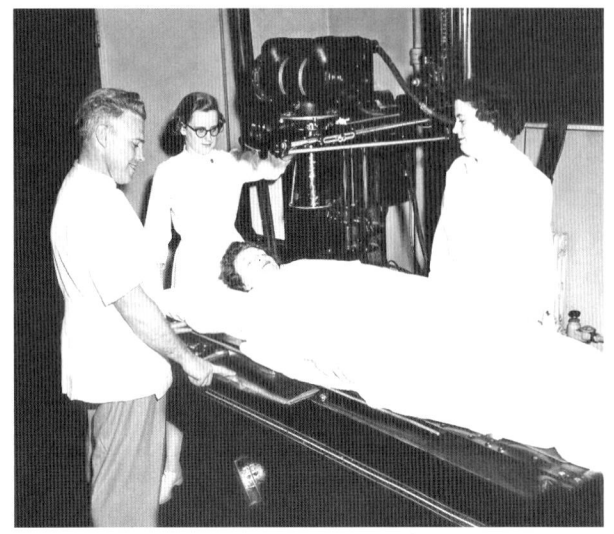

Hospital staffers demonstrate their new x-ray equipment.

In the 1940s, Indiana Hospital's Dr. John Lapsley was one of those physicians hired by a coal company. Though he was in general practice, according to Dr. Waldo, Dr. Lapsley "delivered more babies than anybody else" and was famous for his proficiency with the internal podalic version (the process of turning a fetus in utero), a procedure he taught to Dr. Waldo.

Dr. Lapsley told Dr. Ralph Waldo and his wife Jo of one occasion shortly after becoming a physician for the mines. When the phone rang in the middle of the night, he arrived at the alleged patient's home, only to be told he was being tested to see if he would come when summoned. A few years later, Dr. Brown had a similar experience as a coal company physician. Part of his agreement with the coal company was that he would not be required to treat anybody that he did not like or that did not like him. The first week he got his phone call at 1:00 a.m., and when he arrived, he also was told that no one was sick, that they just wanted to see what he looked like. This time, though, the plan backfired, and Dr. Brown had their name removed from the list. "By noon that day," Dr. Brown recalled, "every coal miner knew not to mess with me."

In the 1940s, the coal miners got a little more assistance when a group of local mine leaders organized the Employees Hospital Committee Fund. Started by the District 2 United Mine Workers Association members, the fund was used as a supplement to their usual UMWA health insurance, particularly during layoffs or when hospital expenses exceeded their coverage. Participation in the plan was voluntary, and for another three dollars per month, they were assured of total hospital coverage at a time when a bed in the ward cost about eighteen dollars per day and the doctor received three dollars per day for each day of the patient's stay. The fund was only applicable to Indiana Hospital, and the monies went directly to the hospital, creating a win/win situation for everyone. The hospital was able to minimize its losses, and the miners and their families enjoyed a measure of peace, knowing they could receive the medical care they needed without incurring crippling debt.

As Indiana Hospital's history is being prepared, the fund is set to finally close out as of June 30, 2013, having served a very valuable service to the hospital and its community.

THE HOSPITAL TURNS THIRTY-FIVE

On Saturday, October 29, 1949, the hospital celebrated its thirty-fifth anniversary by holding a banquet in the social hall of the First Methodist Church. The evening opened with group singing and words of welcome from C. Gilbert Wolfenden, president of the board of directors; Dr. F. J. Kellam, senior surgeon of the medical staff; and Nettie E. Bealer, director of the school of nursing.

More than three hundred people associated with the hospital attended. Members of each class of nurses graduated from the School of Nursing between 1918 and 1949, 110 in all, were present as were Dr. Wetzel and Dr. Buterbaugh, members of the first medical staff of 1914. The hospital's first superintendent, Mrs. Charles Leventry (Sara Morgart) of Johnstown attended as did Mrs. Ethel Reed, then president of the hospital alumnae association.

O'Donnel Iselin of New York City, the nephew of Adrian Iselin Jr., attended, recalling the hospital's dedication in 1914. Since that day, more than 103,000 patients had been treated during the hospital's thirty-five years, and its original forty-patient-bed capacity was now at two hundred. Heath S. Clark of the Rochester and Pittsburgh Coal Company was the featured speaker for the occasion, referring to Indiana Hospital as "the biggest little hospital in the state."

THE AUXILIARY

In September 1947 the Junior and Senior Auxiliaries merged to form the now unified Indiana Hospital Auxiliary. They continued raising money by holding benefit dances, rummage sales, and the annual charity ball. Of all their numerous contributions to the hospital, none have become as much of a fixture at the hospital as the Pantry. Originally a three-stool lunch counter, the Auxiliary established the Pantry in 1951 for the convenience of both visitors and personnel. The first person to be served was Dr. Frederick J. Kellam, chief of surgery, who was served a cup of coffee.

A TEN-YEAR PLAN

In 1954, the hospital devised a ten-year plan to again expand and upgrade the hospital's facilities. Outpatient visits had risen by 205 percent over the preceding ten years from 3,750 visits in 1946 to 11,497 in 1955. X-ray services alone increased by 104 percent. There was no question—additional clinics and diagnostic treatment rooms were desperately needed.

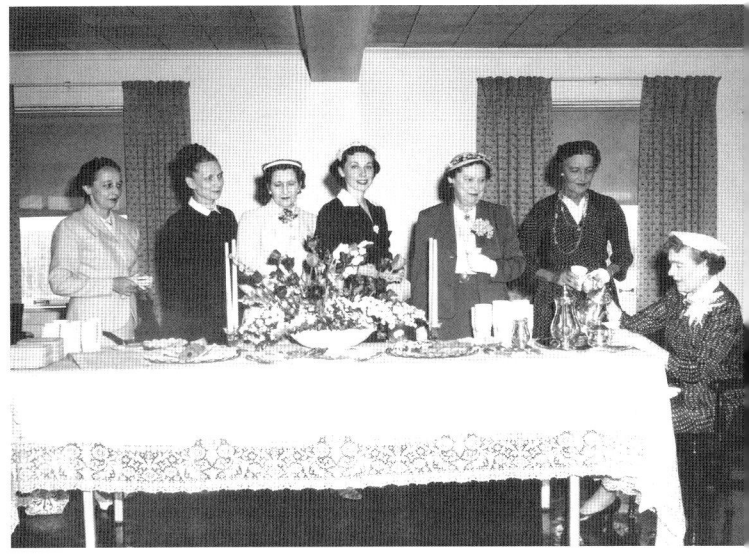

In the 1950s, the ladies of the Auxiliary dressed in their Sunday best for meetings.

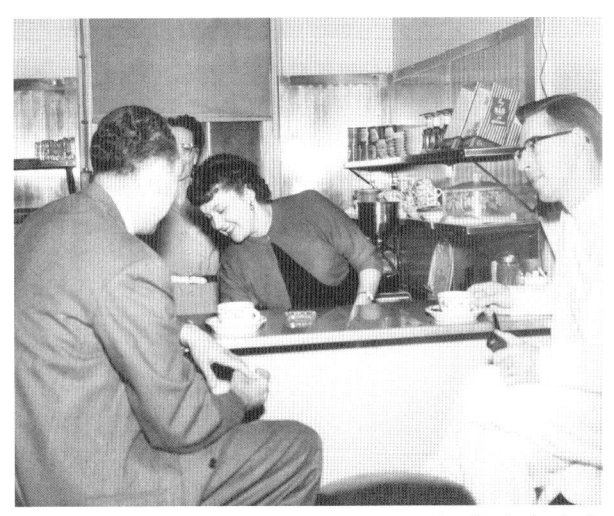

Dr. Herbert Long and Dr. Ralph Waldo enjoy a cup of coffee in the Auxiliary's original Pantry.

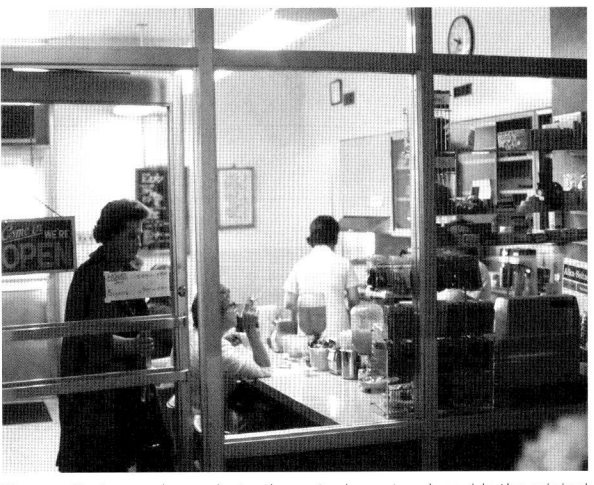

The new Pantry—no longer just a three-stool counter alongside the original elevator.

The Physicians

As of 1952, the following Indiana Hospital physicians were also members of the Indiana County Medical Society:

Dr. Joseph W. Gatti of Indiana Hospital's surgical staff graduated from Homer City High School in 1928 and from St. Bonaventure College in 1932. After receiving his medical degree from Jefferson Medical College in 1936, he interned at St. John's General Hospital in Pittsburgh.

Dr. H. B. Buterbaugh, at the time the oldest member of the hospital staff, was born May 12, 1871, in Cookport, Pennsylvania. He was a graduate of the Purchase Line Academy, Western Reserve Medical School in Cleveland, Ohio, and New York University postgraduate school. Through his association with Dr. Frank Ehrenfeldt, he came to Indiana to begin his practice in 1896.

Dr. Thomas Watkins Kredel was born June 20, 1908, in Johnstown. He received his medical degree at Jefferson Medical College in 1932 and did his internship and surgical residency at Germantown Hospital in Philadelphia. He began his surgical practice at Indiana Hospital in 1936.

Dr. William H. Eastment graduated from the University of Pennsylvania Medical School in 1949 and interned at St. Luke's Hospital in Bethlehem. He joined Indiana Hospital's surgical staff in 1945.

Dr. Daniel Harold Bee was born in Summit Station, Ohio, received his medical degree at Temple University, and did his graduate work at Tufts Medical College, Emory University, and the University of Michigan.

Dr. William Charles Vernocy was born in Oakmont and received his medical degree at the University of Pittsburgh School of Medicine in 1936 where he also served his internship. Dr. Vernocy spent five years from 1941 to 1946 in the army as a major and saw three years of overseas duty in the South Pacific Theatre. As of 1952 he was president of the hospital staff.

Dr. Harry B. Neal Jr. was born in Indiana. Following his premed work at Princeton, he received his medical degree from the College of Physicians and Surgeons of Columbia University in New York City in June 1942. Following his internship at Mercy Hospital in Pittsburgh, Dr. Neal entered active service with the Army Medical Corps in 1945 and for one year served aboard transports in the Southwest Pacific and European Theatres. Dr. Neal returned to Indiana in 1946 where he became associated with his father in the general practice of medicine.

Dr. Frederick J. Kellam was born in Princess Anne, Virginia, on July 21, 1891, and graduated from the Medical College of Virginia in 1915. He practiced in Virginia until 1921 and then practiced in Ernest from 1921 to 1926. After a year specializing in surgery at the New York Polyclinic Hospital, New York, he came to Indiana in August 1927. He took postgraduate work at Tulane University, Massachusetts General Hospital in Boston, Harvard Medical School, Cook County Hospital in Chicago, Boston City Hospital, and Post-Graduate Hospital in New York City.

Dr. J. W. Campbell is a native of Elderton in Armstrong County. He received his medical degree from Baltimore Medical School in 1909 and interned at Columbia Hospital in Pittsburgh. In 1915 and 1916, he took postgraduate work at Harvard University and Cook County Hospital. He took over the Gates Hospital; when it closed in the early 1950s, he joined the staff at Indiana Hospital.

Dr. C. E. D'Zmura received his medical degree from the University of Pittsburgh Medical School. His practice is in Homer City.

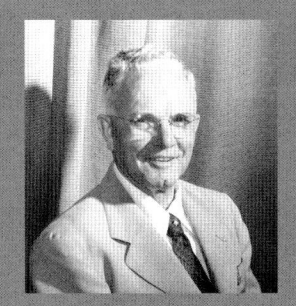

Dr. J. W. Campbell, pictured here in 1953, took over operation of the Gates Hospital in 1935.

Dr. H. B. Neal Sr. was born in Indiana where he lived his entire life, his ancestors coming to the county in 1777. He graduated from Indiana Normal School in 1901, took postgraduate work in 1902, and received his degree from the University of Pittsburgh Medical School in 1906. Along with Dr. George Simpson, Dr. Neal started the Simpson-Neal Hospital. The Hospital Association of Indiana County, which was organized in 1912, contracted with Dr. Simpson and Dr. Neal in February 1913 to care for state aid cases until the new Indiana Hospital opened. In 1952, he was the only remaining physician among the original staff.

Dr. George W. Hanna received his medical degree from Georgetown University after attending there from 1934 to 1938. He served his internship at McKeesport Hospital in 1938 and 1939 and his residency at Sewickley Valley Hospital from 1939 to 1940. He located in Homer City in 1940 and joined Indiana Hospital's surgical staff. He was a surgical associate of the late Drs. G. E. Simpson and G. C. Martin of Indiana from 1940 to 1951. From 1951 to 1954, he did his postgraduate surgical work at the University of Pittsburgh Medical Center Hospitals.

Dr. R. G. Ellis received his medical degree from Temple Medical School in 1936 and served his internship at St. Margaret's Hospital in Pittsburgh in 1937. For eleven years, he was in Brush Valley before he came to Indiana in 1950.

Dr. Dorsey R. Hoyt graduated from Jefferson Medical College in 1933. He served with the US Army from July 1943 to January 1945. In 1952, he began his practice in Indiana and joined the medical staff of Indiana Hospital.

Dr. John Lapsley took his premed work at the University of Pittsburgh and the University of West Virginia, graduating from Temple University Medical School in 1930. Dr. Lapsley served his internship at the South Side Hospital in Pittsburgh from 1930 to 1931 and spent two years in general practice in East McKeesport. In 1934, he went to Waterman where he spent six and a half years. In 1940 he went to Ernest where he spent eleven years as a union doctor. In 1951 he opened a general practice in Indiana and became a member of the medical staff of Indiana Hospital.

Dr. Harold L. Edison, general practitioner, came to Indiana in 1949, a graduate of the University of Pittsburgh School of Medicine. He spent two years in Indiana before being called to the service and returned from Korea in 1952 to resume his practice.

Once again the hospital turned to the community with another capital campaign for a diagnostic and outpatient wing to be added to the east side of the hospital. Again, the community responded, generously raising $665,000. The Auxiliary gave $25,000 to the cause, 80 percent of which came from Pantry profits. The hospital also had $700,000 from foundation, corporate, and individual gifts as well as federal funds they received under the Hill-Burton Act, which Congress had passed in 1946 expressly for the purpose of providing grants and guaranteed loans to improve the physical plant of the nation's hospital system. By 1958 the new $1.3 million building was added to the hospital complex.

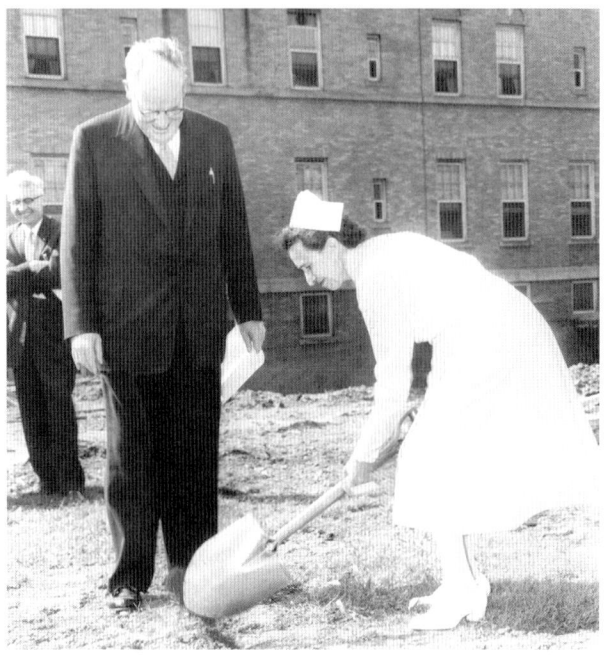

Nurse Bertha Manner is given the honor of breaking ground for the 1958 expansion as Judge Clark (background) and Gilbert Wolfenden, former state senator and chairman of the board, look on.

The Farm
Since its beginning, the hospital maintained a small farm on the hospital grounds using the fruits and vegetables grown there to help feed both patients and staff. In 1953, the farm was discontinued.

Indiana Hospital's First Female Physician
Indiana Hospital's first female resident physician was Dr. Margaret Oakes Strawn, born and raised in Clymer. She graduated from Clymer High School in 1944, took her premed studies at Penn State, and then entered Women's Medical College of Pennsylvania in Philadelphia from which she received her medical degree in 1952. She did her internship at Montgomery Hospital in Norristown and in 1954 joined the staff at Indiana Hospital. Her term there, however, was short-lived. After a year when her husband completed his master's degree, she moved to Virginia to set up private practice.

The basement of the new wing contained the kitchen and cafeteria plus areas for a receiving dock, purchasing offices, and storage. At the entrance to the new wing, an updated Pantry greeted visitors. The first floor was dedicated to radiological and fluoroscopic services, diagnostic and treatment rooms, and administrative offices. Surgical facilities and recovery rooms were on the second floor along with a new laboratory, centrally located to provide easy access to the new operating and recovery rooms. With three times the workspace as the previous laboratory, the hospital was now able to increase its laboratory staff and modernize its equipment. The June 11, 1958, *Indiana Evening Gazette* proclaimed, "The hospital may now perform many new tests previously done only in the larger city hospitals."

Commenting on the addition to the hospital in the May 13, 1958, edition of the *Indiana Evening Gazette*, Nettie Bealer, Director of Nurses and Nursing Services, cited the recovery room as the most signifi-

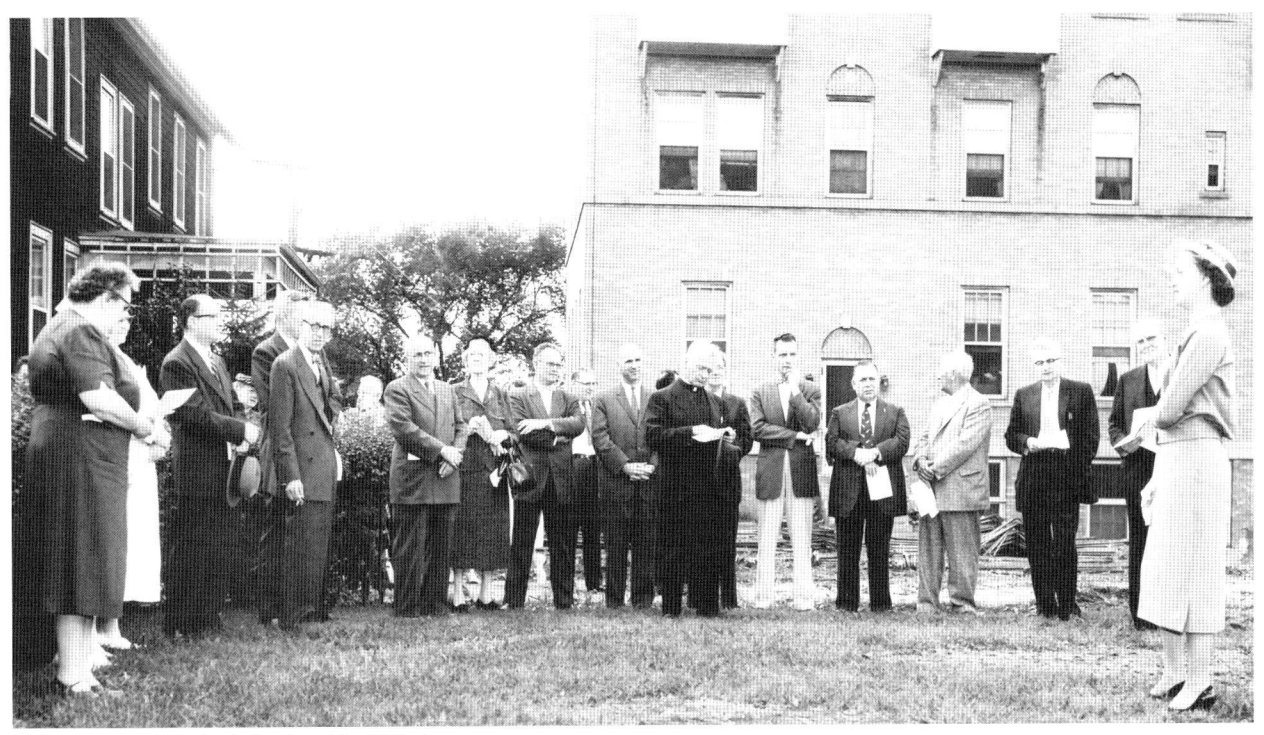

Marge Nolan speaks at the dedication of the 1958 wing.

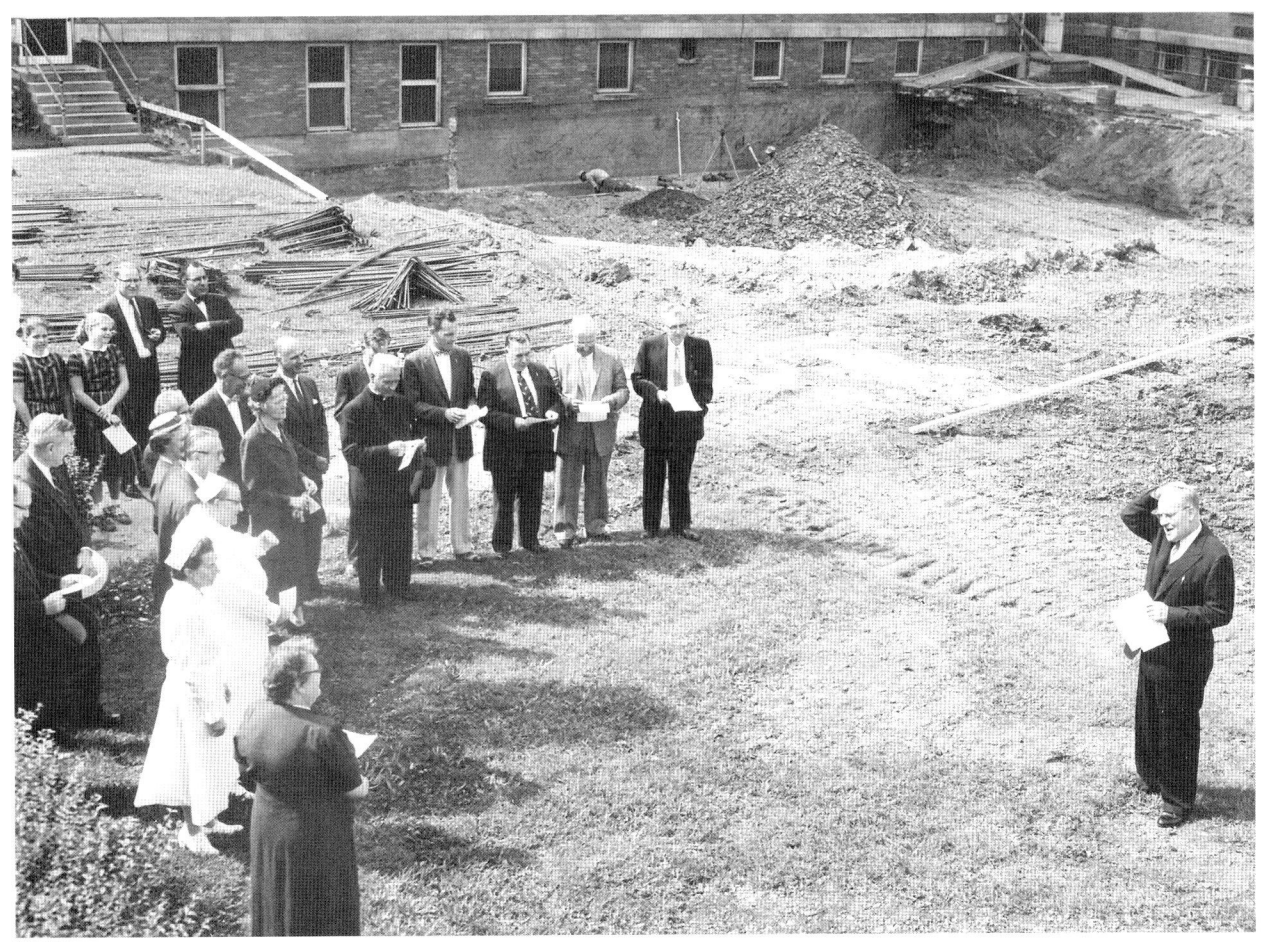

At the dedication of the 1958 wing, three of Indiana Hospital's most notable women were at the forefront—Nettie Bealer, Bertha Manner, and Adeline Hawxhurst.

Chapter 4: The "Hospital on the Hill" Matures — 47

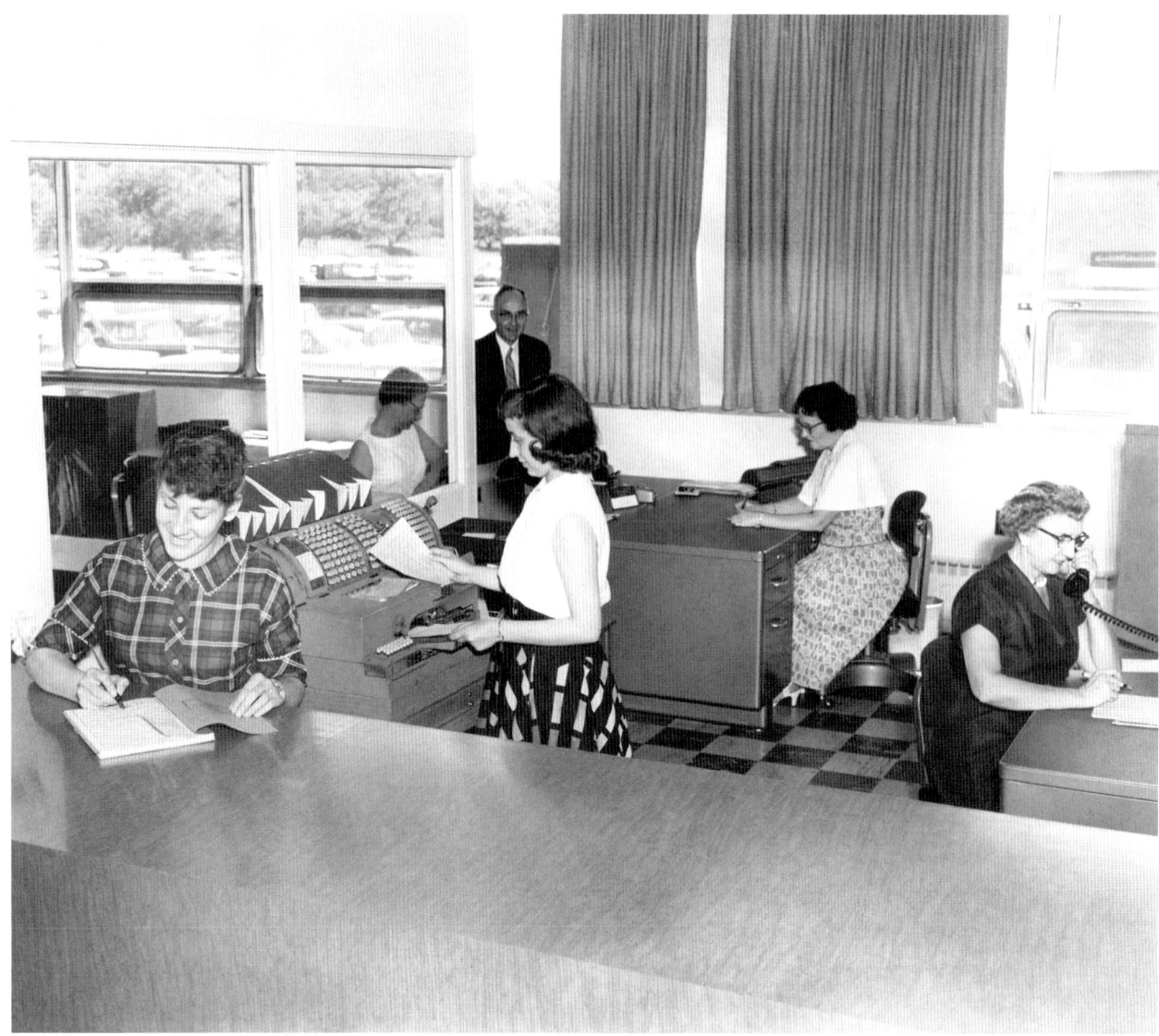

The business office staff, mid-1950s.

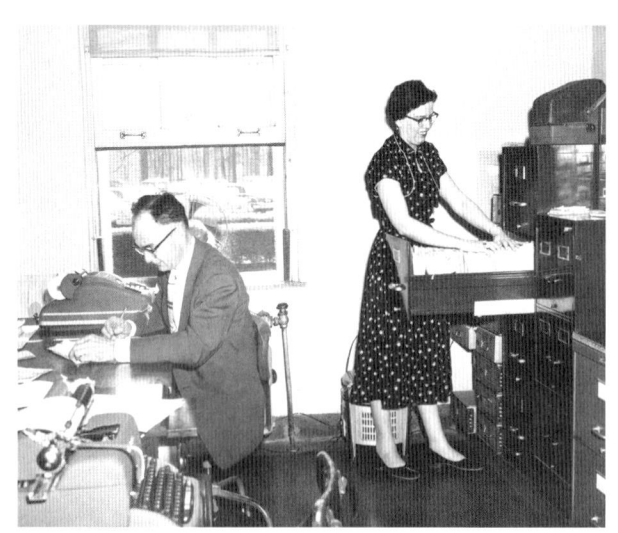

An open window and a fan provide some relief in the pre-air-conditioning days of the 1950s.

cant aspect. "The recovery room is an efficient four-bed surgical unit used as a treatment area following an operation, where constant observation can be made by the doctor, anesthetist, and nurse supervisor. This room is in close proximity to surgery, pharmacy, central supply, and laboratory." Homer G. Harris, hospital accountant, spoke of the new quarters, new equipment, and accounting machines installed to modernize the accounting department. The updated equipment would help alleviate the bottlenecks in payroll and bookkeeping and make it possible for them to compile the statistics necessary for state appropriations eligibility.

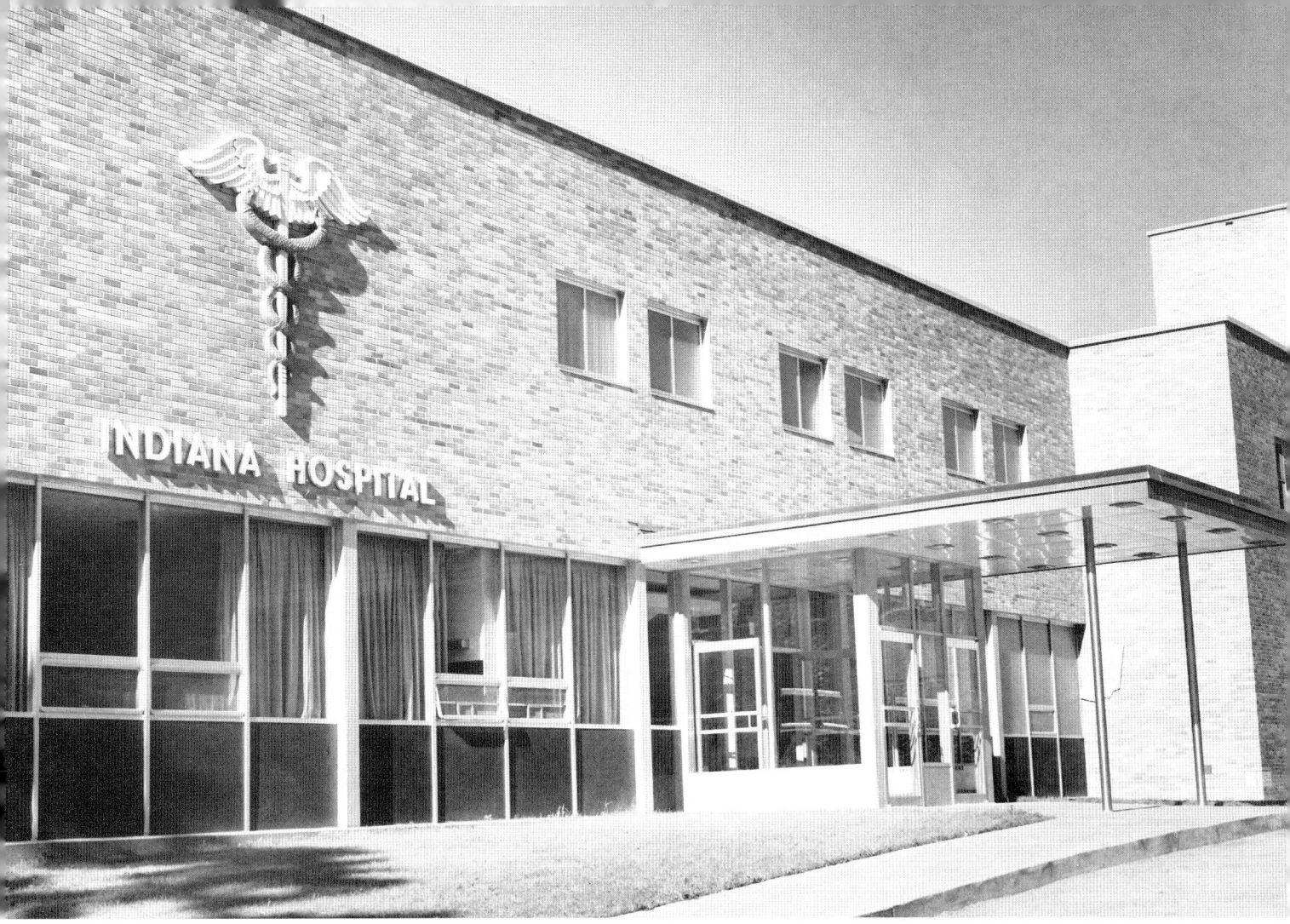

After the 1958 addition to the hospital, the main entrance was on the north side of the hospital.

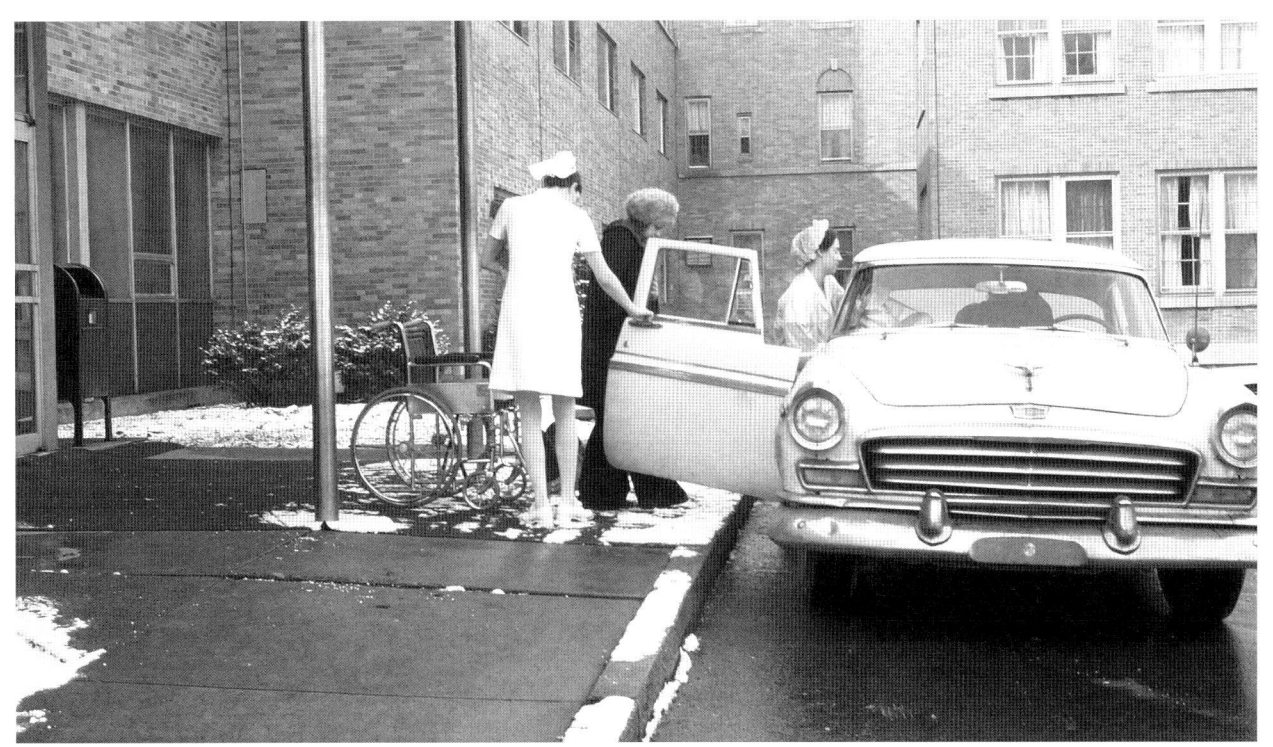

Nurses help a patient with the best part of their hospital stay . . . going home.

Chapter 4: The "Hospital on the Hill" Matures

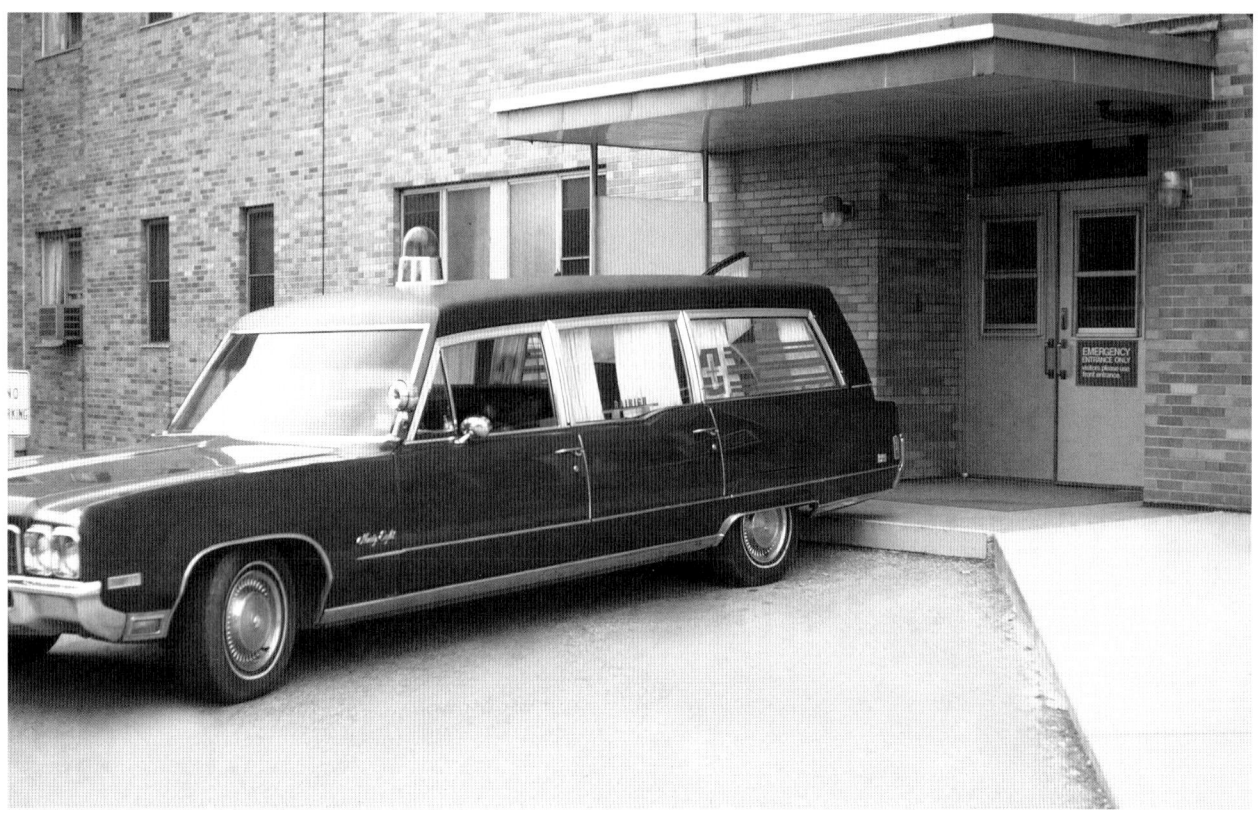

An ambulance pulls up to the entrance to the emergency room in the mid-1960s.

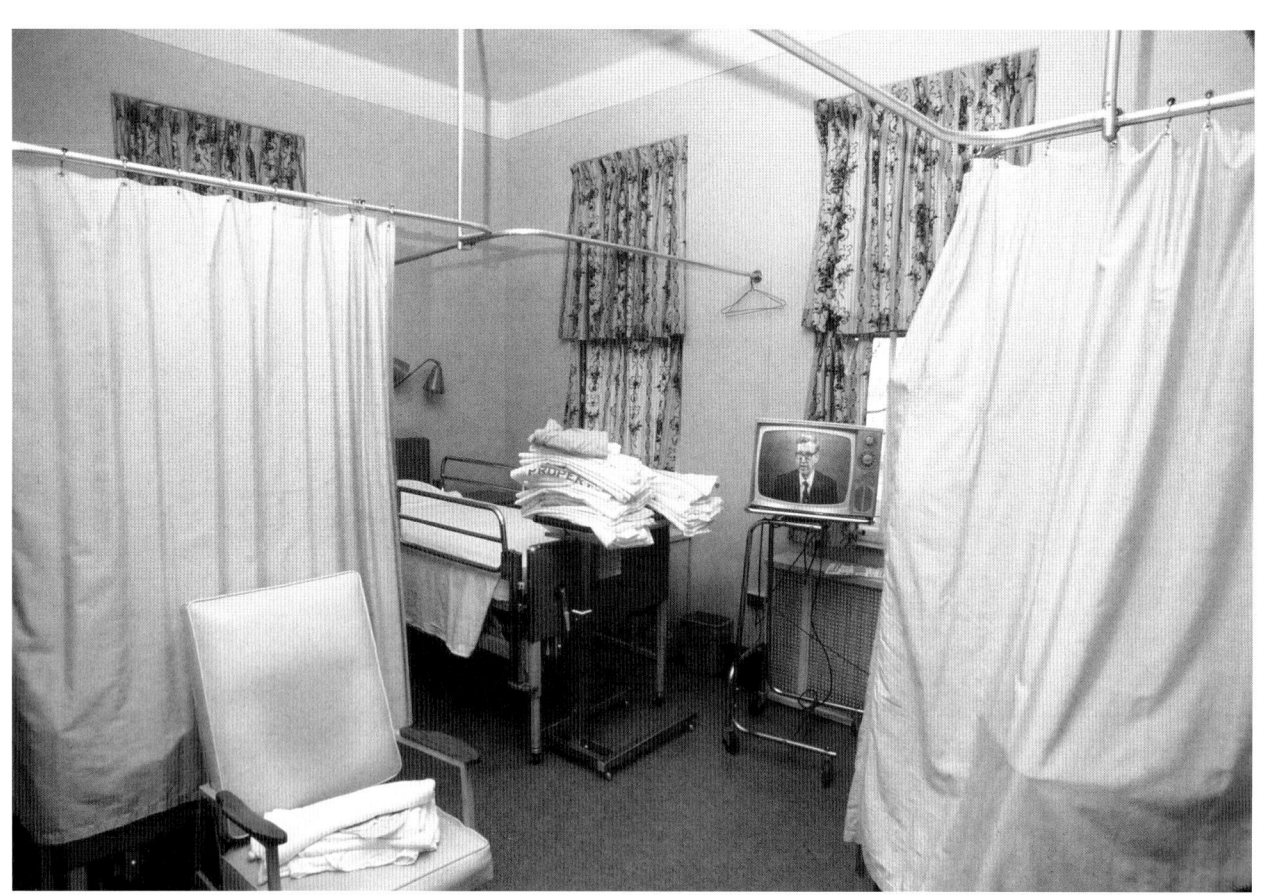

Television service in patients' rooms did not start until 1971. Before that, patients sometimes brought their own.

50 — Indiana Regional Medical Center

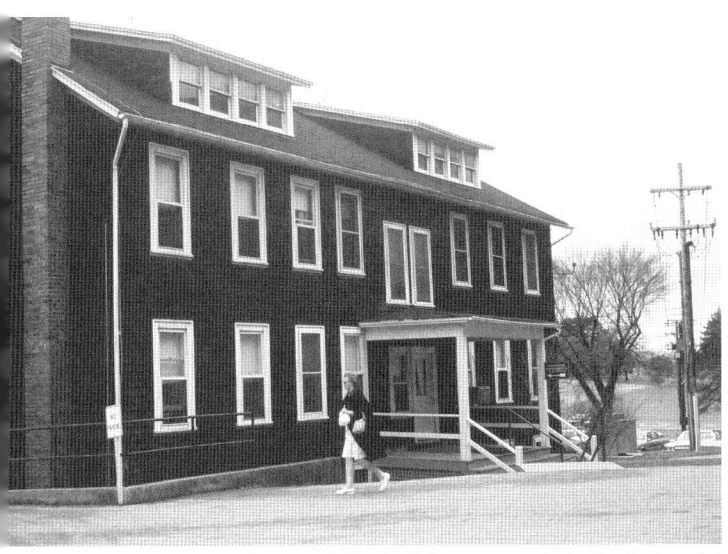

Just as many who came before had done, a nurse dashes to the hospital in starched uniform, white shoes and stockings, and a cape.

An Open House for inspection of the new two-floor wing was held on June 19, 1958. Proud to welcome patients and visitors to the new wing and the updated hospital, the Auxiliary began its guide and escort service to welcome people and provide them with directions and escorts throughout the hospital. They also began their hospitality cart service providing magazines, snacks, and personal care items to patients and visitors at each nursing unit. And though the Auxiliary continued operating the Pantry, it now had its first paid manager.

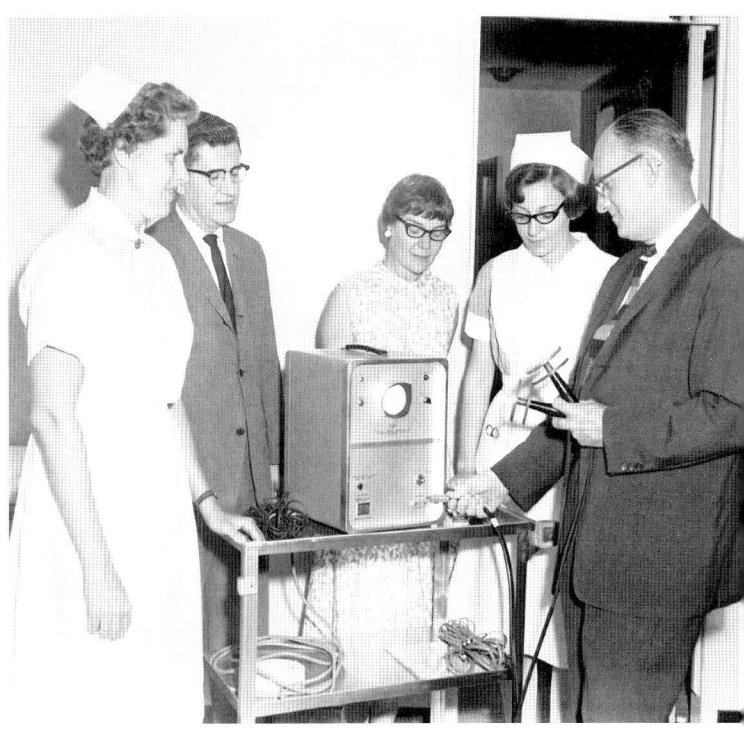

Dr. Bee, far right, demonstrates a defibrillator donated to the hospital in 1965. Photo courtesy of *Indiana Gazette*.

Dr. Campbell's House Calls

The privately owned Gates Hospital at 923 Philadelphia Street in Indiana continued with Dr. J. W. Campbell caring for its patients until the early 1950s. At a time when most physicians were weaning their patients away from house calls, Dr. Campbell never did. Dr. Brown, who himself confessed he never managed the feat, recalled that after closing the Gates Hospital, Dr. Jessie Campbell continued making house calls even when he was ninety years old. "They would go to his house and get him," said Dr. Brown, "take him to see the patient and then take him back home."

Chapter 4: The "Hospital on the Hill" Matures

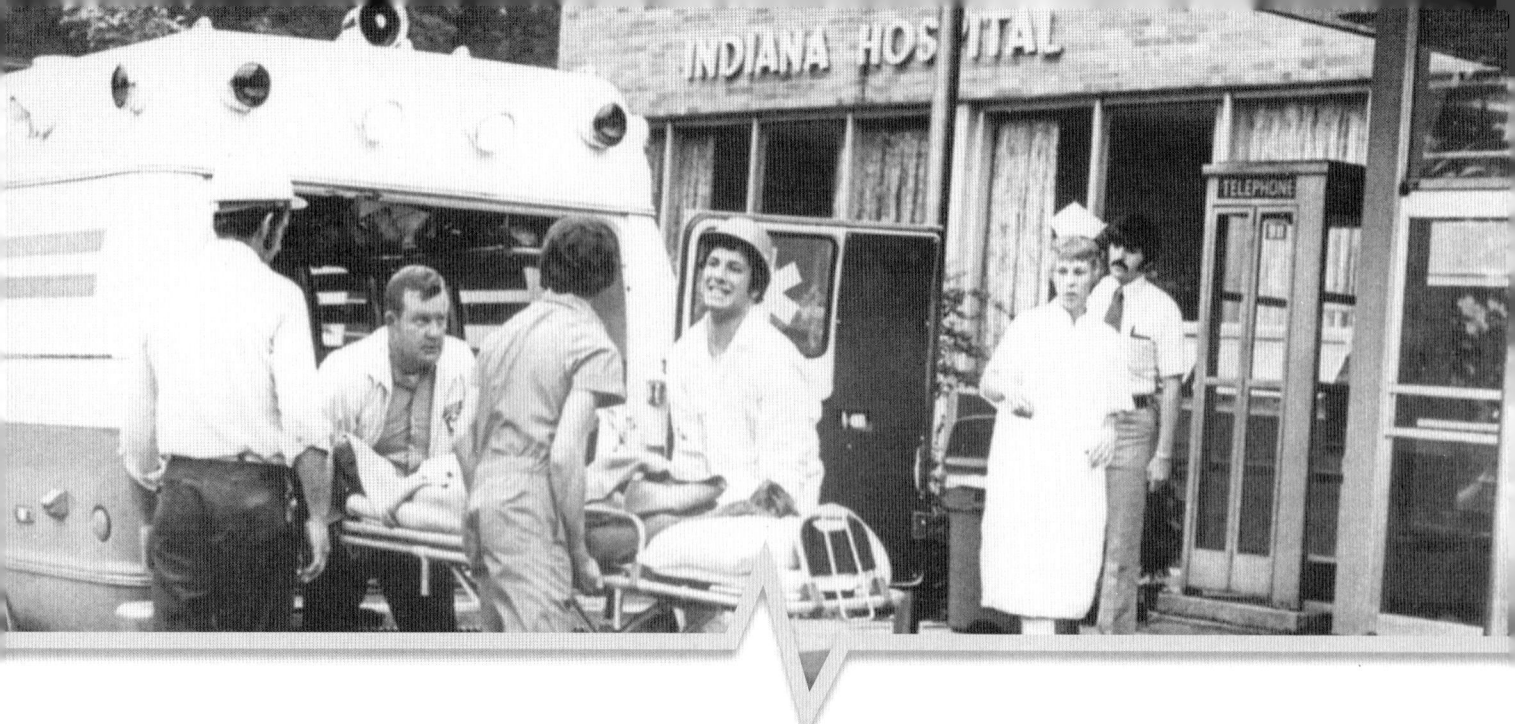

CHAPTER 5
Turbulence, Tradition, and the Tower

The 1960s was a time of turbulence across the United States. The decade would ultimately be marked by three major assassinations—President John F. Kennedy, his brother Senator Robert F. Kennedy, and the Rev. Dr. Martin Luther King—racial tension, and a counterculture of rebellious youths known as "hippies" whose protests of the Vietnam War became famous more for their use of psychotropic drugs than their political prowess. The shaggy-haired Beatles from London changed American rock and roll music forever and brought with them the fashions of Carnaby Street: miniskirts, bell-bottom pants bearing outrageous floral designs, and the psychedelic art of Peter Max.

Amid all this evolution and revolution, Indiana Hospital remained a bastion of traditional values. Nowhere is that more evident than in the standards to which the nurses, student and graduate, were held.

Bernice Leslie graduated from the School of Nursing in 1960. She originally set out to become a flight attendant, but learning that they also had to be nurses at that time, her parents' illnesses caused her to cut her career goals short and stick to nursing, a career to which she dedicated herself for the next forty-one years.

Fortunately for Bernice, an anonymous donor paid for her education, having reviewed the applications and taking note of Bernice's grades. Much later, Bernice learned that a lady named Wanda Wyatt was her educational benefactor. "It was a blessing for me," Bernice said, "because then my parents just had to give me a little bit of spending money."

At that time, the nurses' three-year education consisted of two semesters of classes at Indiana State Teacher's College, three-months-long on-site stays at both a pediatric hospital and a psychiatric institution, and the remainder within the walls of Indiana Hospital. The nursing students were granted two weeks of vacation time during the summer. "We began our freshman year with morning classes at Indi-

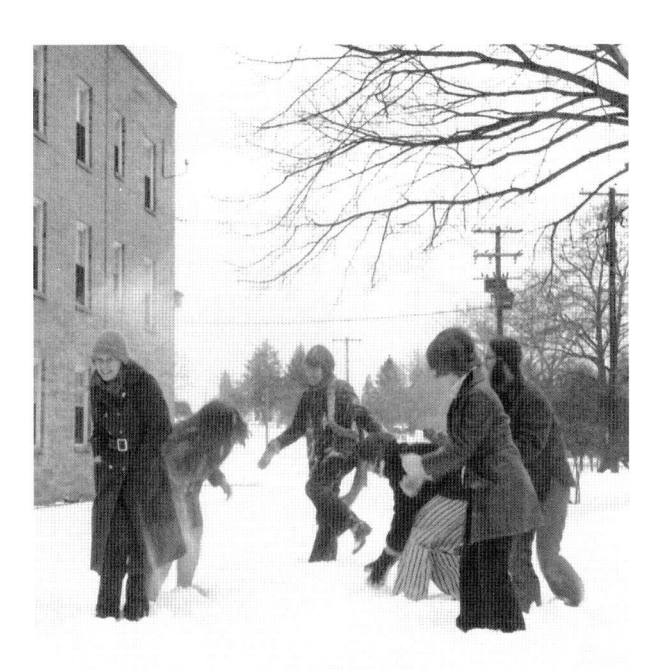

Nursing students take a break from studies to play in the snow.

Opposite page: Nurse Bernice Leslie goes into action as a patient arrives by ambulance.

ana State Teacher's College," Diane Petras recalled, "followed by hospital assignments in the afternoons." Students were transported from the hospital to the college and back again in a station wagon, requiring the driver to make numerous trips to get the nurses back and forth. Once past their probation period, the students participated in a "capping ceremony" during which they received their student caps and a small Nightingale lamp, and were required to recite the "Nightingale Pledge."

During their second and third years, the students were on full-day hospital assignments, alternating with formal classes held in the basement of the nursing building. They were also assigned weekend and holiday shifts at the hospital as well as night shift assignments during their senior year.

As it was when first begun, the School of Nursing was known for its strict discipline, a tradition upheld by its director, Nettie Bealer. "She put the fear of God in

1961

1962 The hospital receives cobalt capsules for the treatment of cancer.

1963 In March, the Auxiliary launches the baby picture service for mothers and newborns.

1964 $550,000, $25,000 from the Auxiliary alone, is raised for the addition of a third floor to the 1956 wing, as well as for renovation of existing facilities. Additions and renovations include new maternity facilities and a modern Dietary Department among others.

The Children's Ward moves to Mack III and becomes the Pediatrics Unit.

1965

A cardiac defibrillator is donated to the hospital.

A radio service connecting Indiana Hospital and Citizens' Ambulance Service Inc. is installed, allowing ambulance attendants to communicate with staff in the hospital's Emergency Services Department. The radio service is one of the first in the country and the first in Pennsylvania.

The Adeline W. Hawxhurst Memorial for nursing students is established to honor her fifty years of service.

1966

Medicare takes effect at hospitals across the nation.

The Candy Striper Unit of the Auxiliary begins for teens interested in the nursing profession.

The School of Nursing receives its first married student and its first male student.

1967

The Inhalation Therapy Department is formed for the diagnosis, treatment, and prevention of lung diseases and disorders.

Forty percent of the total patient days are those of Medicare patients, whose average stay is thirteen days.

1968

The Council of Churches of Greater Indiana begins a volunteer chaplain service at the hospital.

A five-bed Intensive Care Unit opens. The Auxiliary donates $28,000 toward equipment.

1969

The School of Nursing receives its first national accreditation from the National League for Nursing.

The Sixth Street entrance road to the hospital is completed.

Timeline

1970
- The Department of Nuclear Medicine is formed.
- The medical staff organizes the preceptorship program for medical students.
- The Auxiliary begins mail service to patients and departments.

1971
- In August, improvements are made in the Radiology Department, television service for patients begins, and a chapel, furnished by the family of Dr. Hoyt in his memory, is added.

1972
- With a telemetry unit, a patient's electrocardiogram is now transmitted from the ambulance to the hospital.

1973
- James A. Garrettson, MD, performs the first flexible endoscopy at Indiana Hospital.

1974
- A $10 million expansion to the hospital is announced.

1975
- The hospital's Development Fund raises more than $2.6 million from the community for expansion.
- The Indiana County Hospital Authority is established.

1976
- Fire severely damages the 1937 nursing school, which is now set to close when the current freshmen class graduates in the spring of 1979.
- The first paramedic trauma-equipped unit of Citizens' Ambulance Service Inc. begins full operation after 480 hours of instruction at the ambulance service and the hospital. The first class of paramedics volunteered their service to Indiana and surrounding communities.
- Indiana Hospital is honored by the American Hospital Association for marking fifty years as a member institution. In September Indiana University of Pennsylvania's (IUP) Department of Nursing begins its affiliation with Indiana Hospital, with student nurses being assigned to the hospital's clinical areas of pediatrics, obstetrics, and gynecology.

1977
- The first hospital blood drive is held in cooperation with the American Red Cross.

---

all of us," Bernice said, "but she made us nurses." A very large lady with extremely short hair, Nettie Bealer was known for her starched long-sleeve uniforms that were nothing less than meticulous even in the dead of summer before the days of air conditioning.

As with herself, her standards for the nurses were unrelenting. Even in class they wore a blue-and-white-checkered dress with a white bib and white hose, shoes, and cap. Their pockets had divided spaces for a pen, a scissor, and a notebook, items they were required to have with them at all times.

Breaking the rules, no matter how small, was only for mavericks, and Bernice recalls two such students who brazenly shortened their uniforms to just above the knee. When Miss Bealer spotted them, she took out her scissors and cut the stitching from the hem to restore the skirts to their proper length. Students who were engaged were not allowed to wear their ring, and if someone dared to, Miss Bealer quickly confiscated the treasured object.

As unrelenting as she was in her discipline, Nettie Bealer was also steadfast in defense of the nurses in her charge. "We could have made the biggest mistake known to man and she'd be right there with us," Bernice recalled. "Privately, she'd say, 'You know what you did; you made a mistake,' but never to the doctors. She would not give us up . . . ever. We were like her children."

Diane Petras, who started at the School of Nursing in 1960, also recalls the exacting standards of the day. Students were expected to be at breakfast at 6 a.m., and, on occasion, they were inspected. "We couldn't have our nails over the tops of our fingers," she said. "We had to hold our hands up, and if they could see our nails above our fingertips, we had to go back." Uniforms, starched by the hospital laundry, were so stiff they could stand by themselves and were pressed so tightly together the nurses had to peel them apart to get into them. "When we walked, we made all this noise because of all the starch in our uniforms," Diane said.

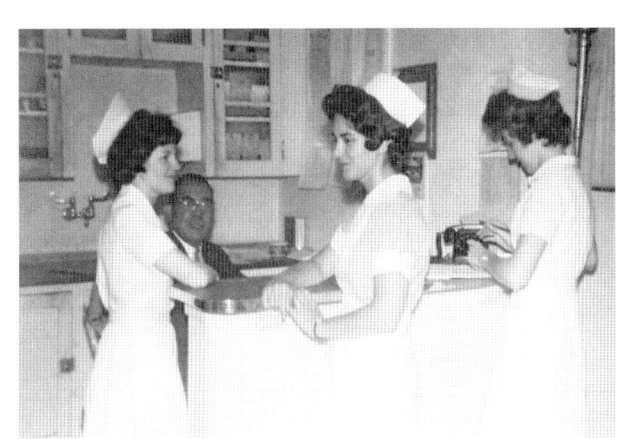

Dr. Dills chats with nurses, 1963.

The nurses' quarters had only one telephone, which everyone shared along with the one television that received only one channel. Study hours, when the use of both the telephone and the television was forbidden, were from 7 to 9 p.m. every night except on weekends. Housemothers walked through the hallways to make sure the students were at their desks. Lights went out at 10 p.m., and everyone had to be in bed. Between 9 and 10 p.m. the nurses were allowed out of the dormitories, but the distance to town posed a challenge. "There was a restaurant in town called the Capitol Restaurant," Diane recalled, "and they had the most wonderful rolls there. We would be ready to run out the door at 9 p.m. and we would run, literally run, to the Capitol and down one of those rolls and a Coke and then run back up the hill so we could make it by ten o'clock."

Strict as she was, Miss Bealer provided some fun as well and was known for holding impromptu ice cream parties with the students, serving up huge banana splits. She also arranged for dances with the members

1978

Indiana Hospital gets Life Flight helicopter service for the transport of critically ill or injured patients who need specialized care. The helicopter lands on the doctors' parking lot to the west of the hospital.

The Respiratory Therapy Department acquires a pediatric/neonatal ventilator.

The new laundry facilities begin operation in the basement.

1979

In February, the seven-story addition is completed and renovation gets underway on three floors of the Mack Wing and the fourth floor of the Iselin Wing.

Dr. Alex Juhasz performs the first colonoscopy at Indiana Hospital.

The nineteen students of the sixty-first and last nursing class graduate.

of Demolay from Indiana University of Pennsylvania, keeping an eye out to make sure they danced with plenty of space between them.

Diane's education at Indiana Hospital—three years of tuition, books, uniforms, and room and board—cost $350, and she was guaranteed a job when it was completed. Like the nurses before Diane and her classmates, however, they provided part of the hospital's workforce. Their only other expense was the pair of scissors they were required to purchase and which the hospital engraved with their name, their red and royal blue wool nursing cape with their initials sewn inside, their shoes, and hose.

In addition to becoming nurses, part of their training was learning how to look and behave like a lady. They were not allowed to wear pants of any kind in public though there were ways around that rule. "We rolled our pant legs up," Bernice Leslie recalled, "and put on our coat. When we got off campus we rolled them down." She also recalled the day Miss Hawkshurst called them into the auditorium to chastise them for buttering their bread a slice at a time instead of

Chapter 5: Turbulence, Tradition, and the Tower

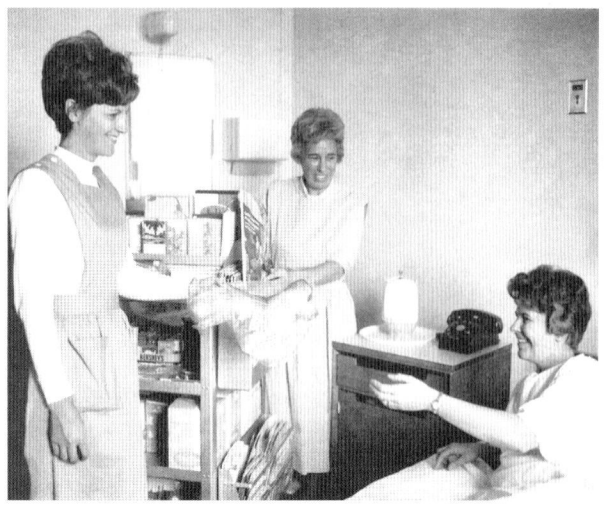

Auxiliary volunteers bring cheer to the patients with their smiles and the hospitality cart.

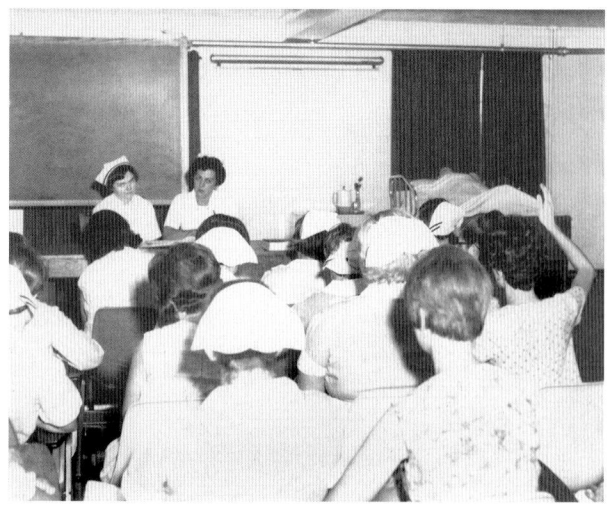

A full classroom at the Indiana Hospital School of Nursing. Photo courtesy of *Indiana Gazette*.

breaking each slice into fours and buttering the quarters separately. "We were confined to campus until we learned how to eat like ladies," Bernice said. "I remember sitting there thinking, 'I can't believe this.' If I recall, we were confined to campus for a month."

Following three years of hard work and diligent study, the students arrived at Indiana State Teacher's College for graduation ceremonies wearing identical graduation uniforms purchased for the occasion, their coveted school of nursing pin, and their new Indiana Hospital graduate nursing caps. Diane Petras recalled, "Miss Nettie Bealer presented each of us with a white handkerchief with an embroidered edge to be worn in our upper front uniform pocket." At the time, graduate nurses could go to work as a nurse immediately; starting salary for a day shift graduate nurse was $300 per month with a $10 per month raise once she passed her state board exams.

As archaic as some of their rules seem by today's standards, so does the equipment they used. Glass thermometers, filled with mercury, were used both orally and rectally and were sterilized in alcohol—in separate containers, of course—between uses. Reusable glass syringes had reusable metal needles that the nurses had to sharpen to remove burs. Every unit had bedpan sterilizers, round devices shaped like a kettle that, if the nurse neglected to secure the lid, showered her when the flusher was pushed, a mistake that was made only once. Rectal tubes and catheters, also reusable, were cleaned after use and then sent to central processing for autoclaving. Rubber gloves were also sent to central processing where they were washed and repowdered, wrapped and sterilized to be used again and again.

In those days, penicillin came in powdered form in a vial accompanied by another vial containing sterile water or saline. Recalled Bernice, "You pulled the liquid up, put it in, shook it up and then you had penicillin." Morphine, however, came in tablet form and was placed on a spoon over a Bunsen burner. The sterile water or saline was added and heated until the morphine dissolved and could be drawn up into the syringe.

Without question, the nurses of Indiana Hospital earned the respect of the physicians with whom they worked. Dr. Brown recalled the obstetrics nurses in particular who called him at all hours of the night predicting the imminence of the baby's arrival. "Ninety-nine percent of the time they were right," he said.

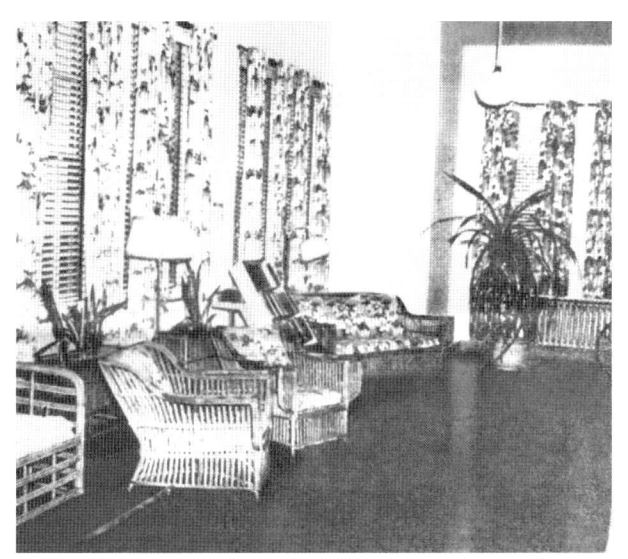

The solarium in the Mack Wing had the look and feel of a tropical oasis.

THE EMPLOYEES
OF THE
G. C. MURPHY CO.
JOIN THE RESIDENTS OF THIS COMMUNITY IN EXPRESSING
THEIR APPRECIATION TO
MR. J. S. MACK
FOR THE GIFT OF THE MACK MEMORIAL WING
TO THE INDIANA HOSPITAL

John S. Mack was president of G. C. Murphy Company at the same time he served on the board of directors for Indiana Hospital.

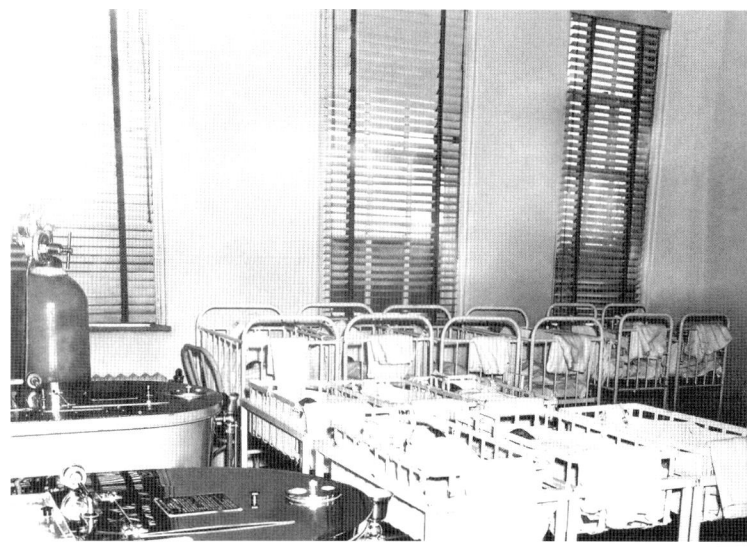

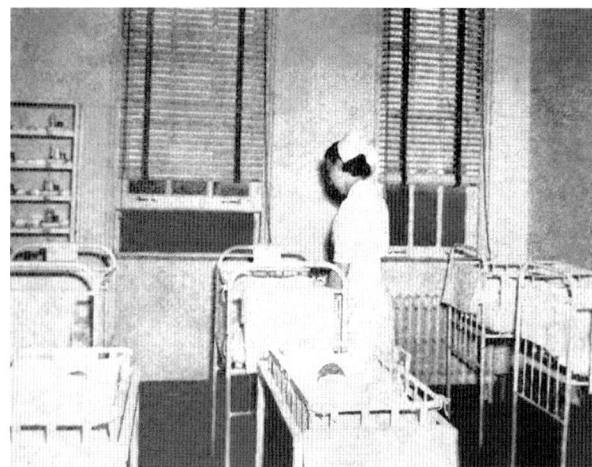

A nurse attends to the infants in the nursery in the Mack Wing, 1939.

appreciation...
WE SALUTE AN OUTSTANDING CITIZEN AND COMMUNITY
BUILDER FOR HIS GENEROUS GIFT OF THE
Mack Memorial Wing
TO THE
Indiana Hospital
WHICH IS DEDICATED THURSDAY, SEPTEMBER 21
WE ARE GLAD TO EXTEND THIS TESTIMONIAL OF OUR
APPRECIATION TO
J. S. Mack
First National Bank
In Indiana
Member Federal Deposit Insurance Corporation

appreciation
•
WE JOIN THE RESIDENTS OF THIS COMMUNITY IN EXPRESS-
ING OUR APPRECIATION TO
J. S. MACK
FOR HIS GENEROUS GIFT
TO THE
Indiana Hospital
•
THE
SAVINGS & TRUST COMPANY
INDIANA, PENNSYLVANIA
Resources Over Six Million Dollars
Member of Federal Deposit Insurance Corporation

Two long-standing supporters of the hospital, First National Bank (now First Commonwealth Bank) and Savings and Trust Company, placed congratulatory ads in the newspaper.

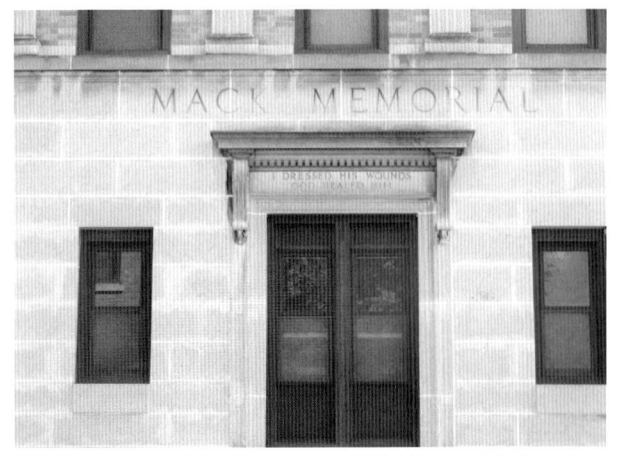

Over the doorway of the Mack Memorial Wing is carved "I dressed his wounds. God healed him." The phrase is attributed to Ambroise Pare, a sixteenth-century French barber surgeon who is considered one of the fathers of surgery.

The first floor was devoted to a complete general medical division, which included five semiprivate rooms, each with four beds. On the second floor was the hospitalization ward for patients whose bills were paid by the John M. and Sara E. Mack Memorial Trust Fund. For patients unable to afford private rooms, a semiprivate section was provided where patients paid a nominal charge for prenatal clinical examinations, delivery, nursing care, and a one-day stay for convalescence.

The six private rooms on the third floor were constructed with sound-absorbing ceilings that eliminated "disturbing noises." A call signal system flashed a lighted number before the nurse on duty to summon help in an instant. Pairs of rooms were connected with sparse but attractive and modern washrooms.

By the time the new maternity wing was dedicated, the annual income of the trust fund, valued then at $300,000, was approximately $13,500. Indiana Regional Medical Center still receives income from that original stock donation to this day. Upon the opening of the new maternity wing at Indiana Hospital, the Brush Valley Maternity Hospital closed its doors.

John S. Mack had completed his goal. Indiana Hospital was now able to apply for interns and could give diplomas to its own nurses. In 1939, the nursing school

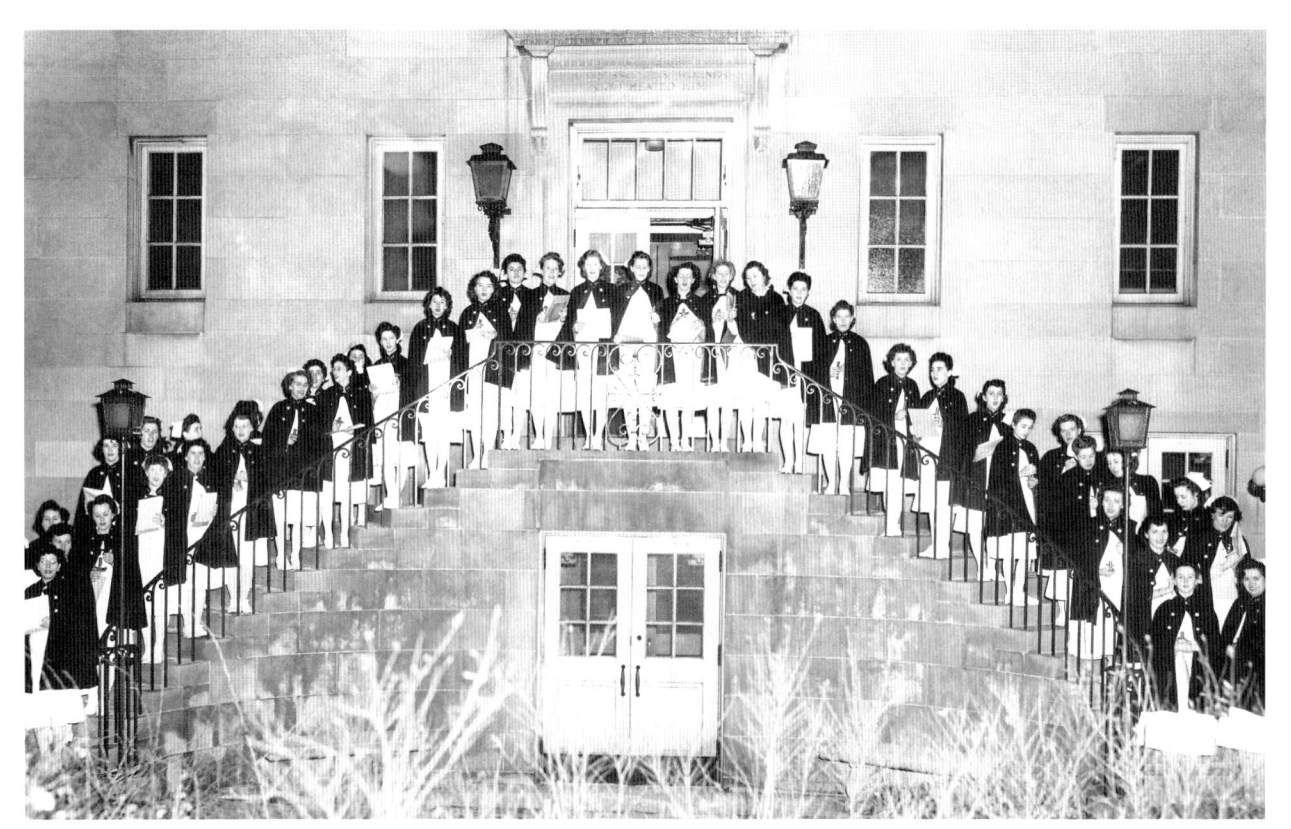

Nursing students pose on the portico of the Mack Wing, Christmas 1947.

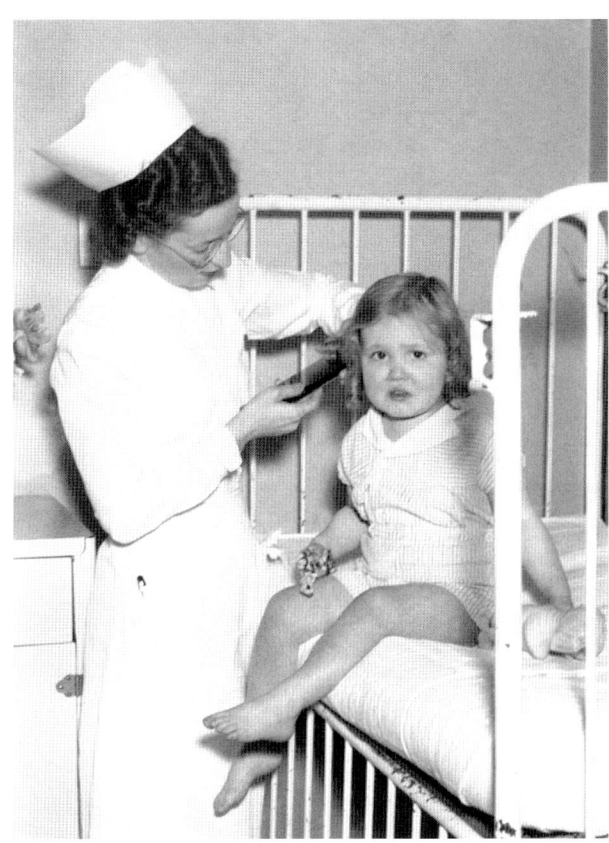

Nurse Anna Jane Bowen Barbor checks the ears of pediatric patient Rosaline Greenlee.

In the wake of Pearl Harbor, Americans across the nation felt truly vulnerable for the first time in recent history and began taking measures against future attacks. Cities held blackout drills and installed air raid sirens. Indiana Hospital representatives met with local officials to arrange a plan for the emergency availability of the medical staff should the necessity arise. The Board of Directors granted permission for the State Council of Defense to use the hospital as an emergency base hospital should civilian casualties occur as the result of enemy action. Once again eager to do its part, the nursing school was one of the first schools to enroll in the United States Cadet Corps program. Under this program, the Indiana State Teachers College cooperated by teaching the basic biological and physical sciences. A total of forty-one cadet nurses were graduated under the program among the graduating classes of January and September of 1947 and January 1948.

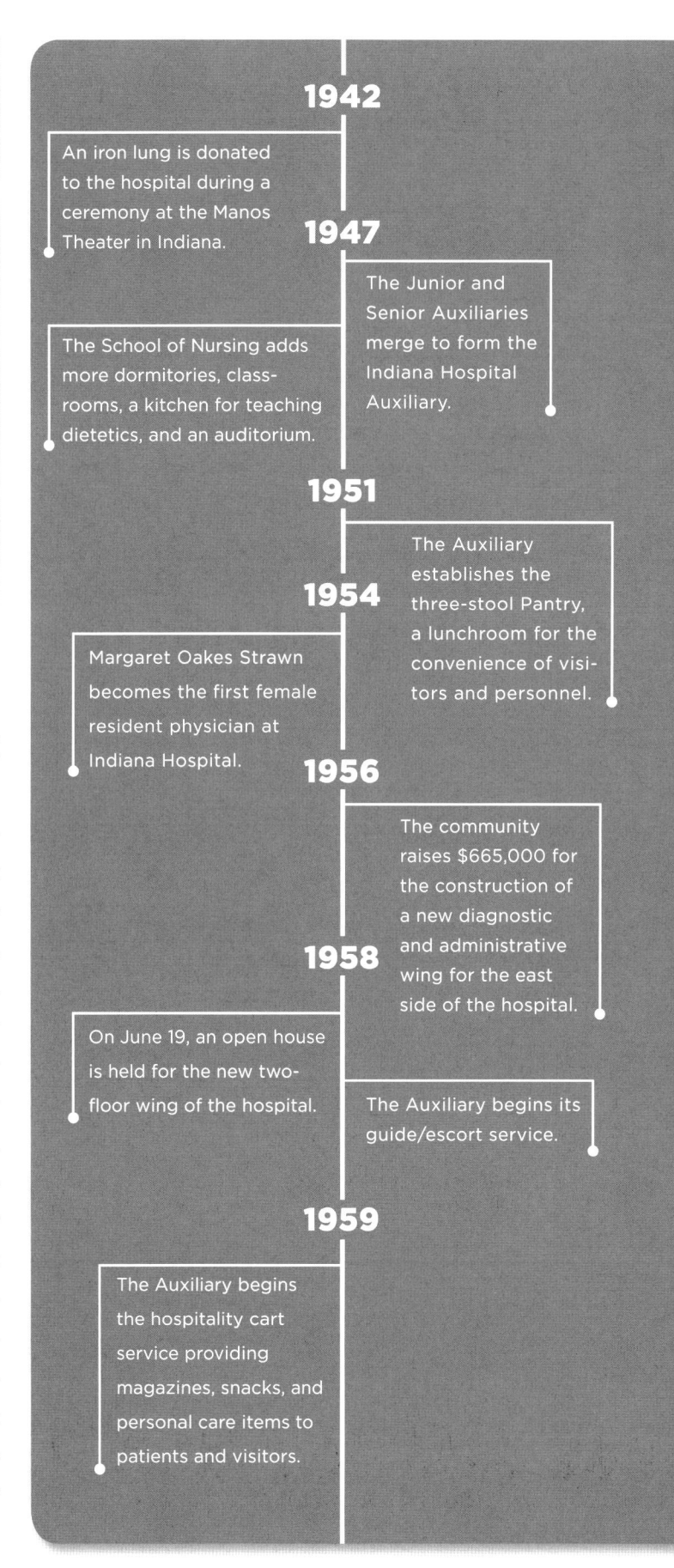

1942
An iron lung is donated to the hospital during a ceremony at the Manos Theater in Indiana.

1947
The School of Nursing adds more dormitories, classrooms, a kitchen for teaching dietetics, and an auditorium.

The Junior and Senior Auxiliaries merge to form the Indiana Hospital Auxiliary.

1951

1954
Margaret Oakes Strawn becomes the first female resident physician at Indiana Hospital.

The Auxiliary establishes the three-stool Pantry, a lunchroom for the convenience of visitors and personnel.

1956
The community raises $665,000 for the construction of a new diagnostic and administrative wing for the east side of the hospital.

1958
On June 19, an open house is held for the new two-floor wing of the hospital.

The Auxiliary begins its guide/escort service.

1959
The Auxiliary begins the hospitality cart service providing magazines, snacks, and personal care items to patients and visitors.

The war years brought other changes for the nurses. Students now had to take an entrance examination to be admitted to the school and had to pay tuition. Additional expenses included approximately $50 for books and $50 for uniforms on top of the $200 tuition for the three years. However, while they now paid tuition, their pay for their work in the hospital was increased. No longer a mere pittance, they received a whopping $50 per month. Their uniforms also changed in 1940. Now, instead of the multiple pieces that created a laundry nightmare, the apron, collar, bib, and cuffs were all one piece.

Victory over Japan did not occur until August 14, 1945, eight days after President Harry Truman unleashed the full force of American military might by dropping an atomic bomb on the city of Hiroshima. For most Americans, however, the end of the war was marked by Victory in Europe Day—May 8, 1945—when German soldiers laid down their weapons and surrendered en masse. Grateful for the service of those physicians who joined the war effort, Indiana Hospital agreed to participate in a welcome home program for the doctors who were now returning from military service.

THE POLIO SCARE

Few things are more frightening for the parents of a child than a life-threatening illness. Poliomyelitis, also known as simply polio or infantile paralysis, is a viral, infectious disease that can attack the central nervous system, occasionally leading to paralysis. Polio epidemics were recorded in numerous cities in the United States since the early 1900s, and in 1928 Children's Hospital in Boston introduced the use of an iron lung, a large, cumbersome machine that artificially created the action of breathing for paralyzed patients. It was not until the 1952 epidemic, during which 3,145 patients, most of them children, died of polio, that the disease captured national attention. Ahead of their time, Indiana Hospital acquired its first iron lung in 1942 through a generous donation presented to the hospital during a ceremony held at the Manos Theater in Indiana. An extremely valuable piece of equipment during the polio epidemic, iron lungs cost as much as an average home, and Indiana Hospital occasionally sent theirs to nearby hospitals for emergency use.

THE SCHOOL OF NURSING

In 1942, the school began its affiliation with Western Pennsylvania Psychiatric Hospital in Pittsburgh, an affiliation that continued until 1947 when Torrance State Hospital was chosen for the nurses to receive their psychiatric training. When the war ended, In-

A Nurse's Recollections

Bertha Manner, RN, put down her recollections of some of Indiana Hospital's earliest physicians in a missive she wrote entitled *Close the Door Gently*. She recalled that Dr. George Martin started the tradition of a Musical Tree in the Children's Ward and that "his aim was to keep the music going twenty-four hours a day." Dr. W. D. Gates, though "gruff as could be," had "tears in his eyes when a little boy had to lose a leg." Dr. H. B. Neale Sr., a quiet and unassuming man, was "deeply concerned with everyone under his care," and Dr. Charles Bee she regarded as not only a wonderful family physician, but a close friend of the families for whom he cared. Dr. W. A. Simpson, who was physician to the nurses, "saw to it that we were sent off duty no matter how busy we thought we were. Some of us were sure we owed our very lives to the gallons of Elixir I.Q. & S. he poured into us." Of Dr. Benjamin F. Coe, she referred to him as "a real treasure."

Miss Nettie Bealer served as director of the nursing school from 1948 to 1965. Upon her retirement, Miss Ruby Dobson became the director of nursing education and Mrs. Bertha Manner Buterbaugh took over as director of nursing services. In 1965 the entire nursing school curriculum was revised. The program was divided into four levels with specific objectives for each of the four levels. All theory and related clinical experience were now to be offered simultaneously.

In 1966 two "firsts" occurred within the School of Nursing as it admitted its first married student, Margaret VanDyke, and its first male student, Lawrence McKlveen.

On June 28, 1968, as the School of Nursing prepared for the fiftieth anniversary celebration of the nursing school's first graduating class, it received its first national accreditation from the Board of Diploma Programs of the National League for Nursing. The accreditation affirmed that the Indiana Hospital School of Nursing had successfully conformed to rigorous academic and curriculum standards for the profession.

Listening to some of Indiana Hospital's earlier physicians, their day-to-day practices also have the feel of some long past era, though it was not so many years ago within the confines of the hospital's history.

Dr. Ralph Brown started his practice in 1958 on Homer City's Main Street where he rented an office for $70 a month including utilities. Unlike today's outlandish malpractice costs, in 1958 his insurance bill was $38. He rented that office until 1966 without a single rent increase. His patients did not come by appointment; he simply had office hours from 9 a.m. to 9 p.m., making house calls after hours and delivering babies in between. Between 1953 and 1985 Dr. Brown delivered more than 5,000 babies. "Looking back, I don't know how I did it," he said.

He kept patient records on 3x5 index cards, and during Christmas and Easter holidays, his patients, whom he considered friends, brought him a variety of baked goods or bottles of homemade wine.

As he recalls, the hospital did not exactly open its arms to new physicians back then. In the two years it took him to join the staff, he could admit patients under another doctor's supervision.

For a variety of reasons, some might say that the doctor/patient relationship was a more personal, old-fashioned relationship back then. Dr. Waldo, who was essentially Indiana Hospital's first hospitalist, always came to the emergency room when one of his patients arrived there. That close relationship, and the insistence on continuity of care, may in fact be the reason Indiana Hospital was so reticent about bringing an ER physician to the staff. Like Dr. Brown and most others, Dr. Waldo also received holiday gifts of freshly baked homemade bread, cookies, and fudge.

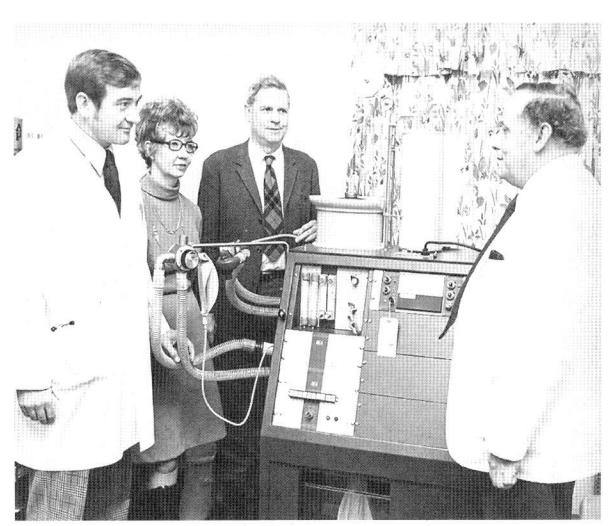

Mr. Croyl (right), a respiratory technician, demonstrates a lung function machine recently donated by the American Lung Association to Dr. Melvin Williams (left). Photo courtesy of *Indiana Gazette*.

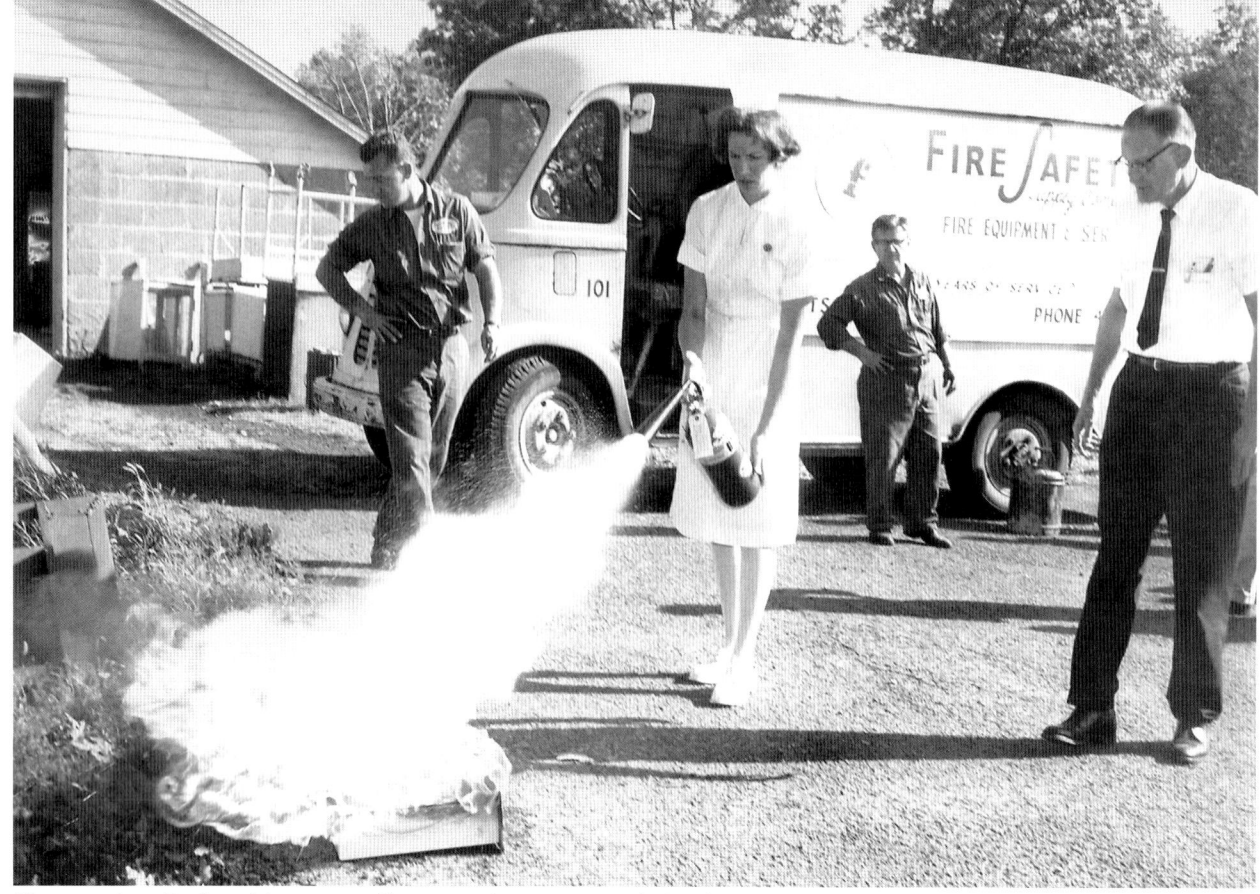

All personnel practice fire safety every year. Here, a nurse learns to operate basic safety equipment. Photo courtesy of *Indiana Gazette*.

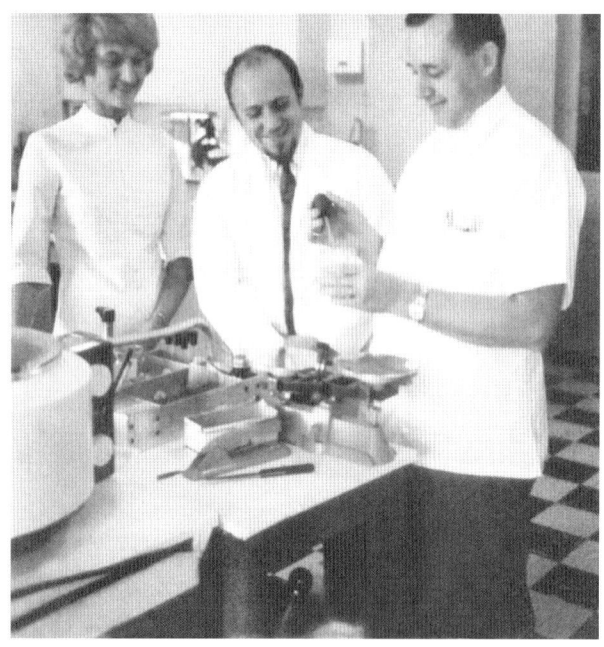

Hospital staffer Betty Coleman and Laboratory Medical Director Dr. Osterling watch closely as Laboratory Director Beatty Dimit conducts a test.

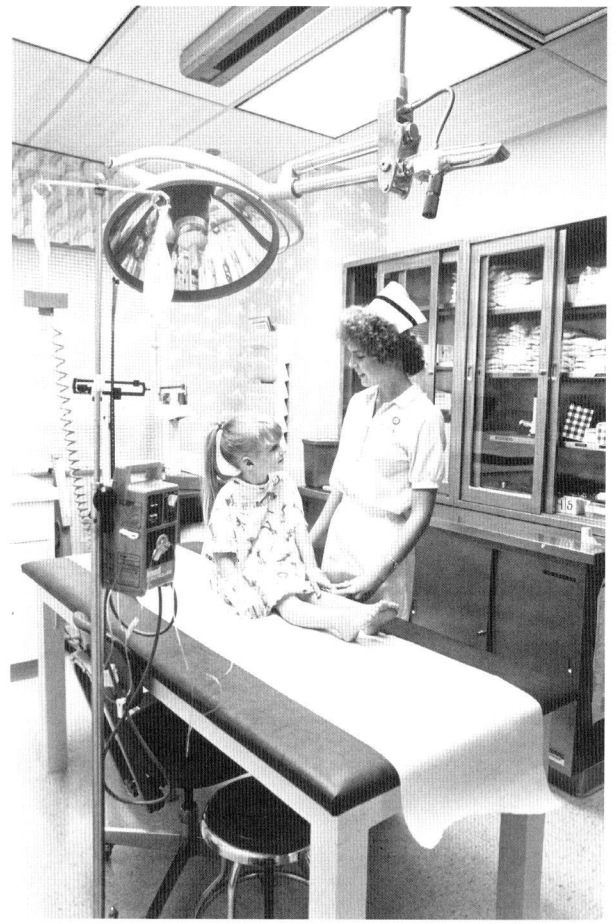

Sometimes a nurse's smile and reassuring touch are the best medicine of all.

When Dr. Melvin Williams, the first board-certified internal medicine physician in the area, came to Indiana Hospital in 1967, there were only eighteen doctors on staff. "It was a pretty rudimentary hospital at the time," he said. "Really sick people went elsewhere." Also qualified in nuclear medicine, it was not

58 —⌁— Indiana Regional Medical Center

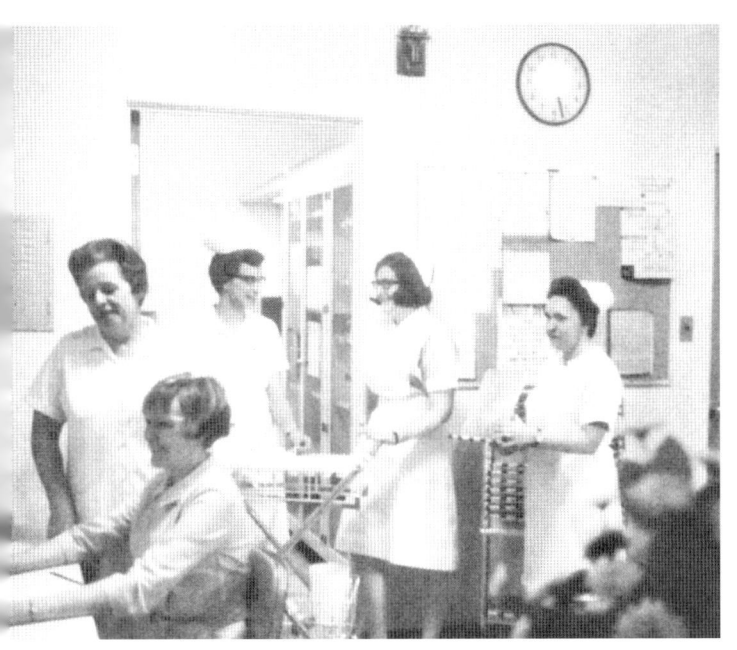

The starched white aprons of the nursing students and the all-white uniforms of the nurses were a source of pride.

until later that Dr. Williams was able to organize a department for it.

The second board-certified internal medicine physician, Dr. James Garrettson, attended the University of Pittsburgh School of Medicine and met Dr. Williams while doing his residency at an army hospital in Tacoma, Washington, and came to Indiana Hospital in 1972. "There were a couple of pediatricians, OBs, an ENT, an ophthalmologist, and that was it," he recalled. "There were no cardiologists, no gastroenterologists, none of that."

Though the medical malpractice insurance issue would not take on great significance until the mid-1970s, Dr. Garrettson's malpractice insurance cost between $300 and $400 per year at the time.

FIFTY YEARS OF SERVICE

After fifty years of service to Indiana Hospital, Adeline Hawxhurst retired in 1965. On October 27, at what was to be the hospital's first employee recognition program, 450 people were present as the Board of Directors honored her with the establishment of the Adeline W. Hawxhurst Memorial Fund for nursing students. Among the honored guests was Mrs. Charles Leventry of Johnstown, the first administrator at the Indiana Hospital.

On the lighter side, Richard Seifert, administrator of Lee Hospital in Johnstown and vice president of the Hospital Association of Pennsylvania, demonstrated the various positions filled by a hospital administrator by donning a variety of hats including a combat helmet, construction engineer safety hat, a politician's top hat, a cook's bonnet, a fireman's hat, a Santa Claus hat, and a fancy ladies hat for meeting the hospital auxiliary.

The board also gifted Miss Hawxhurst with a bracelet, a purse, and a scrapbook. Dr. Henry Mitchell, representing the medical staff, presented her with a check from the physicians. A few days later on November 1, 1965, hundreds attended an open house held to mark the fiftieth anniversary of Indiana Hospital.

As it turned out, Miss Hawxhurst's resignation proved temporary, and she returned as acting administrator

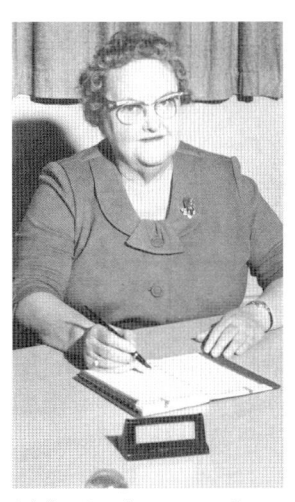

Adeline Hawxhurst was a fixture at Indiana Hospital from 1915 to 1965. Photo courtesy of *Indiana Gazette*.

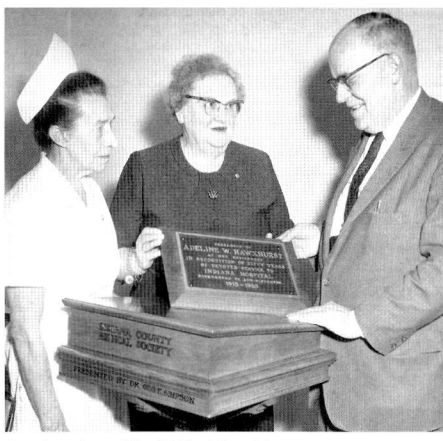

On October 27, 1965, Miss Hawxhurst was honored upon her retirement. Alongside her are nurse Bertha Manner Buterbaugh and C. Gilbert Wolfenden, past board president. Photo courtesy of *Indiana Gazette*.

Chapter 5: Turbulence, Tradition, and the Tower — 59

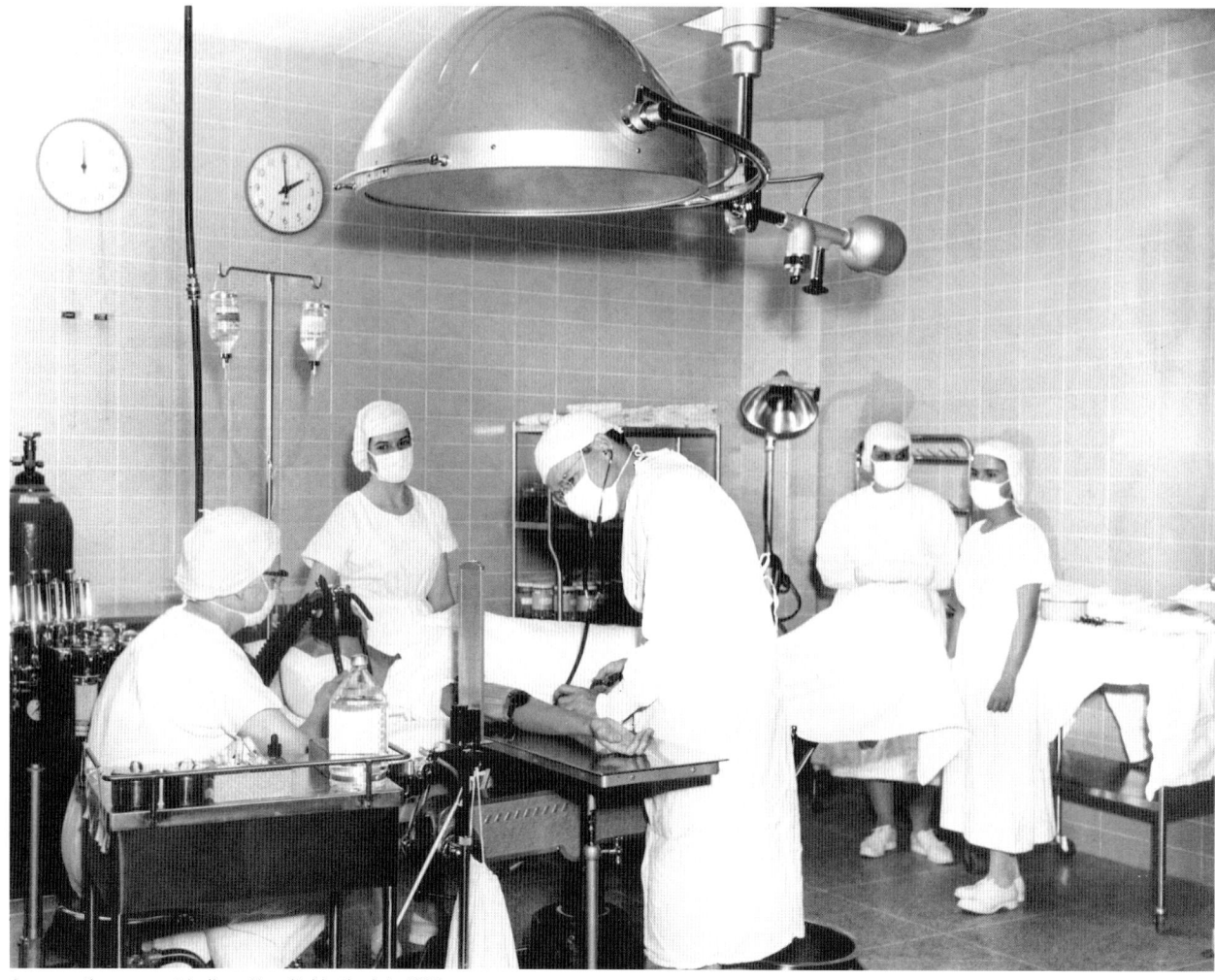

An operating room at Indiana Hospital in the late 1960s.

the following spring upon the resignation of William Peters. At a meeting held June 22, 1966, she proudly reported that up to that moment 224,990 patients had been admitted in the course of the hospital's history. Also during that time, the hospital's physical plant had increased from its original value of $165,000 to more than $4 million. The Auxiliary's donations to the hospital had now surpassed the $60,000 mark.

MEDICARE

The very best of hospital care must be administered with compassion, a vital element that has never been in short supply at Indiana Hospital. Even today, in the midst of mountains of rules and regulations regarding patient care, Dr. Alex Juhasz, retired sur-

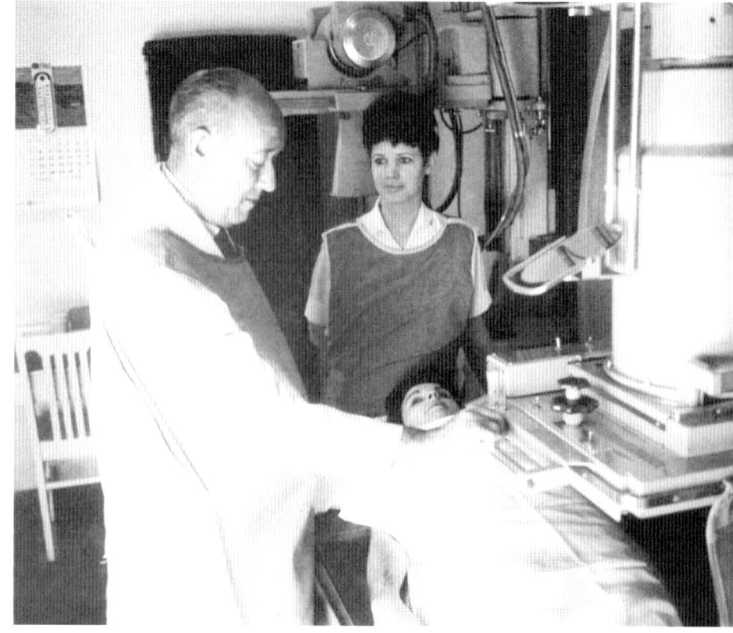

X-ray technician Marsha Wilhelm assists Dr. H. C. Long.

Indiana Regional Medical Center

geon, is proud of the fact that "Nobody is turned away from this hospital."

When the Hill-Burton Act was passed in 1946 to provide funding to improve the nation's hospital facilities, one provision required that a "reasonable" amount of free care be administered, a practice Indiana Hospital adopted from its beginning. It was a simpler time then; most people paid cash for their purchases, including the doctor's bill, and while the miners had excellent benefits through the union, many had no insurance at all. A patient's ability to pay made no difference to the nurses. "It was on the medical record if they were a welfare patient," said Bernice Leslie. "As nurses, we paid no attention to that."

In 1966, the same year Indiana Hospital adopted its "Care and Concern" slogan, Medicare came onto the scene, the first government-assisted program for health insurance. On the date the program went into effect, Indiana resident John Stollotz became the hospital's first Medicare patient.

In May 1968, administrator George E. Ferrey Jr. reported on a number of improvements to the hospital. Three new gas-fired boiler units were installed to replace equipment put in during the 1930s. The x-ray, laboratory, operating rooms, delivery room, recovery room, and emergency room were now air-conditioned.

Electronic accounting equipment and three new clerical personnel were added to handle the increased paperwork caused by Medicare. A new central magnetic recorder made it possible for a doctor to dictate a medical history from any phone in the hospital or from his office phone, providing a faster means of preparing medical records. A new switchboard doubled the hospital's communication capacity.

The hospital was now giving courses in cardiopulmonary resuscitation as part of the Inservice Training Program for nursing service personnel, and new electric beds were installed to assist elderly patients with getting in and out of bed. A department of inhalation therapy was initiated, providing approximately five to six hundred treatments a month.

Most importantly, Indiana Hospital now had an Intensive Care Unit for critical patients. Dr. Melvin Williams, who made the development of the ICU a condition of his hire, worked with Drs. Waldo and Green and nurse Bernice Leslie who visited Good Samaritan Hospital in Dayton, Ohio, to learn everything possible about the needs and operation of an intensive care unit.

They chose the sunporch area in the Mack Wing, quickly got approval, and went to Pittsburgh to select monitoring equipment. The ICU opened in 1968 with five beds, three electric monitoring devices, and

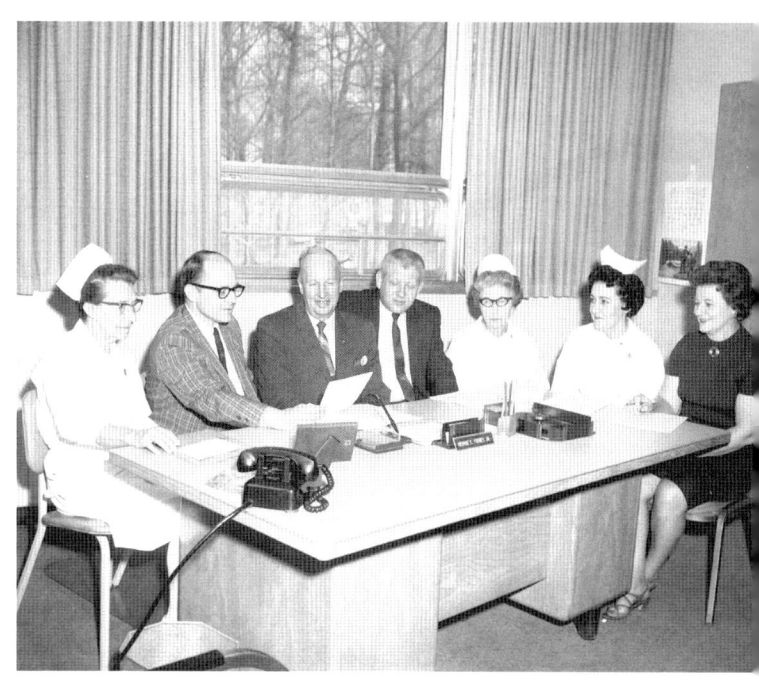

Indiana Hospital's administrative staff at a meeting held May 2, 1968. Left to right: Bertha Buterbaugh, George E. Ferrey Jr., Norman Richardson, Joseph O. Yesh Jr., Mrs. Evelyn M. Sutton, Mrs. Leona Shank, and Martha Copelli.

Chapter 5: Turbulence, Tradition, and the Tower — 61

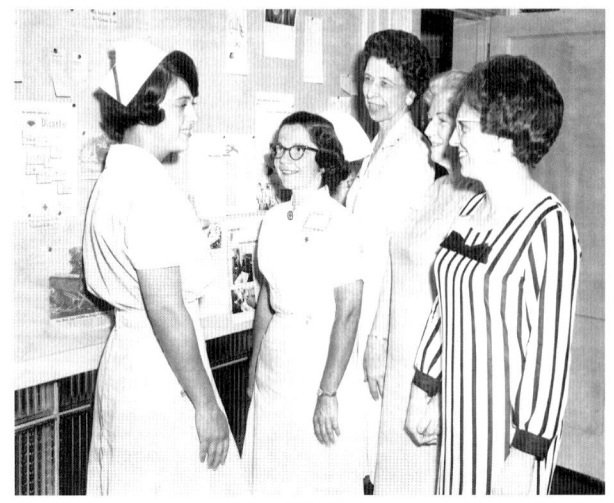

Mrs. Norma Fetters (second from left). Photo courtesy of *Indiana Gazette*.

a crash cart, the hospital's first—all of it provided by the Indiana Hospital Auxiliary. The first patient admitted to the ICU was one of Dr. Williams's, a patient with diabetic ketoacidosis who previously would have been transported to Pittsburgh. "He walked out of the hospital . . . he was fine," Dr. Williams recalled.

According to local historian Clarence Stephenson, in 1970 there were forty-two medical doctors in Indiana County, one for each 1,892 persons in the county. Only sixteen were general practitioners, twenty were specialists, five were based at Indiana Hospital as resident physicians, and one was an osteopathic physician. The hospital's staff numbered 455 workers, who were supported by student nurses, practical nurse students, and auxiliary volunteers.

Also in 1970, a native New Yorker, Donald F. Smith, became the administrator of Indiana Hospital, replacing George Ferrey, who resigned to accept a job elsewhere. Prior to coming to Indiana, Mr. Smith served eight years as administrator of the Children's Hospital of Columbia in Washington, DC.

The Sixth Street entrance road to the hospital was completed with the cooperation of the Mack Foundation, and the hospital's Department of Nuclear Medicine was organized. The recovery room was expanded to eight beds.

VISITING NURSES ASSOCIATION

On July 30, 1970, the Visiting Nurses Association of Indiana County was officially organized under the sponsorship of the Nursing Alumnae Association of the Indiana Hospital School of Nursing and the Women's Civic Club of Indiana. The effort to organize this vital community service began as early as 1962 when Dr. Daniel Bee gave voice to the idea brought forth by nurses Evelyn Sutton and Bertha Buterbaugh. At the time, it received little support. In January 1967, Dr. Bee again brought the idea to the forefront by holding a public meeting.

It was clear there was a need for visiting nursing services, particularly in a rural area like Indiana County where many elderly and chronically ill people were being hospitalized out of a lack of alternatives. A visiting nursing program, Dr. Bee argued, could dramatically improve the general health and welfare of such people and could maintain them longer at home where they would be more comfortable, without hospital or custodial care.

Interest continued growing over the next few years until the Nursing Alumnae Association of the Indiana Hospital School of Nursing offered to underwrite the cost of incorporation and serve as a sponsoring organization. The estimated cost of $30,000 per year would cover the services of a director, two registered nurses, two part-time nurses, and the cost of operation. Funds continued to be raised for the program through benefit events.

In 1972, Indiana County physicians Dr. Melvin Williams and Dr. James Garrettson, and Jerry Esposito of Citizen's Ambulance Service worked with Dr. Peter Sa-

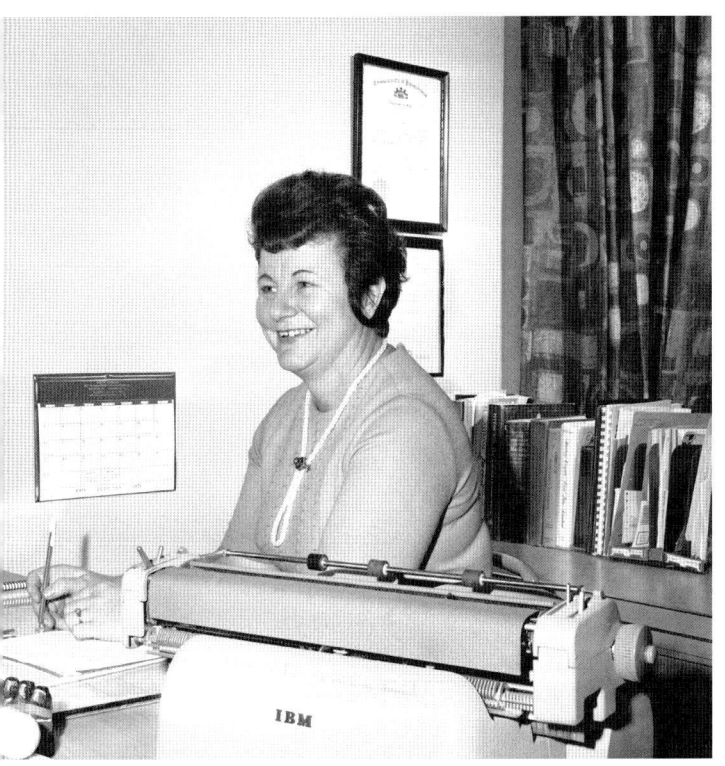

Martha Copelli, pictured here in 1971, worked at Indiana Hospital from 1948 to 1996 and was the CEO's assistant for many of those years.

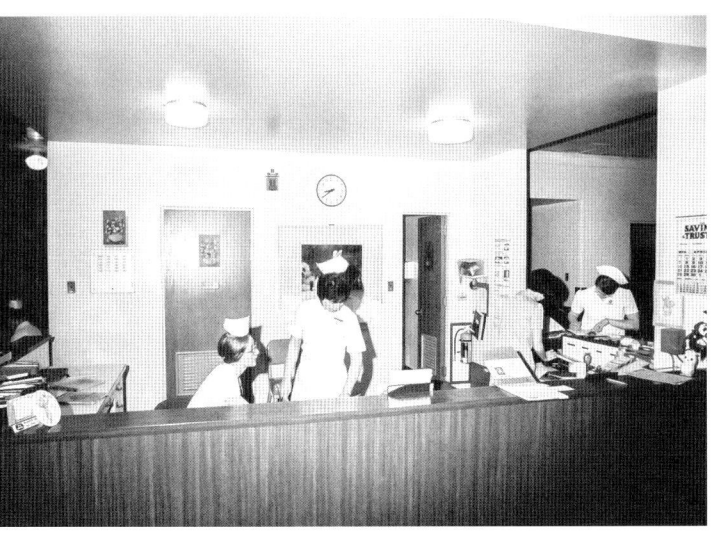

A nurses' station in Mack II, 1974.

An Auxiliary Christmas

In December 1970 the Auxiliary held its annual charity ball at the Indiana Country Club. For a $15 donation, couples could dance from 10 p.m. to 2 a.m. surrounded by a Winter Wonderland theme. That year the Auxiliary gave Christmas stocking receiving blankets and matching tassel caps to babies born during Christmas week. A group within the Auxiliary knitted bed slippers for all the pediatric patients, and the party committee planned and carried out parties for the children on several holidays during the year.

The following October the Auxiliary began making mail deliveries to patients and departments.

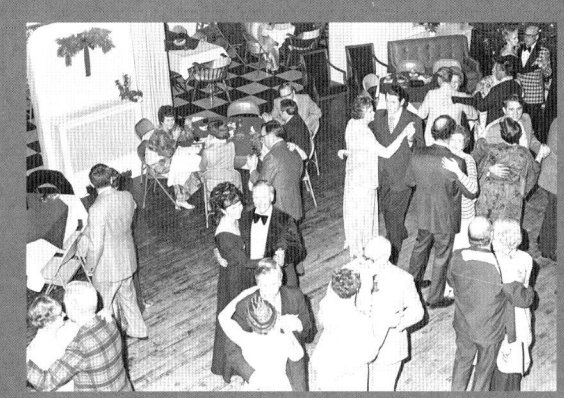

Staff members and their spouses enjoy the Auxiliary's Christmas Dinner Dance, December 1976. Photo courtesy of *Indiana Gazette*.

far, known as the "Father of Modern Day CPR," to lay the foundations for EMS Medical Command in Indiana County through the use of a suitcase-sized electrocardiographic telemetry device. At the same time, the Commonwealth of Pennsylvania was establishing an EMS system that provided rules and regulations for EMS providers and medical commands across the state.

The device made it possible for paramedics to transmit data from a heart monitor at the scene of an emergency across radio waves to the physician's "suitcase" phone. "In the 1970s," said Dr. Garrettson, "this type of training program was not well received until it was proven that it saved lives; then it became accepted." Prior to 1972, Dr. Williams pioneered the program working with Citizens' Ambulance Service and provided medical command from his office and home. In 1972, Dr. Garrettson shared those duties with Dr. Williams until 1975 when Dr. Williams's role was transferred to Dr. Strunk upon his arrival at Indiana Hospital. In 1978, EMS Medical Command moved from the "suitcase" method to a permanent home in the emergency room at Indiana Hospital.

THE END OF AN ERA

In September 1976, Indiana University of Pennsylvania's Department of Nursing began its affiliation with Indiana Hospital, with student nurses being assigned to the hospital's clinical areas of pediatrics, obstetrics, and gynecology.

Sadly, after sixty years, the Indiana Hospital School of Nursing came to an end when fire erupted in the basement lounge area of the 1937 brick nurses' home on Thanksgiving eve in 1976. Fortunately, because of the holiday, none of the nurses were there at the time of the fire. Ironically, only ten minutes before the fire was discovered, the hospital had conducted a routine fire drill.

> The School of Nursing's first graduating class boasted twelve members in 1918. From 1919 to 1930, the classes ranged between four to nine members. From 1932 until the last graduating class in 1979, the classes ran anywhere from fifteen to twenty-six students, the largest being the class of 1962, which graduated twenty-six students.

The decision was made to close the school upon the graduation of its current freshman class. On March 23, 1979, nineteen members of the sixty-first and final class graduated from the Indiana Hospital School of Nursing at a ceremony held in the Pratt Auditorium of the IUP Campus. Mrs. Bertha Buterbaugh, RN, alumna of 1924 and staff member for forty-six years, commented:

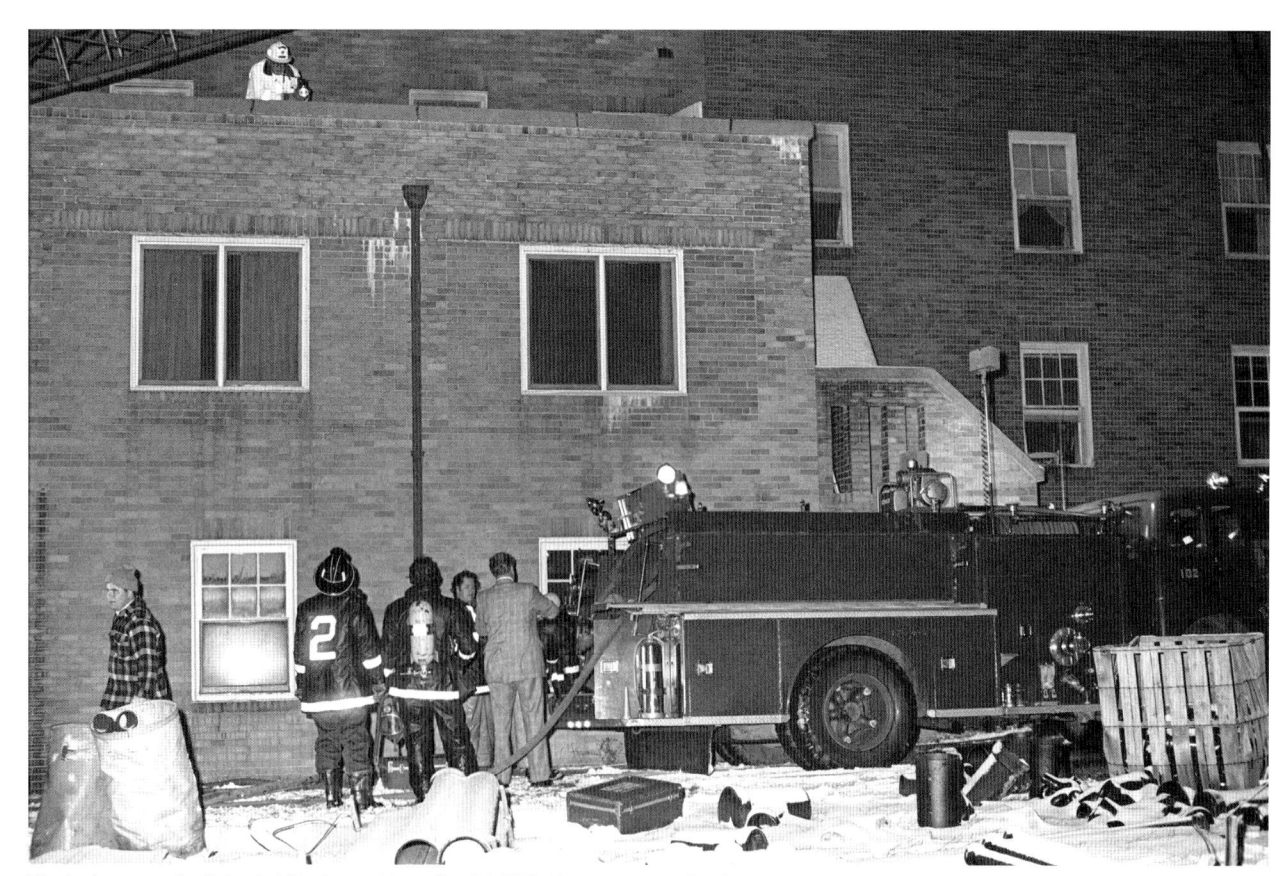

Fire broke out at the School of Nursing on November 24, 1976. Photo courtesy of *Indiana Gazette*.

64 — Indiana Regional Medical Center

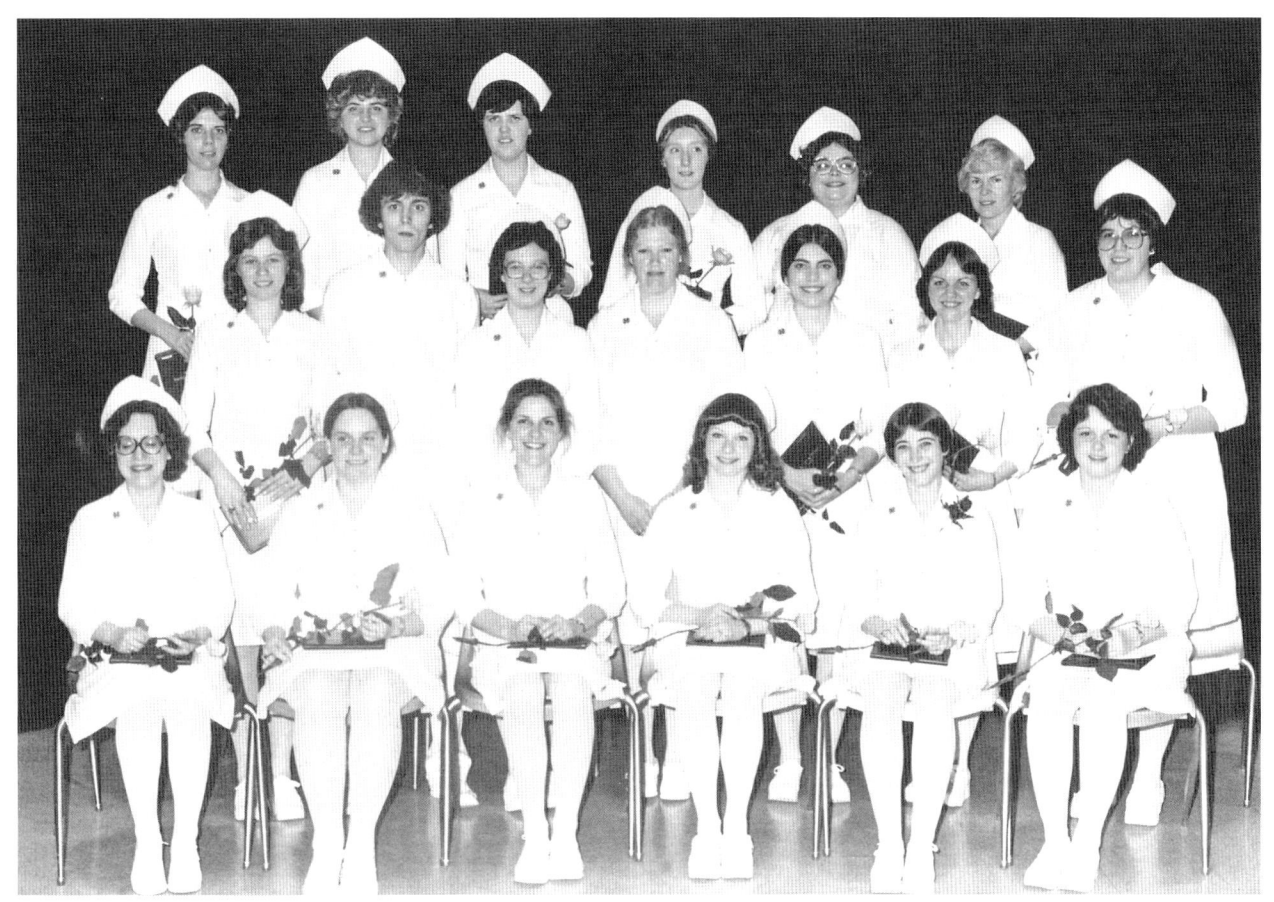

The last group of nurses to graduate from Indiana Hospital School of Nursing, 1979.

"I think the spirit of nursing has remained constant. The desire to serve humanity is the very heart of nursing."

More than 900 nurses graduated from the Indiana Hospital School of Nursing throughout the years under the supervision of only four directors: Nettie E. Bealer, Ruby Dobson, Betty Mallory, and Carol Curey. During the summer of 1977, the original frame building that housed the nursing school was demolished to make way for a new hospital wing.

After the fire, Mrs. Kathleen Cessna assumed the role of librarian to reorganize what was left of the library facilities. Through the hospital's membership in the Laurel Highlands Health Sciences Library Consortium and a grant from the National Library of Medicine, the Medical Staff Library was weeded and then combined with the nursing texts to form the Health Sciences Library. The grant made possible the purchase of $3,000 worth of new texts for medicine, nursing, and allied health specialties.

THE TOWER

For several years, Indiana Hospital had been undergoing continuing modifications to meet Department of Labor and industry requirements. To attract the specialists the hospital needed, in the early 1970s the administration began planning for another major expansion and revamping of the existing facility. While past administrations had remained steadfast in their dedication to patient care, they were perhaps also slow to embrace the technological advances in medical and surgical care and the investment they required.

When Dr. Alex Juhasz began his surgical career at Indiana Hospital in July 1977, he was attracted by the

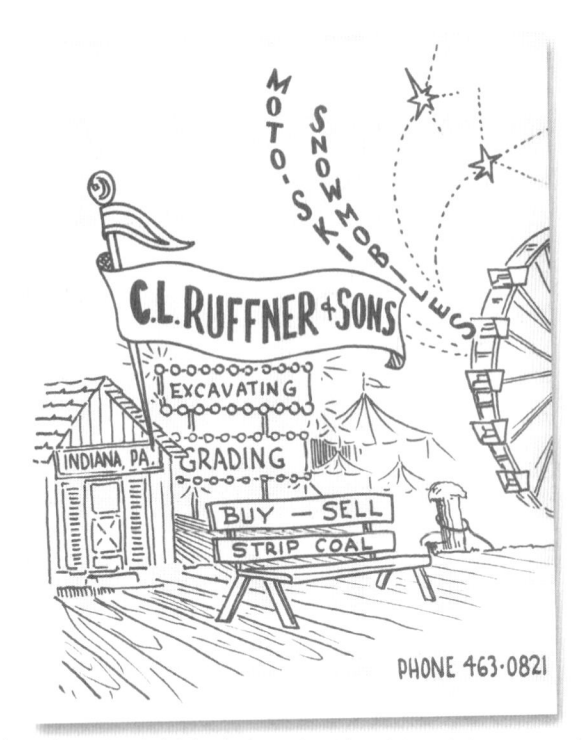

The Indiana Hospital School of Nursing Alumni Association presented *Swells, Ripples and All That Jazz*, a musical revue of Indiana Hospital employees and community members to support the 1979 building fund.

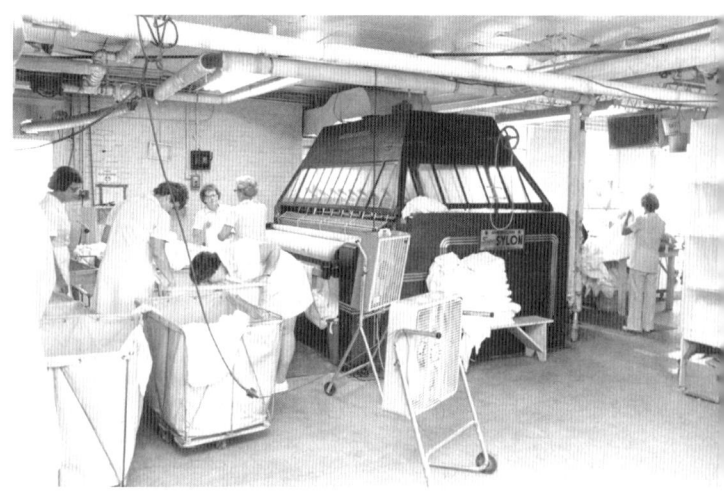

Laundry services were moved to the basement of the hospital in 1978. Photo courtesy of *Indiana Gazette*.

rural area but had doubts about the hospital itself at first. "It was more of a triage station then," he said. "Certainly the more involved cases were transferred out, and I would say back then, the community perception of the hospital itself was not that great."

Following a series of town meetings held throughout Indiana County during 1974, an estimated $10 million expansion was approved by the Comprehensive Health Planning Association of Western Pennsylvania. On February 12 the County Commissioners appointed the five-member Indiana Hospital Authority to supervise the issuance of tax-exempt bonds to finance the project. The Rochester and Pittsburgh Coal Company donated $300,000; a $700,000 grant came from the Appalachian Development Fund along with a Hill-Burton Act grant of $1.5 million and a loan guarantee of $5.56 million. By the time the expansion was announced, nearly $8 million in grants were assured.

Charles J. Potter was named general chairman of the Indiana Hospital Development Fund campaign. The initial goal of $1 million was quickly surpassed, as was a second goal of $2 million. The public response was unparalleled in the history of the county; when all was said and done, 1,249 pledges were received, totaling more than $2.6 million.

The architectural firm of Rea, Hayes, Large and Suckling was chosen to draw up plans for the seven-story expansion. The plans included changes to the public, emergency, and service entrances. The new emergency entrance was planned for the west side of the new building with the Auxiliary's Pantry and Gift Shop at the main public entrance.

The second floor was to include two trauma rooms and observation room beds plus four examination rooms, an outpatient cast room, x-ray with adequate waiting and dressing rooms, and a full-time emergency room physician's office and sleeping quarters.

The new building was to have three times the emergency and outpatient area with intensive and coronary care facilities on the third floor below the surgical suite. Renovations were planned for the third floor of the Mack Wing to provide a "step down" unit for patients coming out of the ICU. The nurses' control

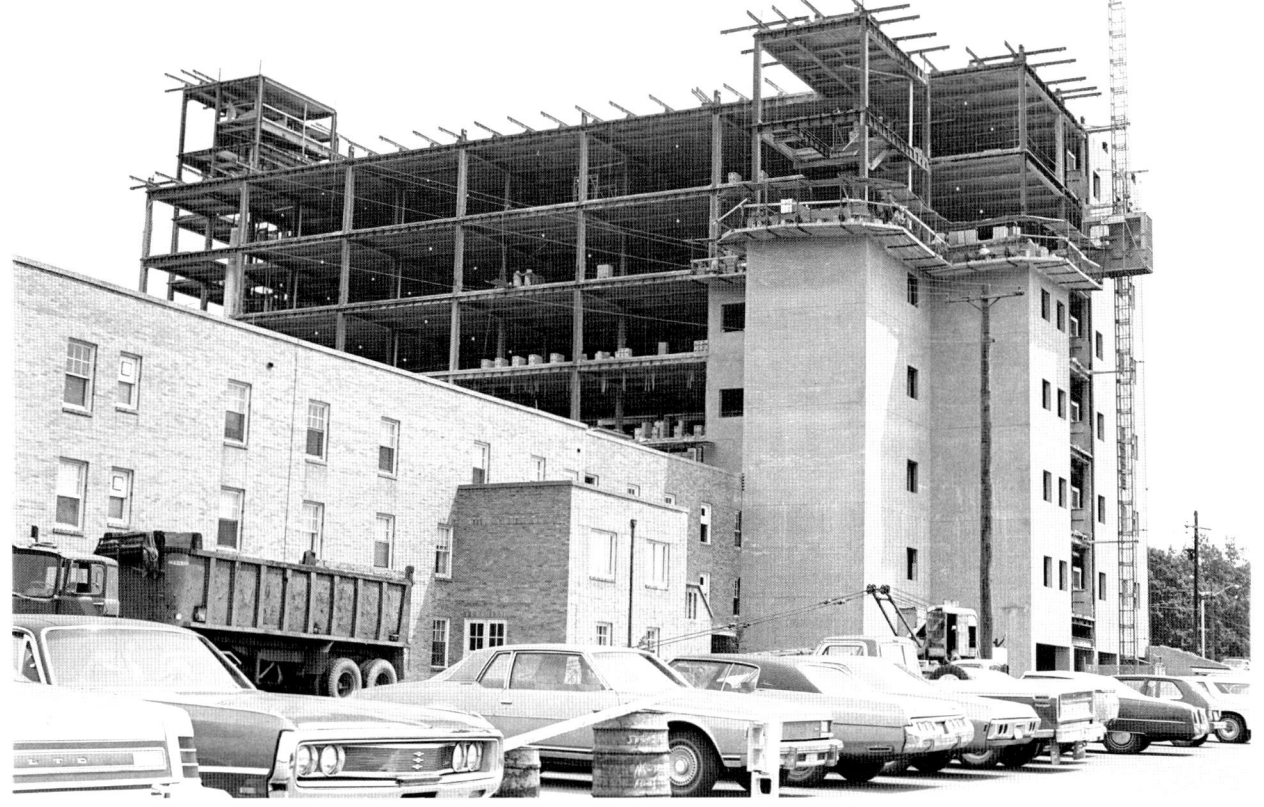

The Tower under construction, August 1977. Photo courtesy of *Indiana Gazette*.

center with equipment for monitoring cardiac patients was to be located in the center of a twelve-bed area.

Central supply was to be located on the third floor for the sterilization of surgical packs and instruments lifted to the surgical floor above by a dumb waiter. The fourth floor was for the surgical suite of five operating rooms and a nine-bed recovery room.

The fifth, sixth, and seventh floors were to be identical nursing units of forty-two beds each with a nurse control station in the center and patient rooms located along the exterior walls of the building.

When the groundbreaking for the new seven-story addition, known as "The Tower," was held on July 3, 1976, the hospital's capacity was at 206 beds. It was the only hospital in Indiana County, serving a population of approximately 83,000. Five hundred and twenty-two full-time, seventy-eight part-time employees, and seventy student nurses supported a fifty-nine-member medical staff.

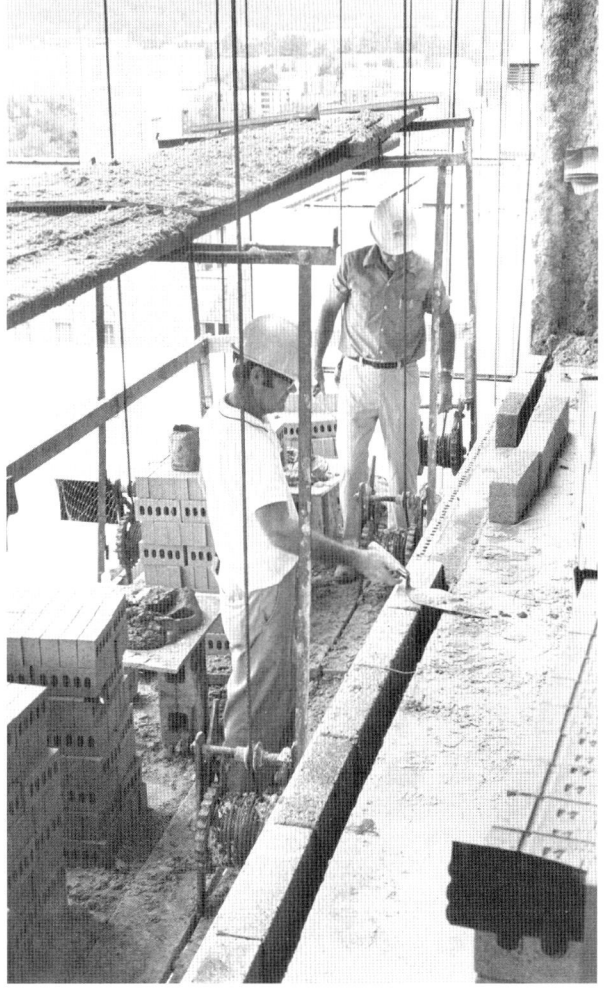

Tom Bebar and Marty Bebar at work on the Tower, 1978. Photo courtesy of *Indiana Gazette*.

Chapter 5: Turbulence, Tradition, and the Tower — 67

The ceremony was held between the Mack Wing and the nurses' home. As hospital board and staff representatives, governmental officials, contractors, and about two hundred interested citizens looked on, Indiana Hospital Board President Henry F. Hild and Indiana County Hospital Authority Board Chairman L. Blaine Grube turned the first shovels of dirt.

Finally, the Tower was completed, and an open house was held February 4, 1979. The new wing became operational on February 11 with the transfer of patients from the old wings. Renovation of the old buildings then began at a total cost, including new equipment, of $1,628,200. It may have been bittersweet for some. For the first time, there would be no separate wards for men and women—the last remnant of the hospital's earliest days. Bertha Manner, RN, and a member of the nursing school's class of 1924, wrote nostalgically, "Close the door gently; if you do, you will hear echoes from the past. Please listen to them." For others, the Tower represented Indiana Hospital's bold move toward its future. Dr. Juhasz credits the upgrading of the physical plant with raising the hospital's standards and profile in order to attract a broader range of specialists to the staff. Said Dr. Garrettson, "This growth in specialties wouldn't have happened unless the administration had been willing to provide them with the equipment they needed."

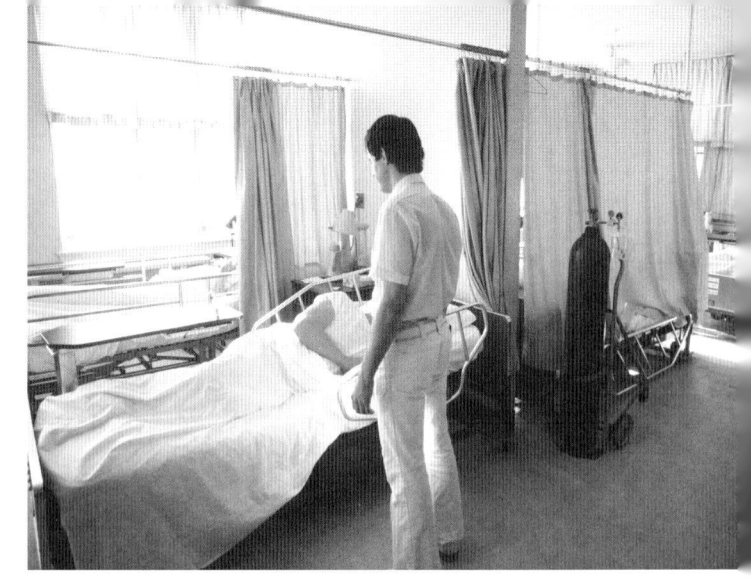

Until the Tower was built, men and women were in separate wards. Pictured here is the men's ward.

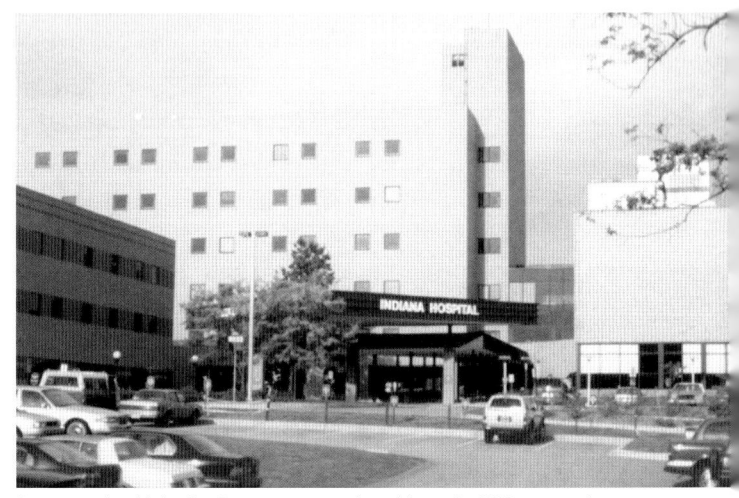

Seven stories high, the Tower was completed in early 1979, a stunning example of community spirit and cooperation.

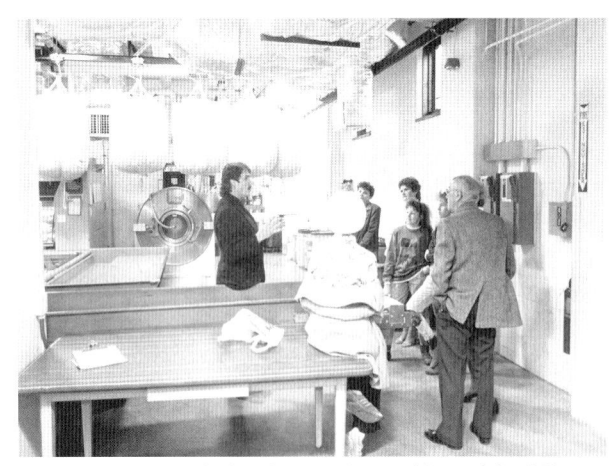

David Perry explains the laundry operation to visitors of the 1979 open house.

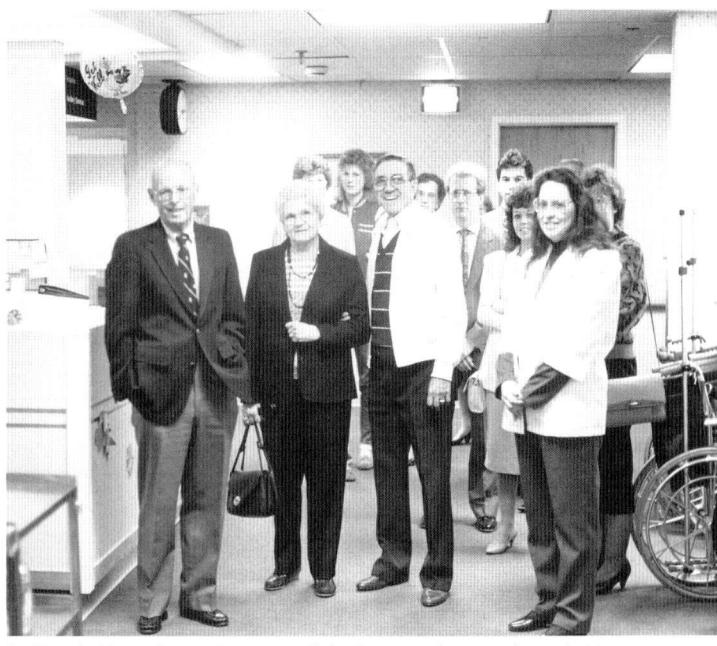

Staff and visitors line up for a tour of the Tower at the open house held February 4, 1979.

68 — Indiana Regional Medical Center

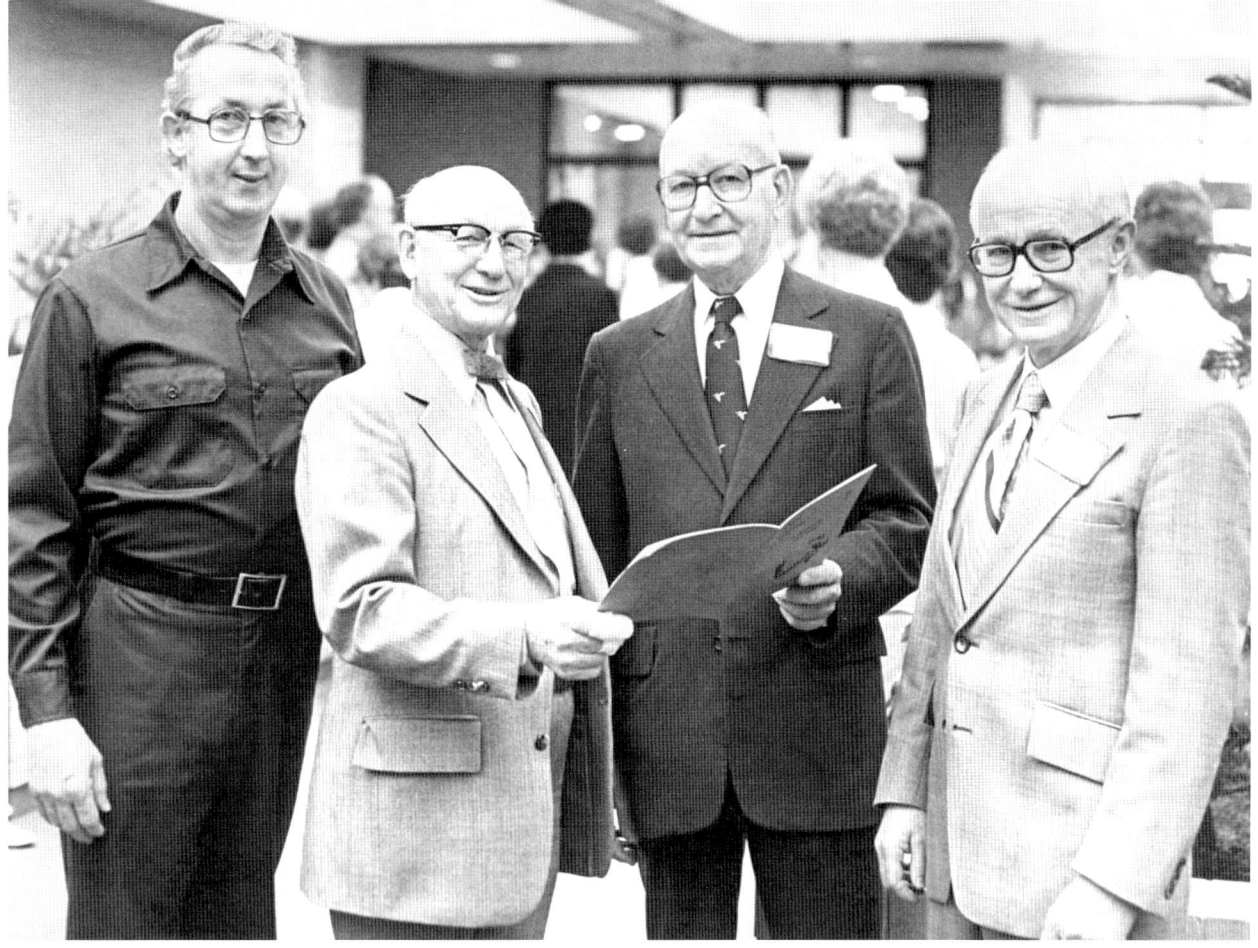

From left, Director of Facilities Ray Swank, County Commissioner Bill McMillian, President of the Board Henry Hild, and Hospital Administrator Don Smith. Photo courtesy of *Indiana Gazette*.

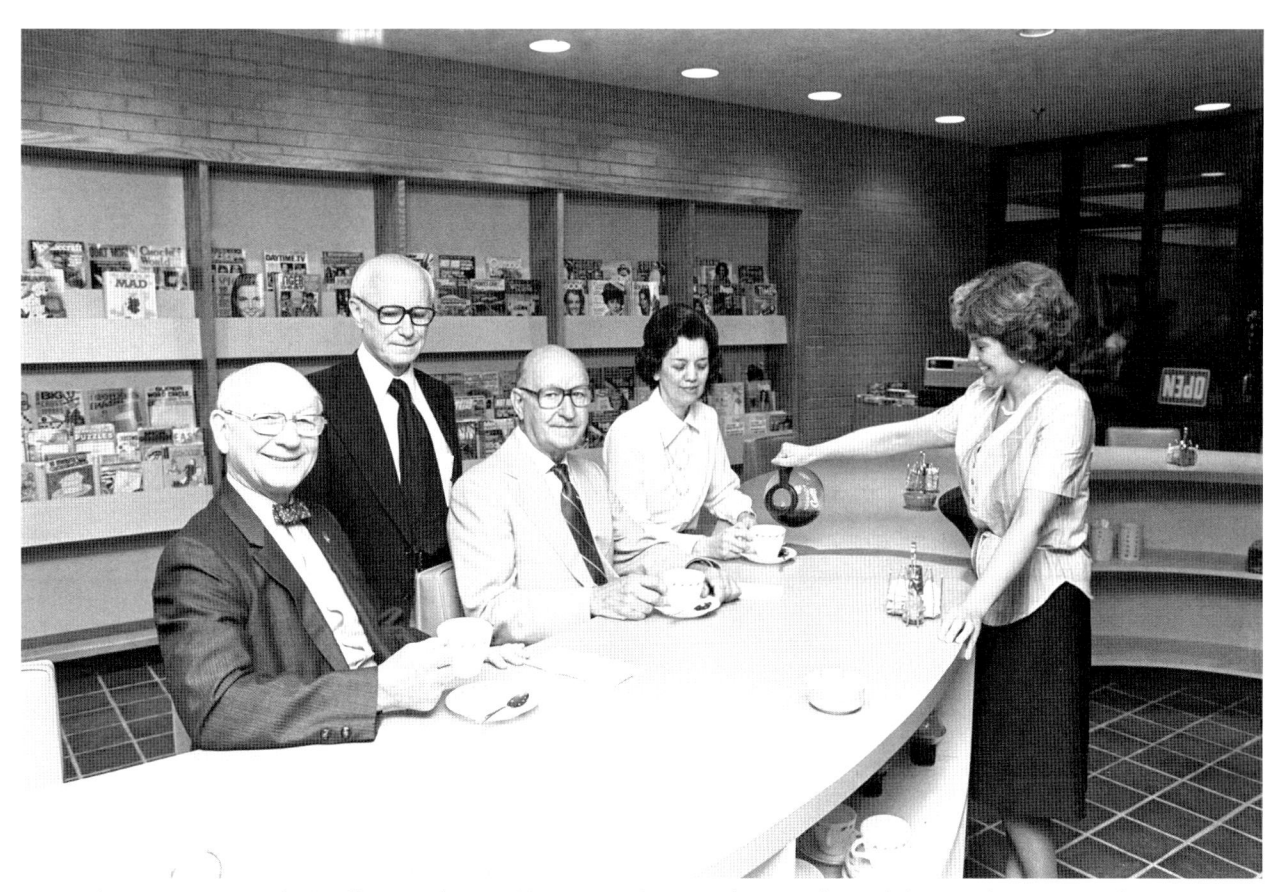

Jan Daugherty serves up some fresh coffee to auxiliary president Marge Scheeren at the new and expanded Pantry. Photo courtesy of *Indiana Gazette*.

Chapter 5: Turbulence, Tradition, and the Tower 69

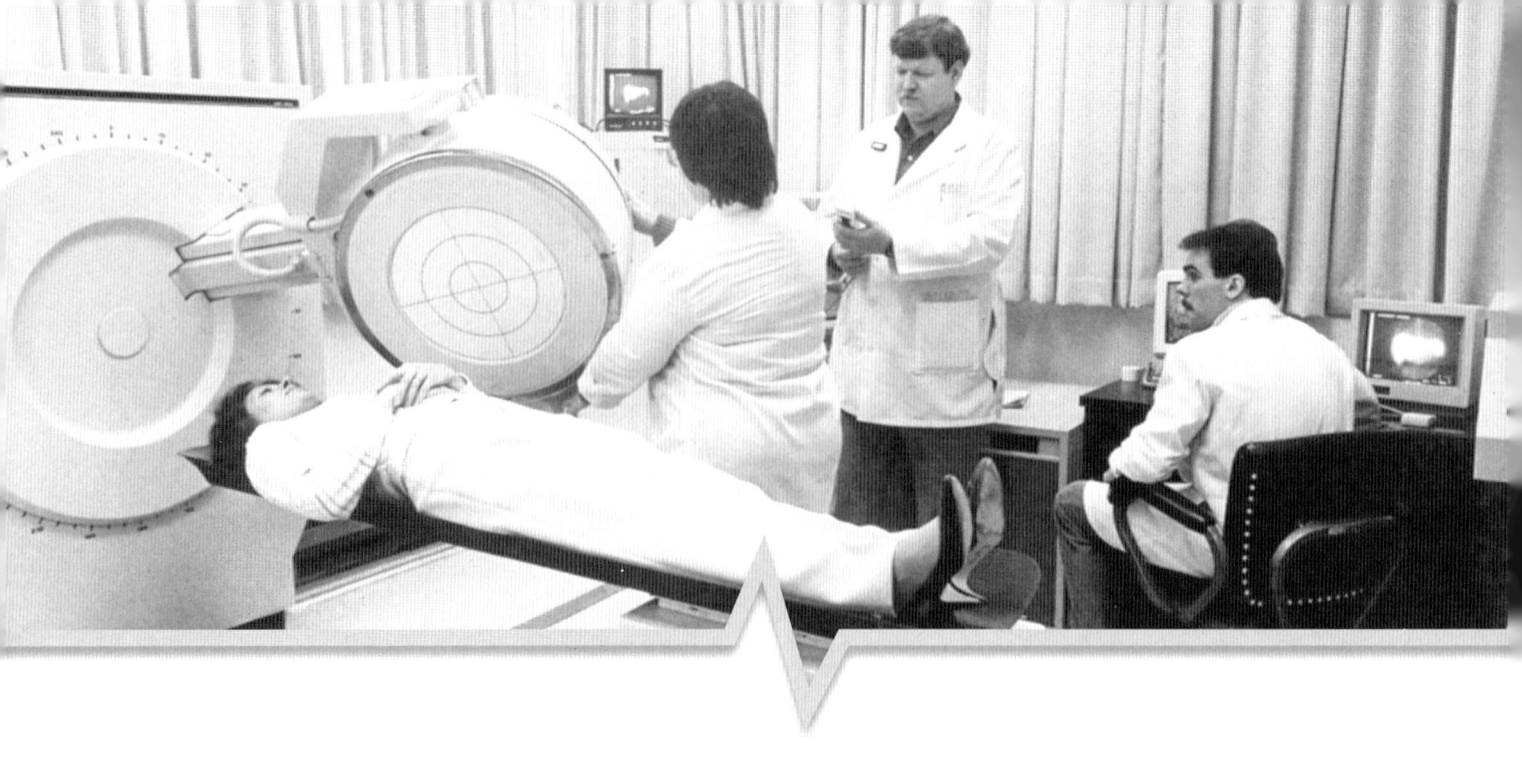

CHAPTER 6
The Preferred Regional Health Services Provider

By 1980, Indiana Hospital had 650 full- and part-time employees. The medical staff's specialties included anesthesiology, general surgery, internal medicine, pediatrics, otolaryngology, ophthalmology, orthopedic surgery, oncology, oral surgery, and urology. During the fiscal year ending June 30, 1980, Indiana Hospital admitted 6,921 patients with an average length of stay of 6.2 days. The Auxiliary with its 550 members celebrated its fiftieth anniversary with a luncheon.

Also in 1980 an eight-bed telemetry cardiac unit was completed on the third floor of the Mack Wing, allowing patients on heart monitors to leave their rooms for a bit of hallway exercise. Mack III, an Intermediate Care Unit, opened to provide medical and surgical nursing care for patients requiring continuous monitoring of cardiac rhythms. The unit's original capacity was twelve patients, but a generous donation from the Auxiliary provided an additional twelve beds with a computerized arrhythmia recognition system.

Finally, the hospital's building program was completed. During late 1980 and early 1981, the accounting and payroll offices, medical staff room, library, Medi-

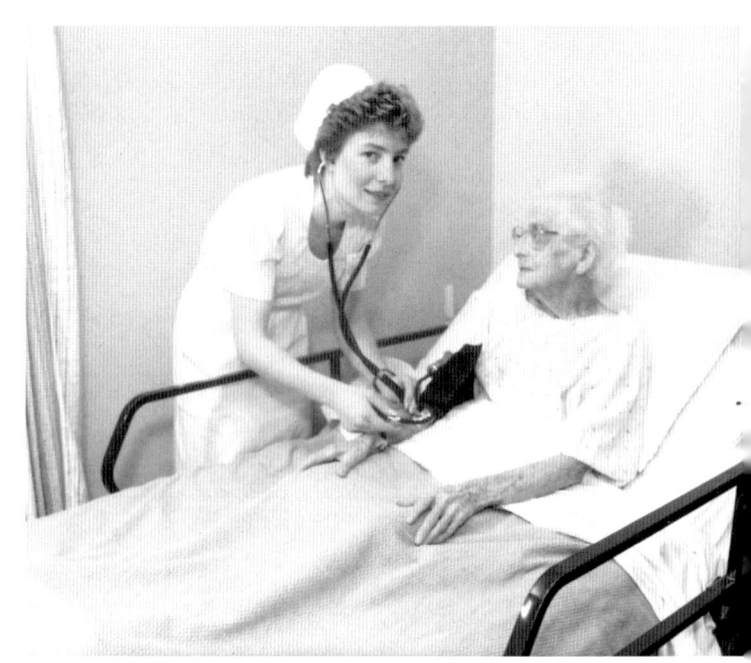

Paula Miller, RN, checks on an elderly patient.

Top: In a demonstration of Indiana Hospital's SPECT Camera, Joan Varnes prepares to screen transcriptionist Shirley Leise posing as a patient as other nuclear medicine technologists Jim Douglas and Barry Deutsch supervise, 1988.

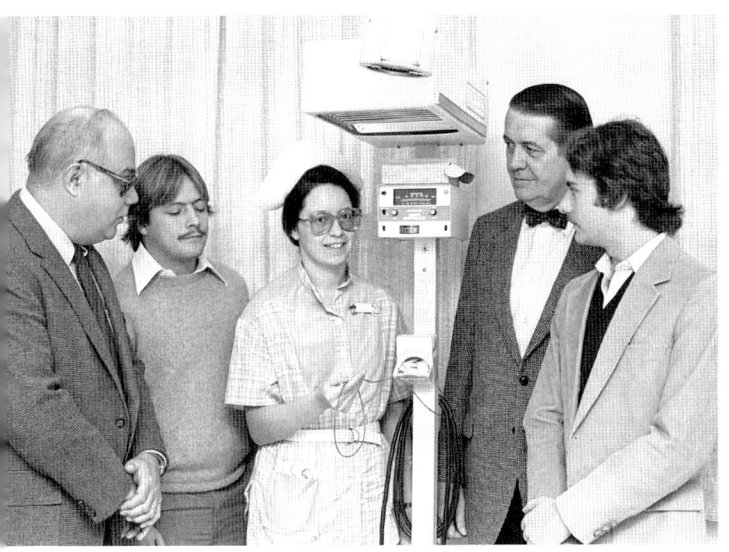

Hospital staff members gather to learn about the latest equipment, 1982.

cal Records Department, and the business offices were completed on the second floor of the Iselin Building. The nursing units on the third floor of the Mack Wing were completed, as was the Materials Management Department on the first floor of the Mack Wing. Renovations were completed in the Medical Office Building on the site of the old nurses' home.

By 1981, the Joint Commission on Accreditation of Hospitals was requiring all hospitals to engage in a formal program of quality assurance. Though the subject was not new to Indiana Hospital, the administration took a major step forward by creating a department devoted to quality assurance. Made up of three sections—infection control, utilization review, and quality assurance—the centralized program was designed to help coordinate activities between departments, enhance problem identification, and ensure follow-up.

MEDICAL DIRECTOR

A major change was made in the hospital's administration on February 22, 1982, when Dr. Henry Mitchell was named the hospital's first medical director to provide medical input in problems that arose either in patient care or between the hospital and staff. "The medi-

1980

Work begins on the renovation of the Medical Office Building at the site of the old nurses' home.

An eight-bed telemetry cardiac unit is completed on Mack Wing's third floor.

1982

The physical therapy department, started in a large room in the basement in 1952 with one small whirlpool, two treatment tables, a mat, and parallel bars made by one of the Rochester and Pittsburgh Coal Company shops, now has five therapists, one rehabilitation nurse, one clerk/receptionist, one aide, and two part-time aides/transporters. They average 120 treatments per day.

Echocardiography is now available at Indiana Hospital.

1983

A landing pad for helicopter patient transport is completed.

Laser equipment for eye surgery is introduced.

1984

The hospital begins offering occupational therapy services.

On July 1, Diagnosis Related Groups (DRGs), aimed at reducing Medicare expenditures, take effect.

On March 9, an installation crew from General Electric Company begins installing equipment for the hospital's new Computed Tomography (CT) Scanner. Over twenty separate pieces of equipment are brought into the hospital. The CT Scanner table and the 5,000-pound circular gantry are brought in through the outside window of the CT Scanner room. A ribbon-cutting ceremony held on April 6, 1984, marks the official beginning of the hospital's new service.

The hospital begins extending laboratory, physical therapy, and electrocardiography services to area nursing homes and begins providing laboratory services to the Blairsville area.

The first birthing room, one room used for both labor and delivery, is added to the Obstetrics unit.

1985

Fifty-nine people who are overcome with chlorine gas fumes at the Homer City Power Plant are treated at the hospital.

On July 27, the newly renovated Pediatrics Unit is dedicated in the memory of the late Dr. John Watchko, the hospital's first pediatrician.

On September 7, the new Citizens' Ambulance Service building, located on hospital grounds, is dedicated.

1986

- The hospital begins Lifeline, a personal emergency response system, funded by the Auxiliary.
- A new diagnostic center opens in Blairsville as an extension of the hospital's outpatient services.
- The hospital lobby's remodeling is completed.

1987

- Forty-five workers at the Keystone Power plant near Shelocta are taken to Indiana Hospital following a sulfur dioxide spill.
- On January 19, the Indiana Regional Cancer Treatment Center opens on hospital grounds.
- Indiana Hospital undergoes a corporate restructuring making Indiana Healthcare Corporation the parent company of four subsidiaries.
- The Healthcare Foundation is established.
- Indiana Hospital begins offering wellness programs to area residents.

1988

- Indiana Hospital receives the American Hospital Association's 1987–1988 Healthcare Administrative Services Certificate of Recognition for cost containment.
- The Laundry Department is enlarged and renovated.
- The Mammography Center opens at the hospital.
- Indiana Dialysis Center, located in the 119 Professional Center in Indiana, opens. It is operated by Allegheny General Hospital of Pittsburgh in affiliation with Indiana Hospital.
- The renovated Obstetrics Unit (Maternity Center) is unveiled with an open house.
- The first corneal transplant is performed at the hospital.

1989

- The hospital begins treating endometrial cancer by implantation of sealed radioactive sources.
- A Stroke Rehabilitation Program, providing patients with an individualized treatment plan, is now available at Indiana Hospital.
- The hospital introduces Magnetic Resonance Imaging (MRI), lithotripsy, and patient-controlled analgesia.

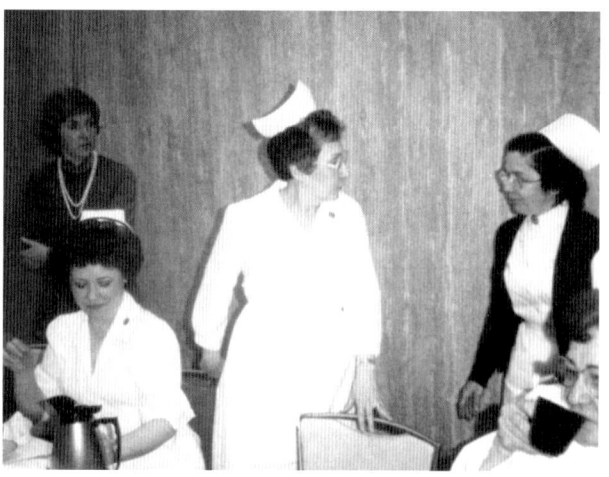

Nurses Dolores Pennington, Beverly Bender, Sylvia Hilty, Norma Fetters, and Leona Shank, 1985.

cal director position was conceived as sort of a medical spokesperson—somebody who was on their [the physicians'] side so to speak," said Dr. James Garrettson.

The other very important function of the medical director's position was to build the hospital's profile concerning specialized services. The completion of the Tower, the expanded and upgraded facility with its state-of-the-art equipment, meant that the hospital could now attract the highly trained physicians necessary to improve the depth and range of services that would attract a greater proportion of the region's patients to Indiana Hospital. Dr. Mitchell's efforts paid off. With support from the Indiana County Medical Society, over the next four years, Indiana Hospital's concentrated recruiting effort brought thirty-one new physicians, many of them in specialized areas, plus seven emergency room physicians to provide quality care to its patients.

MEDICARE, MEDICAID, AND DRGS

Up until now, the government had been reimbursing hospitals retrospectively for the care of Medicare and Medicaid patients based on the actual cost of the care provided. However, a new law went into effect on July 1, 1984, that caused hospitals across the nation to evaluate virtually every procedure they performed. Aimed at reducing Medicare and Medicaid expenditures, the law called for a Prospective Payment Program designed to pay hospitals an established amount based on the patient's diagnosis. In a letter to the employees, Chairman of the Board Henry F. Hild encouraged both doctors and nurses to participate in the success of the program. "Your responsibility is paramount—to literally preserve a vital community resource," he wrote. "Within the community, you are our best link with the public in assuring them that whatever changes occur under the new payment system, this institution's commitment to quality health care will remain inviolate."

The Prospective Payment Program used a system called Diagnosis Related Groups or DRGs that identified specific types of illnesses, their treatment, and the price the government would pay for each. With fully 60 percent of Indiana Hospital's patients either Medicare or Medicaid recipients, swift action was necessary. The hospital formed a DRG committee with Dr. John Mills as director of the program. The committee's job was to integrate Utilization Review, Quality Assurance, and Medical Records and to educate both the community and hospital staff on the implementation of DRGs. Shortly after the law went into effect, the Medical Records Department implemented the Hospital Utilization Project (HUP) Grouper software, a program that assigned patients to DRG categories using medical abstract data.

The challenge, of course, was to find ways to keep costs within or below the fixed rates while maintaining quality care. "In a cooperative effort," Dr. Mills said, "we all must consider the way we use the hospital's resources, continue to increase productivity, and look for cost-effective alternatives to routine procedures." The recommended solutions put forth by Medicare were to decrease the length of stay for patients, to have physicians develop procedural standards among them-

1990

The hospital's Cardiac Rehabilitation Program is initiated, and pacemaker insertion surgery is introduced.

An Organ/Tissue Donor Policy in cooperation with the Pittsburgh Transplant Foundation (PTF).

The first pacemaker surgery is performed at Indiana Hospital.

1991

The Cardiology Department expands its capabilities with vascular laboratory testing.

The Cardiac Rehabilitation Program, begun in December 1989, moves from the Physical and Occupational Therapy Department to an area on the first floor of the Medical Office Building.

Laparoscopic cholecystectomies are now used for the removal of gall bladders.

1992

Brachytherapy for radiation therapy is introduced, provided by Indiana Hospital in conjunction with the Indiana Regional Cancer Center.

Outpatient Services Building opens.

1993

Indiana Hospital introduces endoscopic retrograde cannulation of the common bile and pancreatic ducts (ERCP) and endoscopic carpal ligament release for carpal tunnel syndrome, and lasers are now being used to perform transurethral resection of the prostate (TURP).

1994

The Sleep Disorder laboratory and Transitional Care Center open.

The first Life Flight patient, Karen Rippen, is transported from Indiana Hospital to Allegheny General Hospital in Pittsburgh.

Indiana Hospital Pediatric and Adolescent Dental Clinic opens.

The hospital acquires a Mobile Medical Unit, which will provide health services to county residents and businesses.

1995

The Cherry Tree and Plumville Family Medicine practices open in August to help meet the healthcare needs of residents in northern Indiana County.

1996

On September 3, Indiana Hospital's Fast Track closes.

Affiliation forms between Indiana Hospital and Visiting Nurse Association.

1997

- Indiana Hospital begins offering bone density testing to detect osteoporosis.
- The Ambulatory Surgical Center opens.
- An extended-hour primary care and specialty practice opens in Barnesboro.

1998

- The Geriatric Care Center, an inpatient mental health unit, opens in June.
- Market Square Pediatrics opens in Blairsville.
- Indiana Psychiatry Services opens on South Sixth Street in Indiana.
- Saltsburg Internal Medicine opens in September.
- Jacksonville Family Medicine opens providing primary care and laboratory services.

selves, and to be extremely conservative with the use of diagnostic tests. The net effect of the law was the acceleration of the trend toward increased outpatient services, a trend that would impact the hospital's decision-making process for decades to come.

A NEW ADMINISTRATOR

Chief Executive Officer Donald Smith resigned on September 28, 1981, after eleven years of service to the hospital. Dr. Henry Mitchell served as interim administrator until the hiring of Donald Valentine in 1982. Previously chief executive officer of a Pittsburgh-area hospital, Mr. Valentine held the position until 1983. From there, a committee made up of Dr. Larry Kachik, director of emergency services; Larry Marshall, chief financial officer; and Henry Hild, chairman of the board; served as interim administrator.

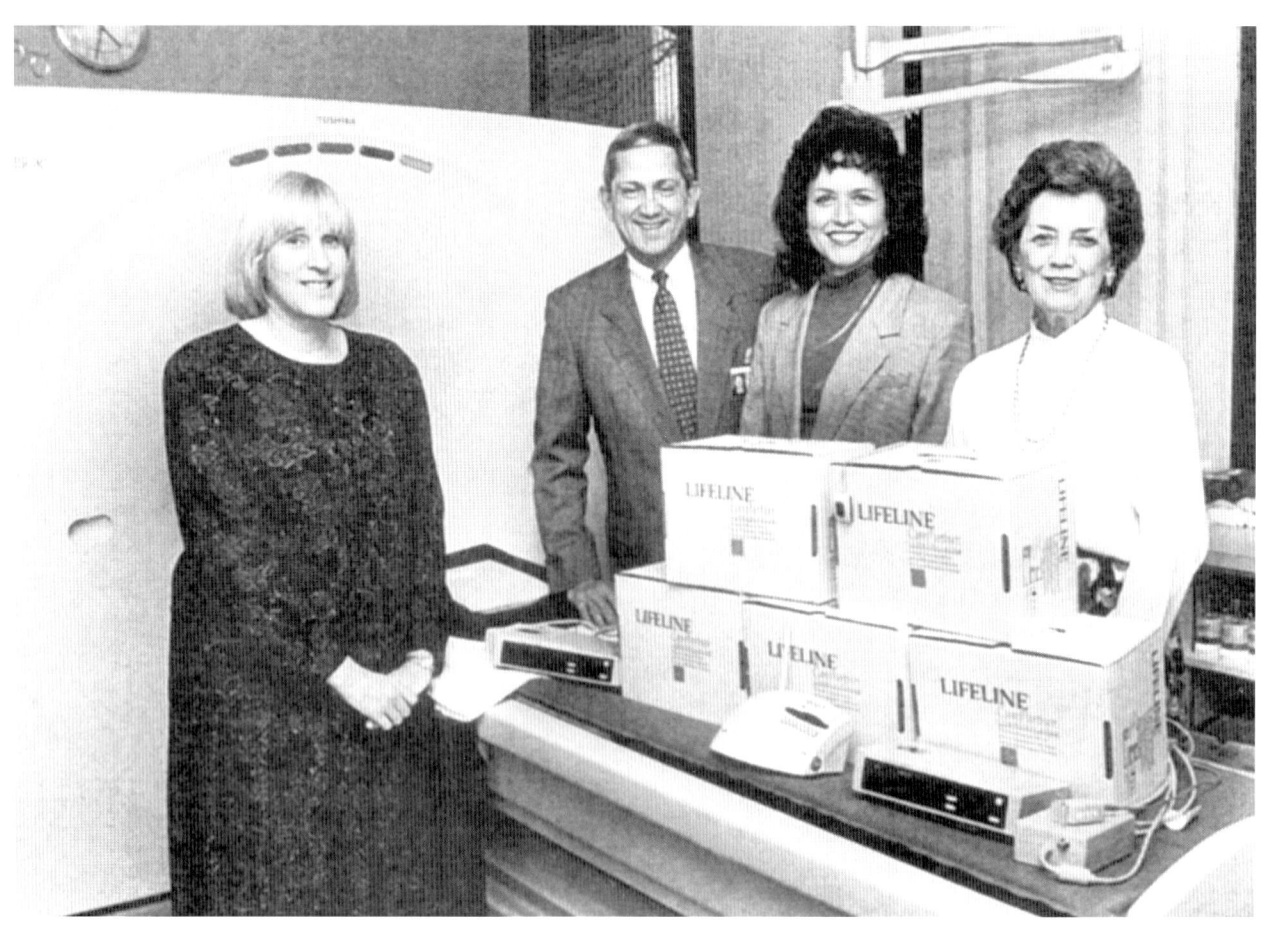

The Auxiliary provided the initial funding of $18,000 to start the Lifeline program, 1985.

After careful deliberation, in April 1985, Indiana Hospital announced the appointment of its new administrator, Donald D. Sandoval. For eight years prior to coming to Indiana, Mr. Sandoval was assistant administrator at Durham County General Hospital in Durham, North Carolina. A native of West Virginia, he was raised in the coal mining town of Mullens.

The upgrades to the hospital's physical plant and equipment during the past decade, however stressful, were reaping rewards. In June 1985, the College of American Pathologists accredited the Indiana Hospital Laboratory. Dr. Steven P. Griffin, pathologist and director of the Department of Laboratory Medicine, applauded his staff: "To go through the accreditation without any deficiencies is similar to getting an A-plus. It doesn't happen very often and we are proud of it."

LIFELINE

In addition to the countless simpler ways in which the Auxiliary contributed to the care and compassion of the patients and their families, they have over the years made some very significant tangible contributions to Indiana Hospital and the community at large. In 1985, their gift of more than $50,000 was used to transform the former intensive care unit and third floor wing of the Mack Building into a pediatric unit. It was dedicated July 27, 1985, in honor of the late John Watchko, MD, the hospital's first pediatrician who, according to his wife Eileen, decided

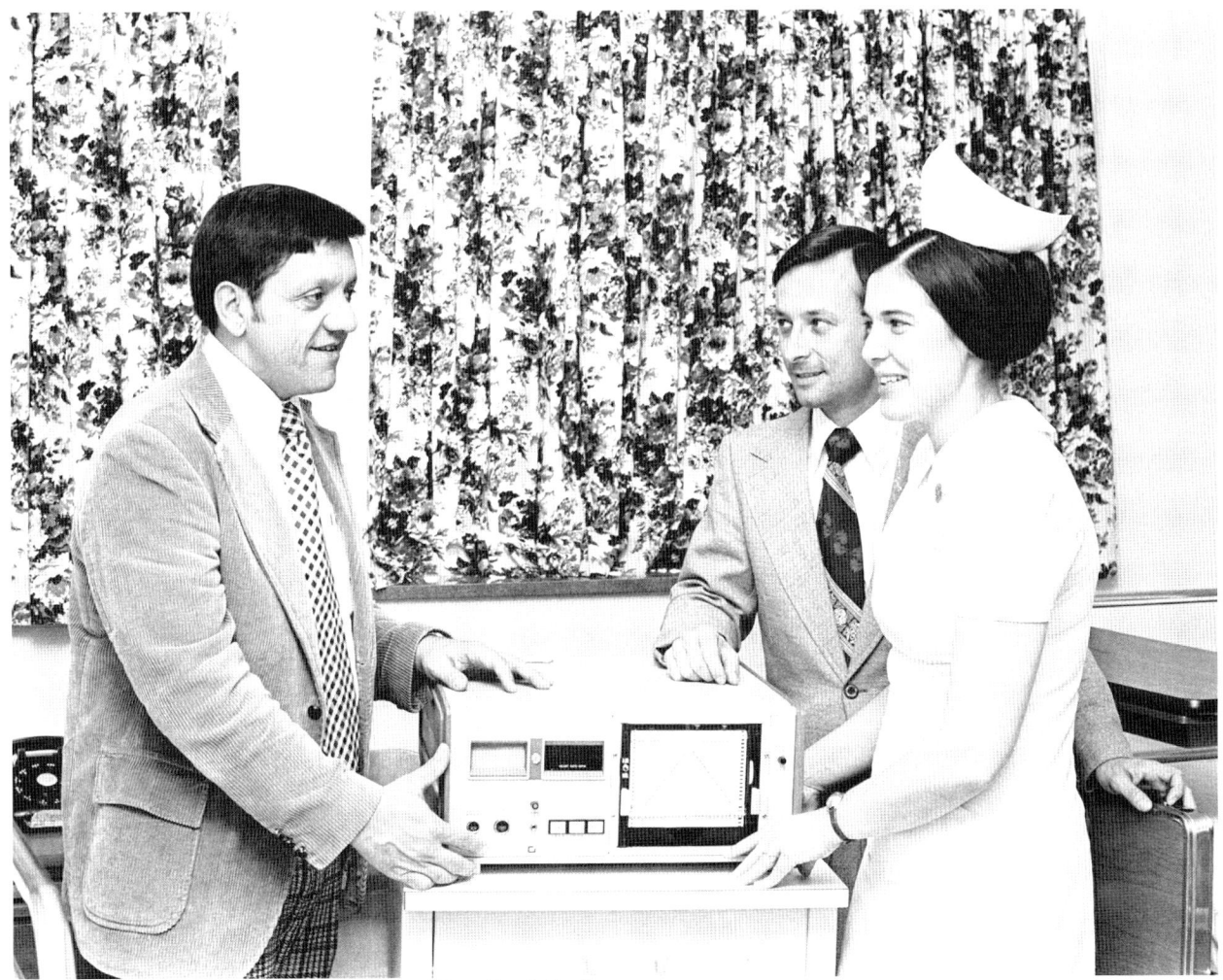

Dr. Freda, OB/GYN physician, with Suzanne Jamison, RN, and Les Gottardi.

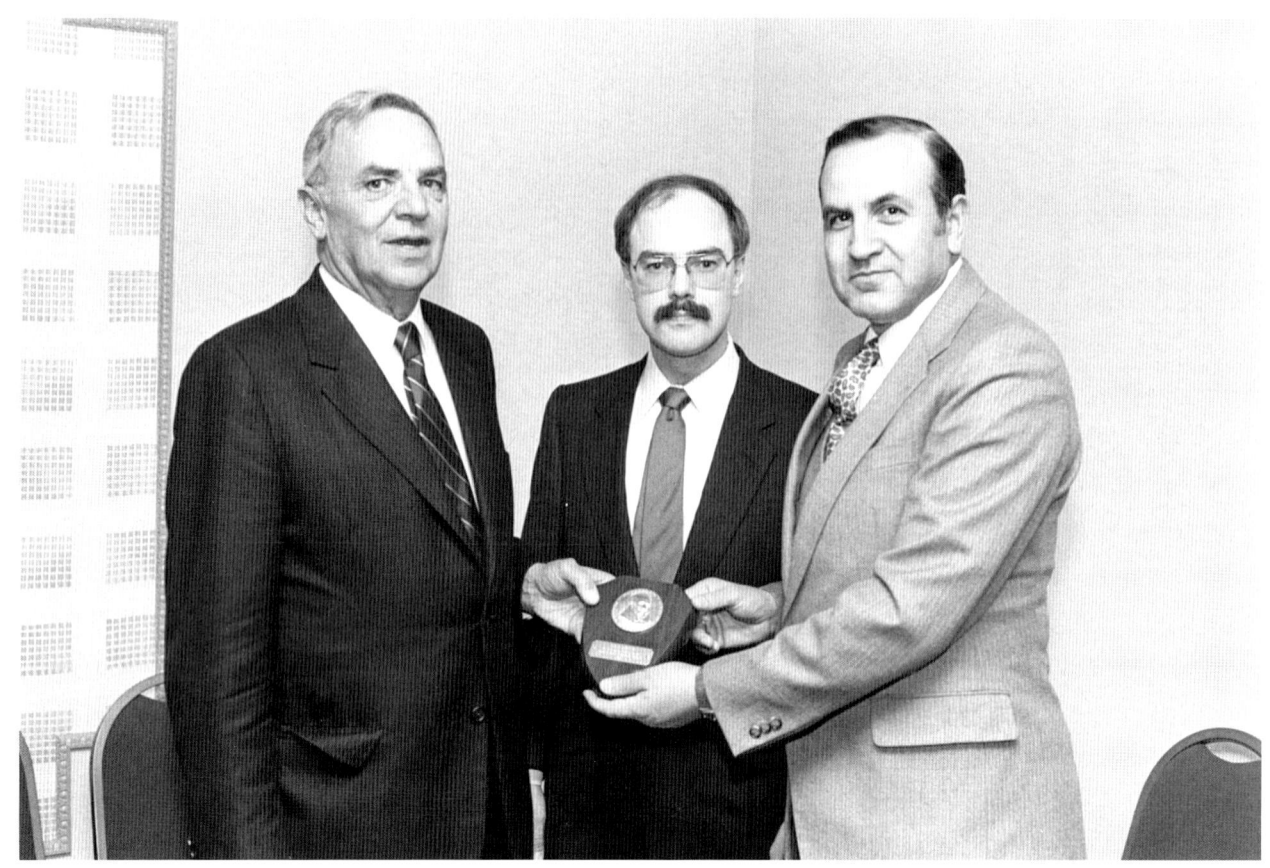

The Benjamin Rush Award was presented to Sam Jack, left, by Dr. Mark Boykiw and Dr. Shafic Twal for his outstanding service to the hospital, 1986.

to go into pediatrics after their first child was born. Adored by both patients and parents, Dr. Watchko was part of a generation of physicians who answered calls all hours of the day and night until his untimely death in 1974.

Extending their care beyond the hospital's walls, the Auxiliary provided the initial funding of $18,000 for the installation of Lifeline, a personal emergency response program that made it possible for senior citizens and disabled persons to live independently with an invaluable sense of security. Electronic equipment installed in the subscriber's home was hooked directly into the telephone system. A portable help button worn around the neck or wrist was used to summon help. The emergency response center was located in the hospital's emergency room where twenty-four-hour coverage was provided to initiate emergency procedures in the event that designated responders—friends, relatives, or neighbors—could not be located. At the 1987 annual meeting, CEO Donald Sandoval announced, "All the Lifeline equipment was a gift from the Indiana Hospital Auxiliary, which has contributed nearly 250,000 hours and approximately $340,000 worth of equipment to the hospital." By April 1990, the Auxiliary's support of the Lifeline program totaled $109,162 and to date exceeds a half million dollars.

CANCER CENTER

For the first time, Indiana Hospital partnered with another health care provider to make essential services more accessible to area residents. Cancer patients receiving treatment often had to travel to Pittsburgh numerous times per week for weeks at a time. Already weakened by their disease or the treatment itself, many patients never completed their therapy. In September 1986, Douglas R. Colkitt, MD, president of

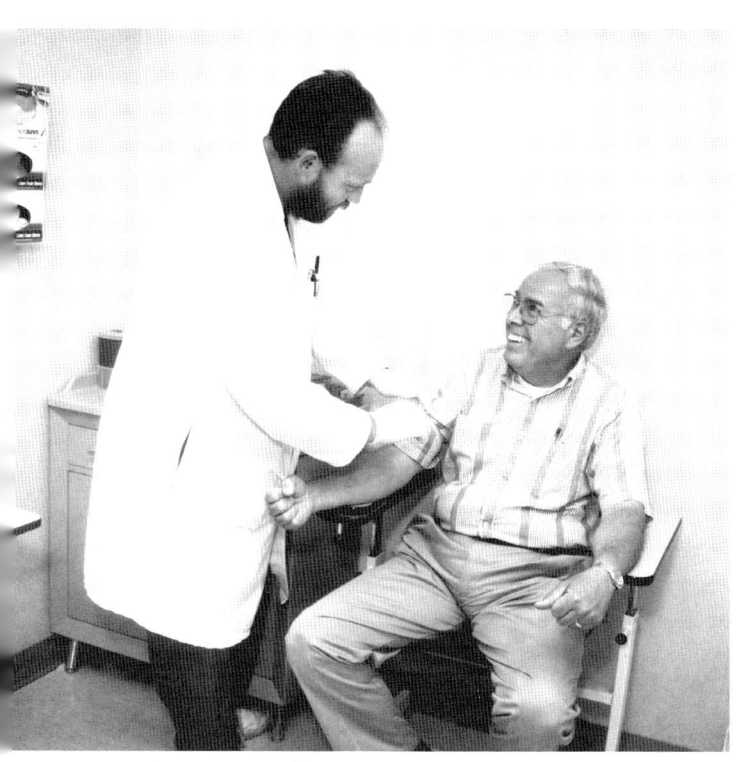

Lab technician Jeff Brown prepares patient Howard Abrams for a blood test.

Oncology Services, Inc., announced plans for the construction of a cancer treatment center adjacent to the hospital. "Indiana Hospital is making land available to Oncology Services, Inc., in support of containing health delivery services at a central site," said Donald Sandoval.

The one-story, 4,000-square-foot brick structure located in the southwest corner of the Indiana Hospital property was owned and operated by Oncology Services, Inc., of State College, Pennsylvania. The new center included a linear accelerator, a machine designed to precisely deliver high-dose, high-energy radiation, approximately sixty times as powerful as the typical chest x-ray. Medical treatment offices were also designed for the delivery of oncology chemotherapy services. Built at a cost of $400,000, the Indiana Regional Cancer Treatment Center opened on January 19, 1987, making the latest techniques in the treatment of cancer readily available to Indiana County residents.

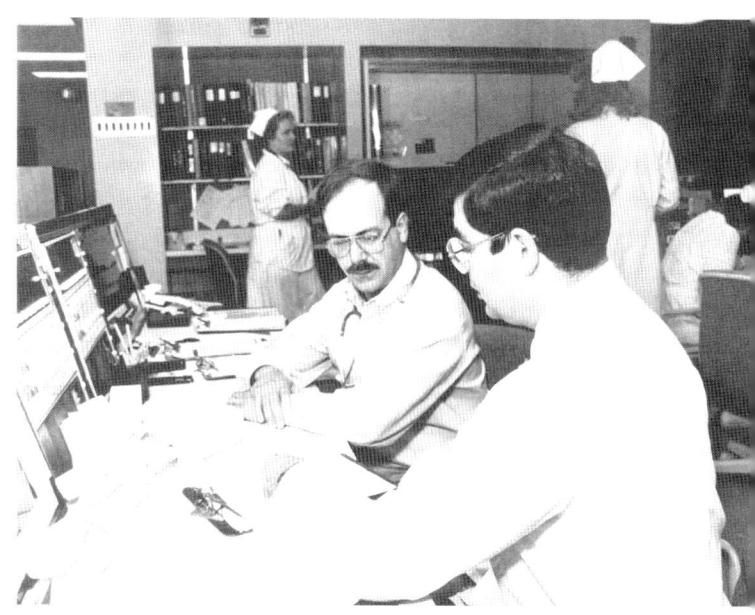

Dr. Russell Drozdiak and Dr. Bruce Bush.

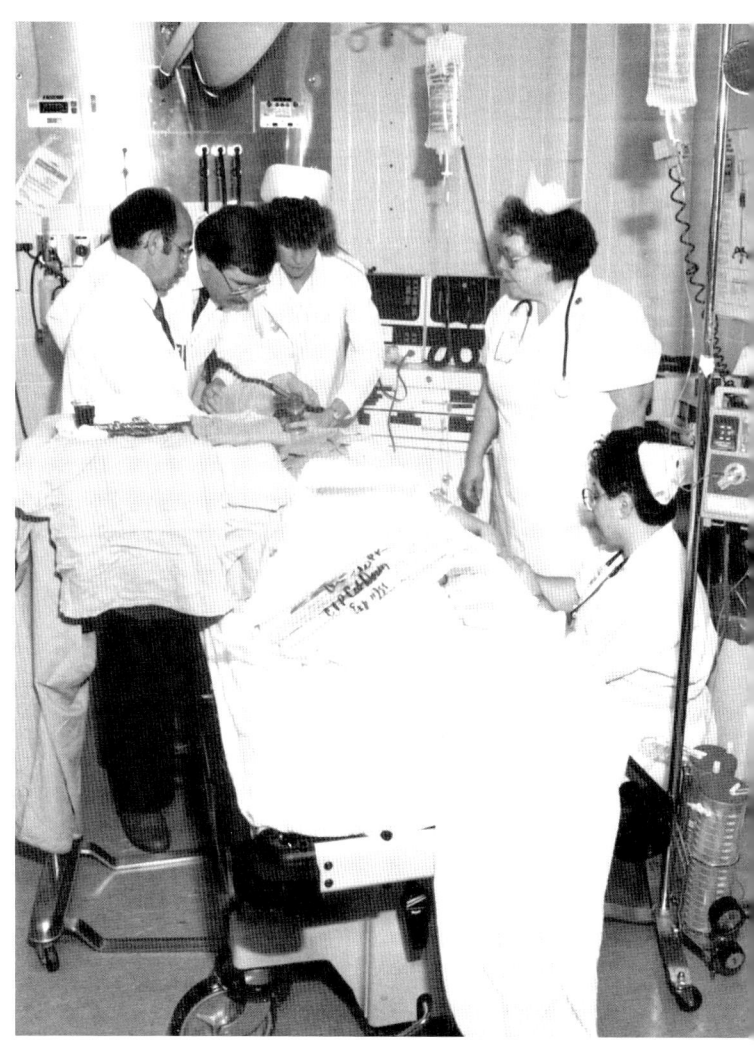

Dr. Campbell, Dr. Kachik, director of Emergency Services, Natalie George, and Nancy Smith give a patient their concentrated attention in the Emergency Department.

Increased government regulations and insurance company demands were just beginning to place unprecedented burdens upon health care providers. Their challenge: to contain costs while providing a broader range of services in order to remain competitive.

The first and most obvious solution was to provide more health care services on an outpatient basis. In 1985 the length of stay at Indiana Hospital was 5.5 days compared to 6.9 days for all Pennsylvania hospitals. Don Sandoval commented, "Big business is becoming more concerned about how to get the most for their health care benefits dollar. We can be very competitive with other hospitals since our current private room rate is $205 compared to $245 in Latrobe, $240 to $250 in Johnstown, $295 in Presbyterian in Pittsburgh, and $352 at Allegheny General in Pittsburgh."

To enhance the hospital's profile within the community, satellite offices and community programs were developed. Indiana Hospital opened a new diagnostic center in Blairsville in July 1986 in Dr. Herbert L. Hanna's office in the Market Square Professional Building to provide local residents with laboratory, x-ray, and EKG services. Another laboratory was opened at 119 Professional Building in Indiana in 1988 where blood samples could be taken, separated, refrigerated, and delivered to the hospital for analysis each day. Wellness programs including weight loss and smoking cessation were offered to residents for the first time.

The hospital found additional ways to cut expenses. David James, director of Materials Management, completed negotiations with People's Natural Gas to provide natural gas for the hospital at a cost savings of $90,000 to $100,000 per year. Said Mr. James, "This gas lease was negotiated as a result of our switch from gas to oil heat last spring, in the first of the cost-saving efforts. As a result of that change, gas companies began making competitive offers to the hospital to reclaim the business." This and other measures paid off. In 1988, the American Hospital Association awarded the 1987–88 Healthcare Administrative Services Certificate of Recognition to Indiana Hospital for its efforts in reducing costs while maintaining quality healthcare services.

The changing healthcare landscape created the need for upgrades to the hospital's physical plant as well. In 1986 the hospital lobby was remodeled, adding modular workstations for patient registrations. The increased number of outpatient procedures increased the hospital's laundry from 900,000 pounds in 1985 to 1.024 million pounds in 1986. A hot water heat reclamation system, along with a heat exchanger, was installed to transfer the heat from the used water draining from the washers to the clean water refilling the machines, thus saving on water heating expenses.

In May 1987, the hospital announced plans for a $2.5 million to $3 million project to renovate and relocate the Obstetric and Ambulatory Care Units. The relocated Obstetrics Unit would now reflect the latest concepts in labor, delivery, and recovery rooms for the approximate 800 babies delivered each year at Indiana Hospital. The home-like atmosphere complete with recliners, private bathroom, and large windows made it possible for the babies and fathers to spend as much time as they wished with the new mother. Congratulatory champagne dinners were served to help the new parents celebrate. All the equipment and furnishings for the nursery were donated by the hospital Auxiliary.

The Ambulatory Care Unit, currently located on the fifth floor of the Tower, was relocated to the fourth floor. A bridge was constructed to connect the unit to the surgery and recovery areas so that patients having one-day surgical procedures, approximately 60 percent of the hospital's surgical cases, were now able to remain on one floor from admission to discharge.

Even the hospital's paperwork demands were changing. In 1988, the Medical Records Department piloted a new computer software program from McDonnell Douglas Corporation, HDC Plus. The new system, mandated by both state and federal law and required by Medicare, Medicaid, and Blue Cross, involved insurance reimbursement for ambulatory care patients and was designed to help with new government and insurance requirements regarding the coding of outpatient procedures.

Computer terminals located in all nursing units and admitting stations were linked to the main computer in the Data Processing Department. Patient histories, including insurance information, were now permanent records, eliminating repetitious information gathering for employees and patients. The hospital's statistics showed that 1–2 percent of provided services were never billed to patients. The new system saved time, minimized errors, and expedited patient registration.

A NEW CORPORATE STRUCTURE

Until 1987 the hospital was managed by the Indiana County Hospital Association, which was formed in 1907 and incorporated as a nonprofit corporation in 1913. New federal Medicare regulations adopted in 1984 accelerated a trend to provide less-expensive outpatient services. As a result, the number of beds for patient care in Indiana Hospital dropped from a peak of 206 in 1976 to 137 beds by 1987.

To combat rising costs and increased competition in the health care field, the hospital underwent a corporate restructuring. Under the new system, Indiana Healthcare Corporation was formed and charged with

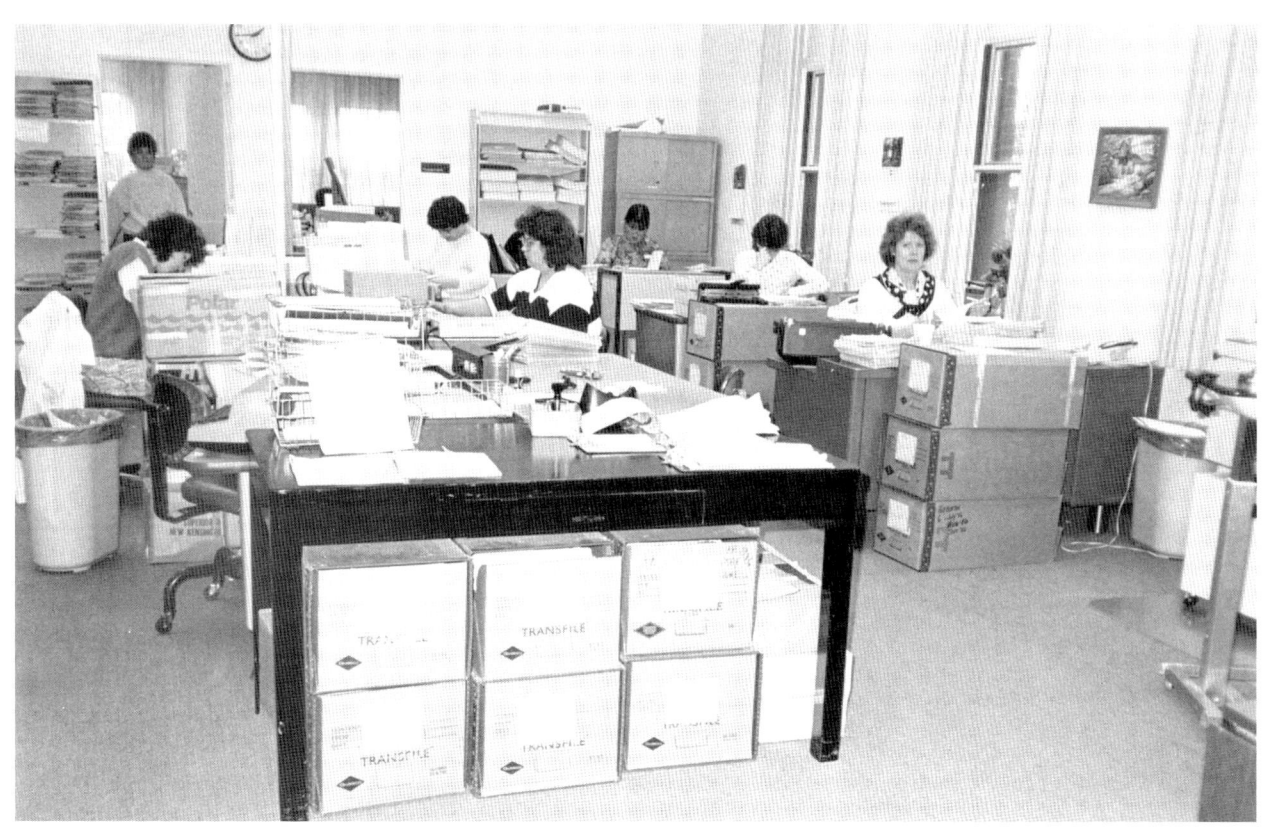

By the 1980s, medical records meant mountains of paperwork.

planning, overseeing, and coordinating the activities of four subsidiaries: Indiana Hospital, Indiana Hospital Properties, Indiana Healthcare Enterprises, and the Indiana Healthcare Foundation.

Indiana Healthcare Corporation was comprised of sixty residents representing various sections of the county. The corporate members were given responsibility for electing the sixteen-member executive board governing the operations of the corporation and appointing the members of the operating boards of the four subsidiaries.

Indiana Hospital Properties was established as a nonprofit corporation with the sole function of holding title to income-generating property. Indiana Healthcare Enterprises, a tax-paying corporation, was organized for the purpose of engaging in and doing health care–related business such as joint ventures with physicians. The primary function of the Indiana Healthcare Foundation was to manage the funds raised by Indiana Healthcare Corporation or transferred from other subsidiaries to assure that funds are allocated to the appropriate use. In announcing the reorganization, CEO Donald Sandoval pointed out that all profits and donations generated by the holding company and all subsidiary corporations were to be used to help offset the operating costs of Indiana Hospital.

With its new structure, the hospital was now in a position to undertake projects that were previously off limits because of various legal and financial restrictions. "The new corporate structure was necessary," said Don Sandoval, "to protect the assets of the hospital and to provide more flexibility for expanding services so the hospital could continue to compete."

The first exercise of the new corporate structure came in September 1988 when Indiana Hospital Properties entered into an agreement with Allegheny General Hospital to provide hemodialysis services to residents of Indiana County and the surrounding areas. Located in the 119 Professional Center, it provided eight hemodialysis stations for the treatment of patients with end stage renal disease. Ashok Chaddah, MD, was the center's medical director.

> In 1988, Indiana Hospital had approximately 740 full- and part-time employees, making it the fourth-largest employer in Indiana County.

The problem of an aging population and decreased government funding added up to shrinking profit margins for hospitals across the country. During the 1988–89 fiscal year, Indiana Hospital provided more than $300,000 in charity care and lost approximately $750,000 to bad debts. Of the patients admitted to Indiana Hospital at the time, 40 percent were Medicare recipients and 10 percent were Medicaid patients. With fully half of its patients receiving government funds, the continued funding cutbacks for these programs resulted in less and less reimbursement for the hospital. "Before this year, Pennsylvania hospitals received eighty cents for every dollar spent on Medicaid patients," said Donald Sandoval. "There is no question that Indiana Hospital loses money on Medicare and Medicaid patients." He and other officials and business representatives from Indiana County met in February with aides to United States Senator John Heinz to express their concern regarding these cutbacks in funding.

In the meantime, the hospital's Cost Containment Committee did its best to ease the situation, teaming up with other hospitals for the purchase of ba-

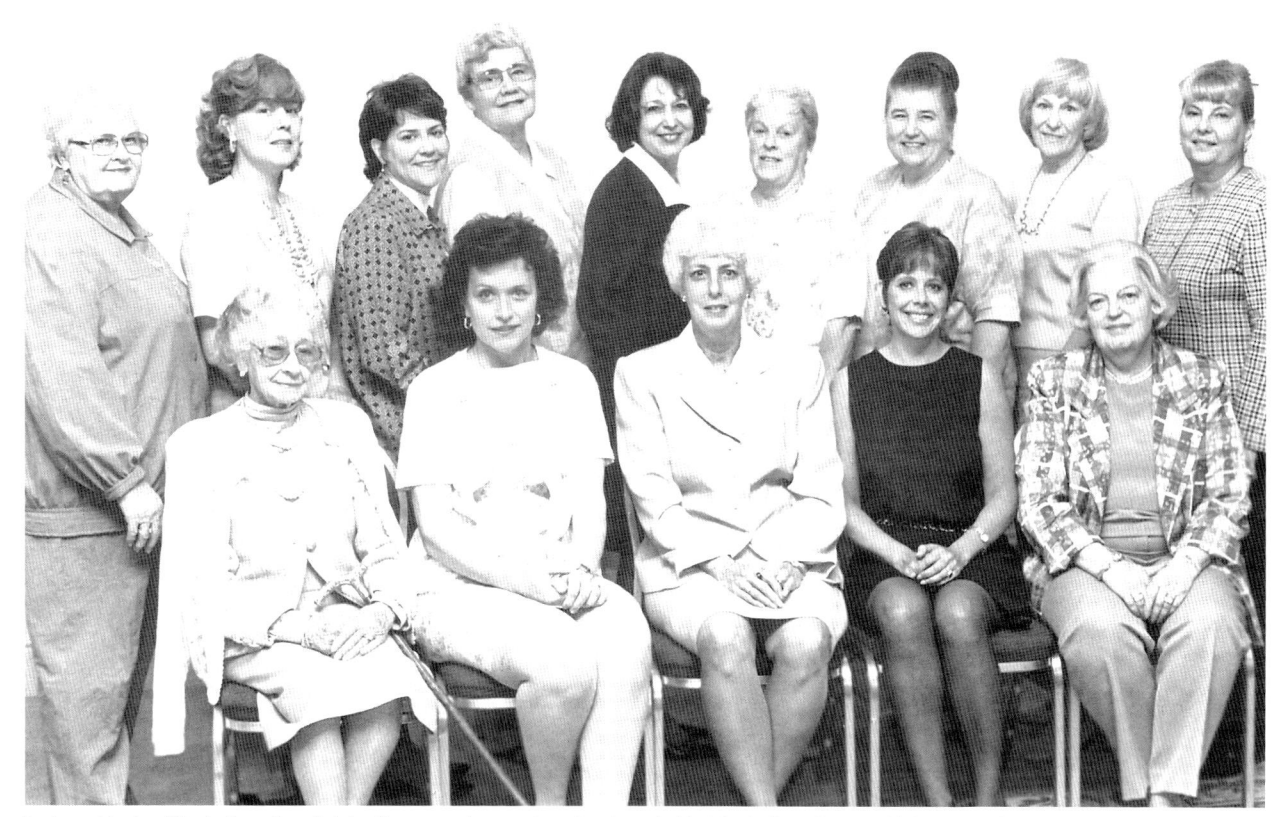

Past presidents of the Indiana Hospital Auxiliary were honored at a luncheon held at the Indiana Country Club. Front, left to right: Dorothy Parnell, Patty Bidwell, Kim Balcerak, Karen Wiley, and Phyllis Patchin. Back, left to right: Nancy Clawson, Maureen Bash, Christine Calhoun, Louise Hildebrand, Marcy Martin, Catherine Pike, Linda Connell, Jenny Williams, and Bonnie Parsons.

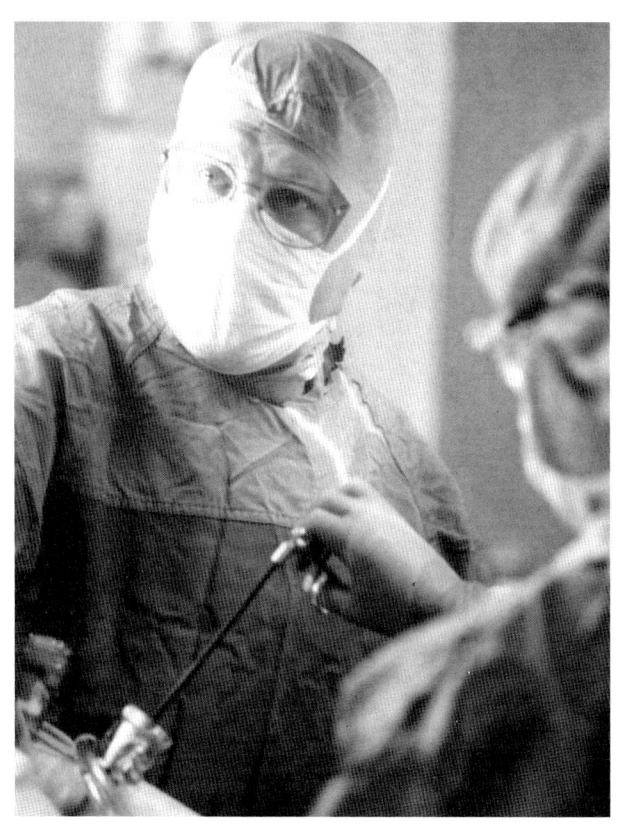

Dr. Alex Juhasz performed Indiana Hospital's first laparoscopic cholecystectomy in 1991.

sic supplies and implementing a policy of changing bed linens every other day when possible. No detail was too small. They managed to save $2,000 annually just by changing the purchase of paper towels from bleached white to brown. In its first year of existence, 1990, the Cost Containment Program realized a total of $624,580 in savings to the hospital.

OUTPATIENT SERVICES BUILDING

Limited space and the increasing demand for outpatient services prompted the hospital's board of directors to approve plans for a new Outpatient Services Building in the spring of 1991. The two-story, 18,000-square-foot brick building cost approximately $1.9 million and housed the ER Fast Track, Chemotherapy Unit, outpatient physical and occupational therapy, two educational classrooms, and the departments of Fiscal Services, Accounting, and Billing.

Chapter 6: The Preferred Regional Health Services Provider — 81

Built near the main hospital building with a thirty-foot covered walkway connecting it to the Medical Office Building, it was completed in January 1992. At the same time, the hospital also expanded the Emergency Services Department so that patients with less serious injuries could receive treatment at the new emergency center, the ER Fast Track, decreasing the wait time for people with noncritical injuries.

TELEMETRY UNIT

By November 1991, renovations were completed on the seventh floor of the Tower, and the telemetry patients were moved from the third floor of the Mack Wing to the seventh-floor Telemetry Unit. While telemetry patients are able to walk, they require continuous monitoring through electronic devices that transmit heart rates, electrocardiograms, and other functions to computer screens located in the nurses' stations. The new unit was now divided into three modules, each with its own nurses' station, giving the nurses fewer patients to monitor, which in turn meant a much faster response time.

During the 1992–1993 fiscal year, Indiana Hospital provided medical care in the amount of $4,880,706 to patients who, for whatever reasons, were unable to pay their medical bills. With mounting unemployment and cutbacks in Medicaid and Medicare, the hospital faced losses nearing $2.3 million for the services they were providing. The hospital's board of directors encouraged everyone to voice their opinions regarding healthcare reform to legislators.

A new trend was emerging: healthcare providers began focusing on the prevention of disease and the promo-

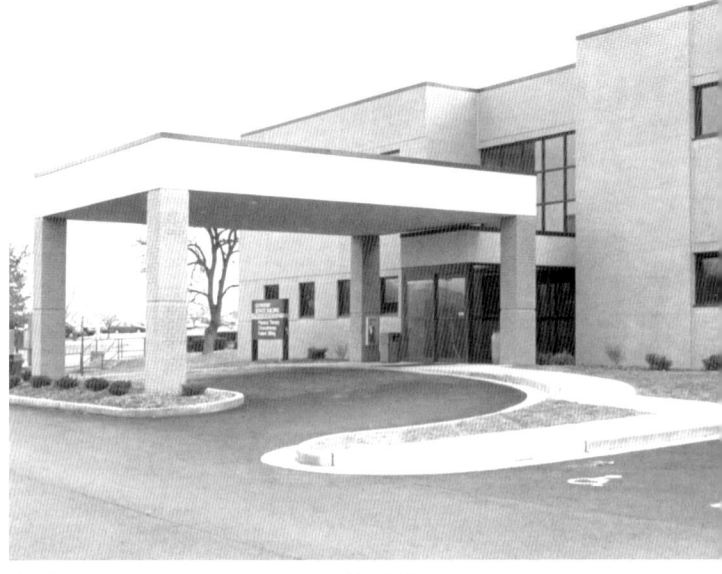

The Outpatient Services Building opened in 1992.

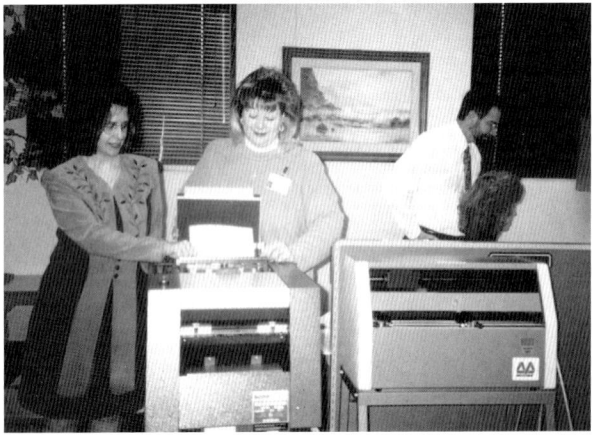

Accounting staff Mern Ruhl, Joni Wolford, Tom Treasure, and Diane Beck.

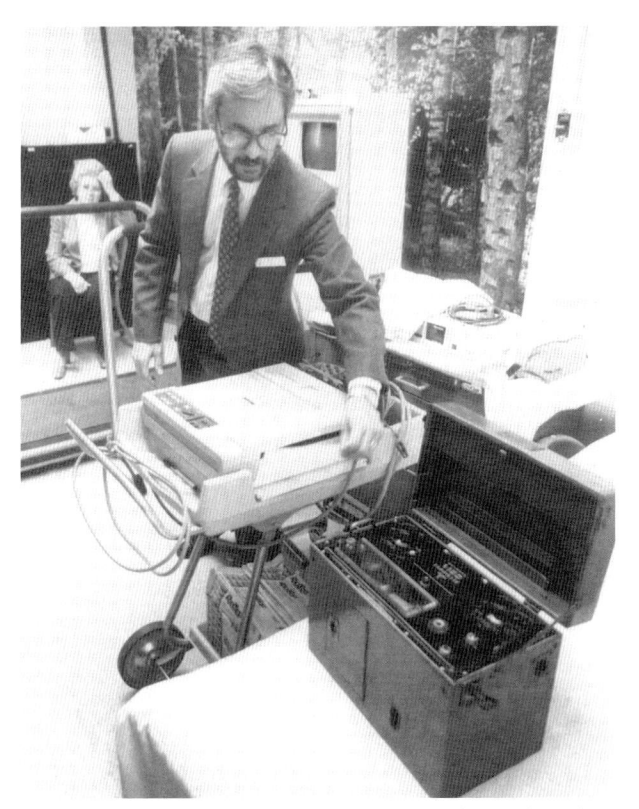

Lancy Brunetto, administrative director of DIS and Special Services, demonstrates equipment at a health fair.

82 — Indiana Regional Medical Center

tion of healthier lifestyles. Indiana Hospital launched a new program for school-age children called Healthy Communities to encourage the development of positive health habits, and more than 3,000 people attended the hospital's first major health fair offering information and free healthcare screenings. Requests from businesses for local affordable services to promote healthy and productive employees led to the development of the Executive Physical Program and the expansion of Occupational Health Services. OHS began offering physicals for new employees, drug screenings, injury management and prevention, health-risk appraisals, health fairs, and on-site wellness seminars.

More than ever before, it was vital for the hospital to identify the particular needs of the community, and several of the hospital's improvements in the early 1990s focused on the ever-increasing senior population.

The Tower's sixth floor underwent renovations in 1993 to address the needs of elderly patients who may be vision or hearing impaired, have special dietary requirements, and have multiple medical issues. The number of patient beds was reduced from forty-six to forty-two, and two nurses' stations were created to provide constant care. The renovations provided a hemodialysis room, inpatient chemotherapy room, two conference rooms, a lounge for patients and family members, an examination room, a kitchen, and utility area.

The Health Alert program was also initiated in 1993. This free service provided patients with a packet containing personal health information and emergency contact numbers upon their discharge from the hospital. Telephone stickers were provided to direct first responders to the packet's location. With this information readily available, patients' and family members' minds were put at ease and paramedics could begin treatment much quicker.

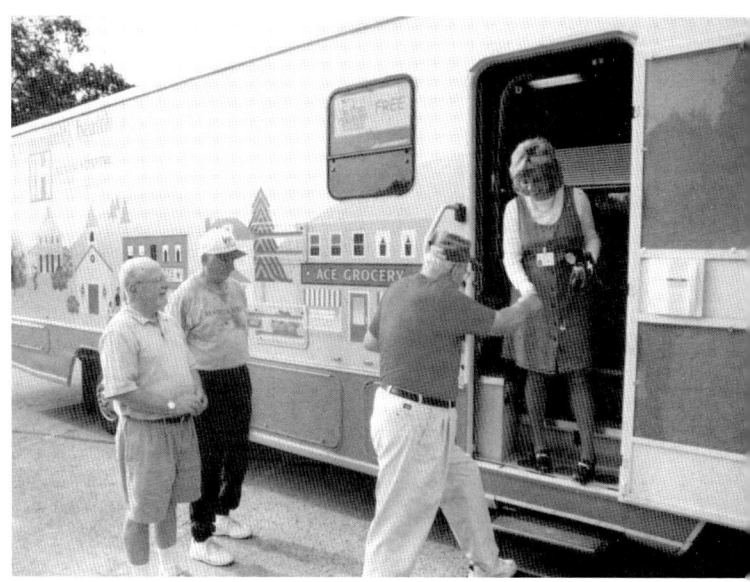

Nancy Smith, director of Community Services, welcomes patients to the mobile van that was purchased in 1994 to extend more services to the rural communities.

Construction began on the Transitional Care Center in early 1994. A skilled nursing facility, it was designed to provide short-term medical care for patients who no longer required hospitalization but were not well enough to return home and care for themselves. The Mack III Surgical Unit was completely redesigned and renovated to accommodate the new center. The Transitional Care Center included eighteen beds, an activity room, a laundry facility, and a dining area for patients. The typical length of stay in the center averaged between fifteen and twenty-five days at a much lower cost than had the patient had to remain in the hospital. In 1997, the Transitional Care Center became the first subacute-care center under a management contract with Diversified Health Services to receive JCAHO (Joint Commission on Accreditation of Healthcare Organizations) accreditation.

Indiana Hospital, like most hospitals across the country, struggled to find ways to meet the challenges brought on by severe reductions in Medicare and Medicaid hospital payments, pressure from insurance companies to reduce lengths of stay, and the growing presence of managed care. Throughout the industry,

Life Flight

Beginning in August 1993, Indiana Hospital entered into a joint venture with Allegheny General Hospital in Pittsburgh to provide Life Flight, a helicopter transport service for critical patients. Dr. James Garrettson recalled the days before such a service existed. "I remember many times jumping in the back of the ambulance with a nurse or maybe an EMT and working [on the patient] all the way to Pittsburgh." Karen Rippen was the first Indiana Hospital patient to be transported to Allegheny General Hospital via Life Flight.

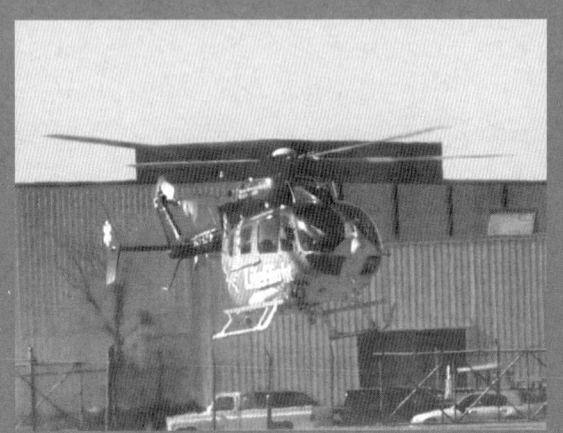

The Life Flight helicopter transport service, a joint venture between Indiana Hospital and Allegheny General Hospital in Pittsburgh, began in 1993.

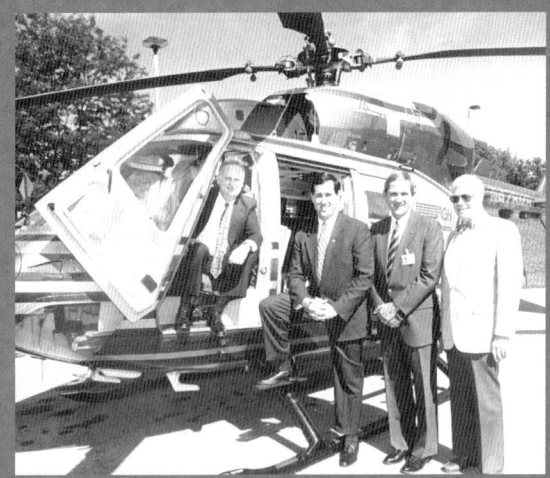

Carson Green, Rick Santorum, CEO Donald Sandoval, and Dr. John Mills pose alongside a Life Flight helicopter.

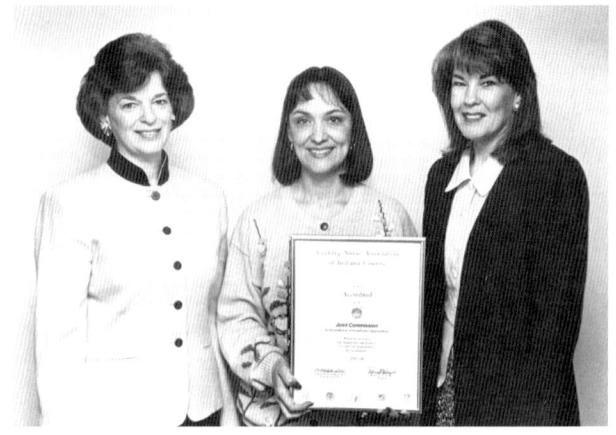

Diane Petras, Debbie Beer, and Linda Bettinazzi proudly display the Visiting Nurse Association's certificate of accreditation from the JCAHO, 1998.

larger medical institutions were gobbling up smaller ones and creating affiliations. The future direction of the hospital was in question. To their credit, the board of directors brought the medical staff leadership into the decision-making process.

That is about the time that Dr. Robert Parker joined the staff at Indiana Hospital. "The hospital had a history of being very financially stable," he said. "They had talented members of the board." A weekend retreat to devise a plan for the hospital's future was held locally and involved medical staff, employees, administration, members from the community, and the board of directors. The conclusion was that the hospital should stay independent.

A Community Health Survey was mailed to more than 33,000 Indiana County households in 1994. The results of the survey would give the information needed to provide the highest quality medical care for every dollar spent.

Among other things, the survey identified a need for basic dental care for children. In response, CEO Donald Sandoval announced the formation of the Indiana Hospital Pediatric and Adolescent Dental Clinic. Located in Fast Track, the clinic provided care for children and adolescents through age eighteen whose families received medical assistance.

The survey also brought to light the challenges regarding the breadth of the hospital's service area. The county's population of approximately 90,000 made it a reasonable service area, but people who lived in the periphery of the county were going to other hospitals. What they needed were some avenues for uniting the entire community.

First among their solutions was the purchase of a Mobile Medical Unit, a 37-foot-long, 11½-foot-high traveling medical center that included a patient registration and waiting area, two examination rooms, a patient information area equipped with a television, and a laboratory collection area complete with restroom. Pat Hillebrand, vice president for Planning, Marketing and Development at the time, echoed the hospital's new direction: "The new healthcare-delivery system is no longer located within four walls or in one spot—it happens where the people are." The Mobile Medical Unit made it possible for the hospital to provide preventive health-care screening services and promote healthy lifestyles throughout the county, particularly in the more remote rural areas, as well as for businesses and their employees in surrounding cities.

Many managed care health insurance plans were now requiring patients to be seen in physician offices rather than hospital emergency departments. As a result, part of the hospital's plan to strengthen the hospital's ties to the community was to create primary care facilities in towns that had not had that resource for a number of years.

First on the list was Cherry Tree, a community that had not had a resident physician for nearly twenty years. Having approached the townspeople, the hos-

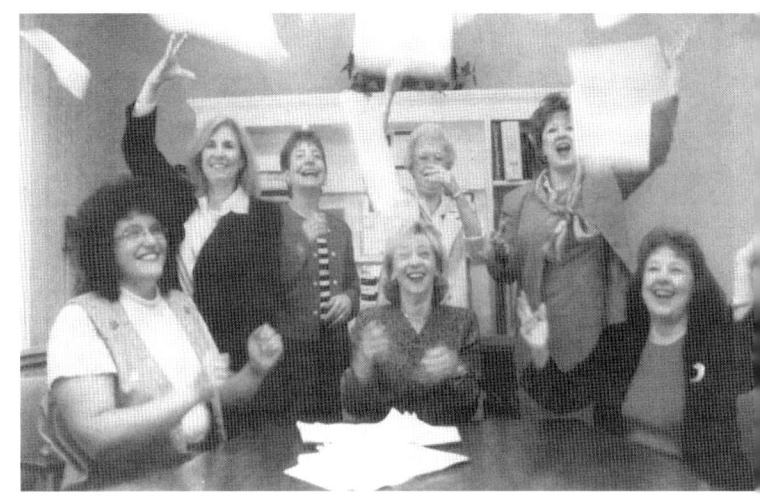

The Quality Assurance Team celebrates condensing sixty-four forms into one, 2000. Back, left to right: Cindy Virgil, Paula Miller, Bernice Leslie, Dawn Zoldak. Seated, left to right: Brenda Bakaysa, Kim Traynor, and Claudia Kepple.

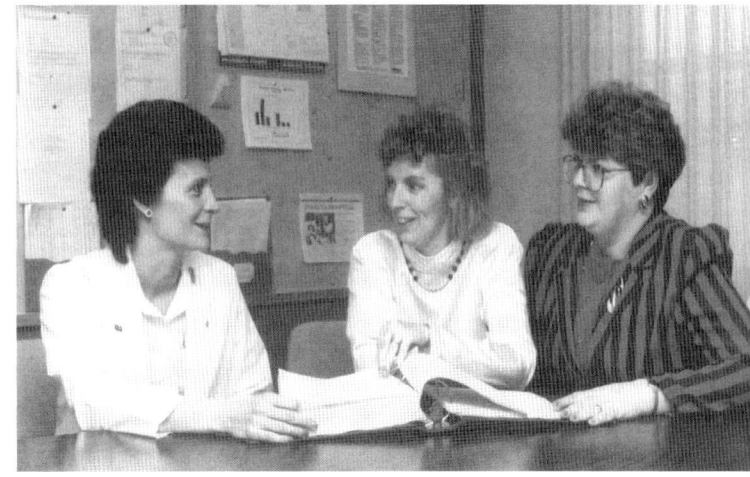

Patricia Hildebrand, center, with Cindy Shirley and Deb Succheralli.

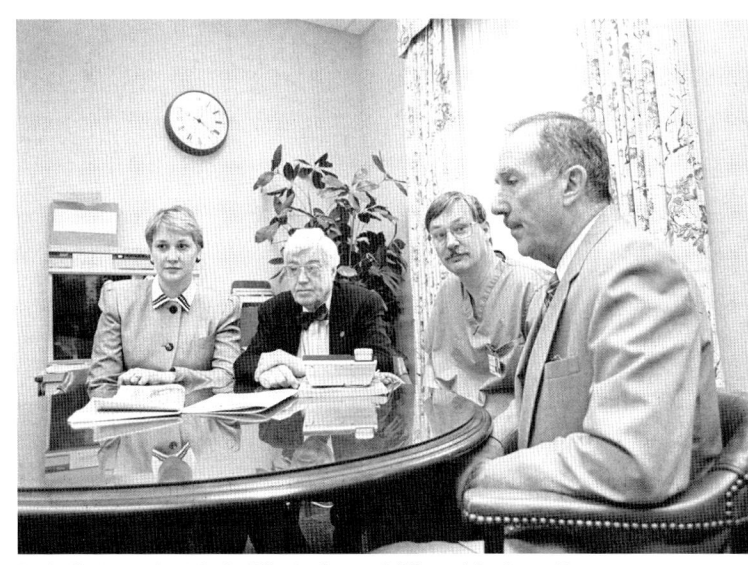

Dr. Stella Boron, Dr. John D. Mills, Dr. Steven Griffin, and Dr. James Bauer grapple with national health care issues.

Chapter 6: The Preferred Regional Health Services Provider — 85

pital found them enthusiastic, but there were some challenges to overcome. "Our major problem was that there was no sewer tie-ins," Dr. Parker recalled, "so we had to rent a facility that already had a sewer tie-in." The only structure that met that requirement, as well as the hospital's requirements, was a building that had previously been an auto repair shop. "In the back of the building there was still a hydraulic lift," Dr. Parker said. "But it had a bathroom. It was an open building, so we essentially built inside the existing building." During the fall of 1995, the Cherry Tree Family Medicine Center opened at 71 South Main Street.

The following year, the Plumville Family Medicine Center opened at 188 Main Street, another former auto repair shop.

The hospital continued to change its focus to meet the demands of the changing health care market. In 1996, 6,000 people turned out for the hospital's second major health fair held at Indiana Mall. The hospital's Occupational Health Services program was expanded to include a Workers' Compensation program to provide follow-up care to workers injured on the job so they can return to work as soon as possible.

After providing area residents with minor medical care for the past four years, Indiana Hospital's Fast Track closed on September 3, 1996. Originally opened to help relieve overcrowding and patient care delays in the hospital's main Emergency Services Department, Fast Track treated approximately eighty patients per day at its peak. However, with managed care insurers requiring their members to have primary care physicians, use of Fast Track services had declined dramatically.

At the same time Fast Track was closing, Indiana Hospital expanded its cardiac rehabilitation services to include a home-based exercise program for people whose schedules or transportation needs hindered visits to the hospital. Transtelephonic Cardiac Rehabilitation (TCR) allowed participants to follow a supervised exercise program in their homes. Par-

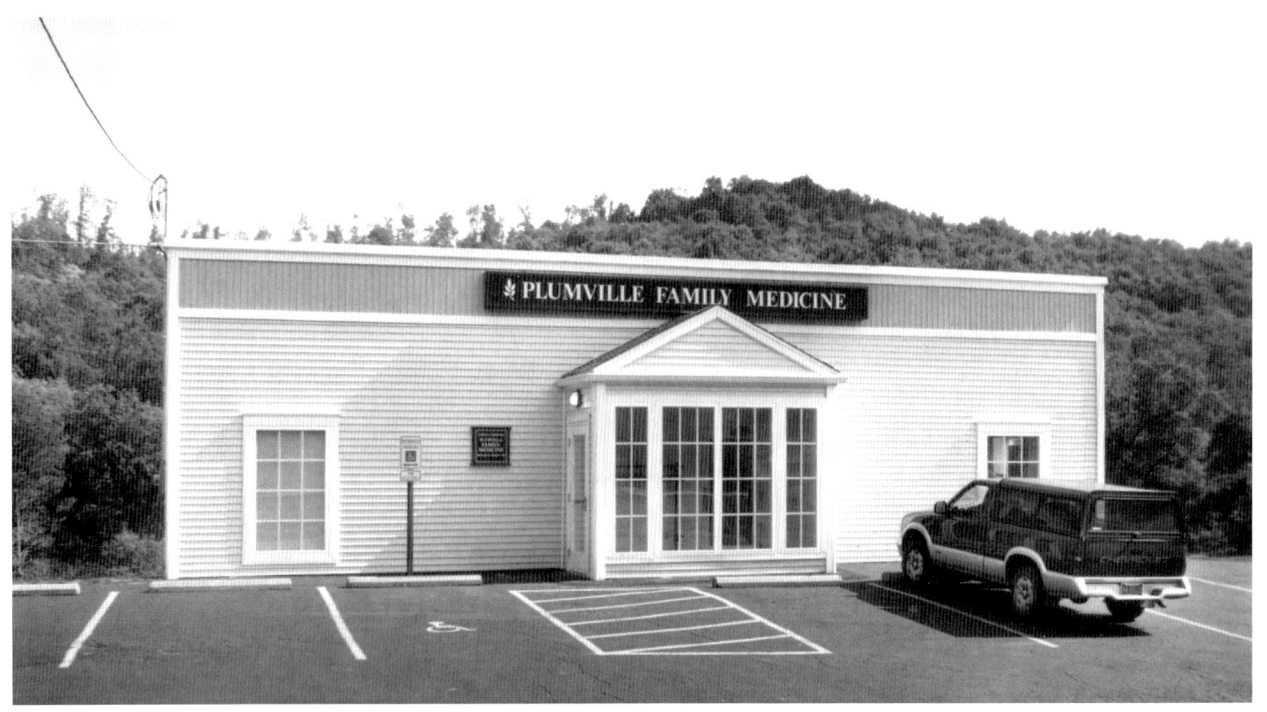

The Plumville Family Medicine Center opened in 1996.

ticipants wore a telephone headset through which they interacted with an exercise supervisor who also checked the participant's heart activity with continuous electrocardiogram monitoring.

In November 1996, the hospital's year-to-date loss on operations soared to approximately one-half million dollars. Managed care insurers stepped up their efforts to decrease inpatient admissions, patient lengths of stay, and the ordering of diagnostic tests and procedures. Declining reimbursement rates and payment of property taxes also contributed to the loss of operating income. However, through the hospital's cost containment measures, they managed to achieve a year-end positive income from operations of $376,000.

The initiative of providing primary care in outlying areas continued through 1997. On October 1, Indiana Hospital opened an extended-hour primary care and specialty practice in Barnesboro. The decision to establish a practice in Barnesboro was largely due to Miners Hospital of Northern Cambria's proposed move from Spangler to Hastings, which left as many as 6,000 people without medical care. Located in the former McCrory's department store building on Tenth Street, Barnesboro Family Medicine was designed to provide primary care and basic radiology and laboratory testing to residents in the Barnesboro and Spangler areas, along the eastern border of Indiana County.

Three more primary care facilities were opened during 1998, in Blairsville, Saltsburg, and Jacksonville. Market Square Pediatrics opened in Blairsville in August, providing a full range of pediatric services. Located in an adjacent office, the Blairsville Outpatient Testing Center was opened to provide laboratory, x-ray, and mammography services. Saltsburg Internal Medicine opened in the cafeteria section of the former Saltsburg High School in September to provide a full range of internal medicine, laboratory, and x-ray services for patients age fourteen or older. Jacksonville Family Medicine opened in October at 29 Saltsburg Road, providing primary care and laboratory services.

Closer to the hospital, Indiana Psychiatry Services opened in July 1998 at 1177 South Sixth Street in Indiana to provide comprehensive psychiatry services for people age eighteen or older. In addition, an inpatient geriatric mental health unit was established

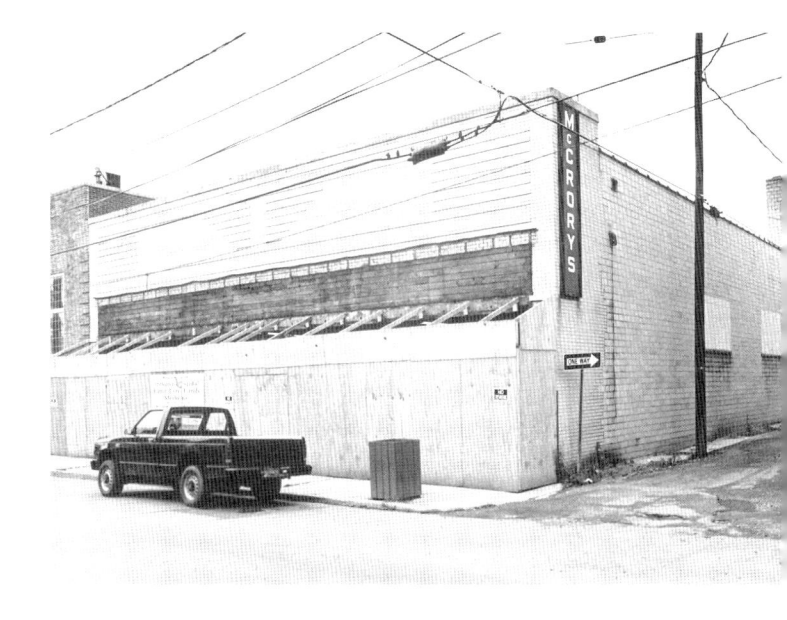

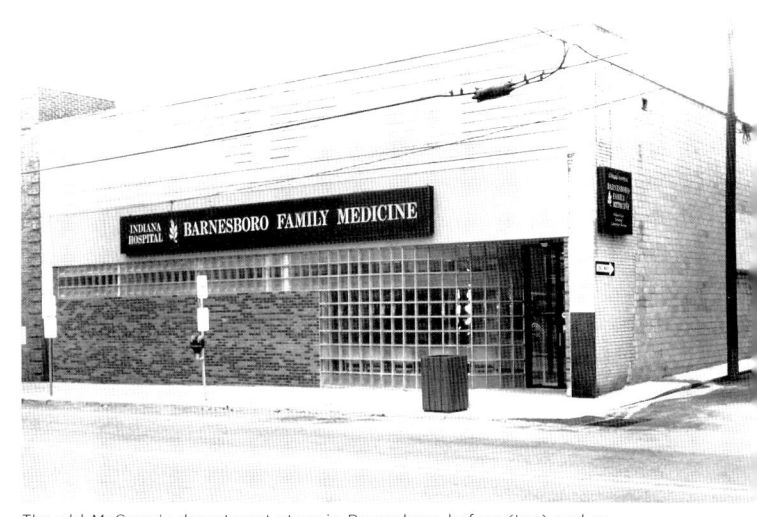

The old McCrory's department store in Barnesboro before (top) and as the new Barnesboro Family Medicine Center, 1997.

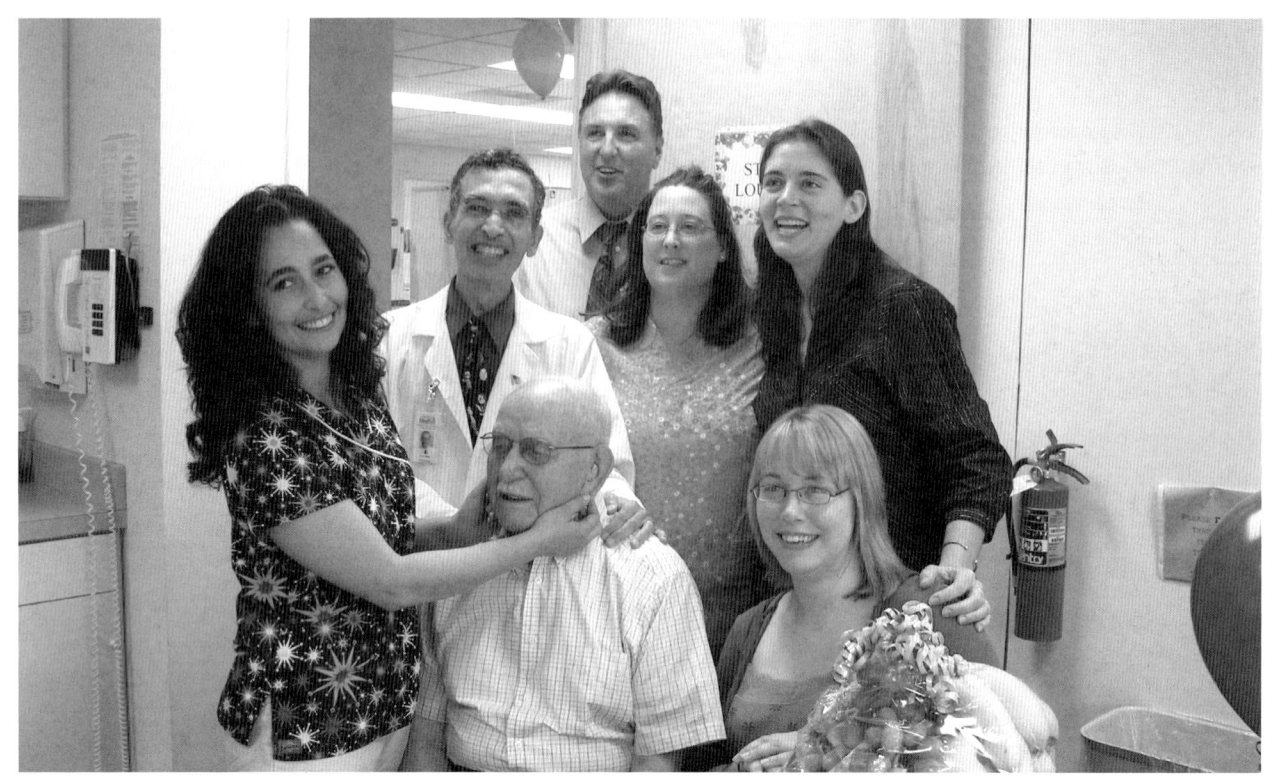

Dr. Wahba and the staff of the Jacksonville Family Practice celebrate the 100th birthday of Mr. Maryai.

in June 1998 to provide short-term comprehensive care to patients age sixty-five or older with serious psychiatric disorders, age-related functional difficulties, or problems with memory, reasoning, or other thought processes.

A NEW MISSION

In the spring of 1997, Indiana Hospital began working closely with physicians, hospital trustees, local businesses, and community leaders to develop a strategic plan that would expand the scope of healthcare services offered to the community. According to Robert C. Parker, MD, MPH, senior vice president for Medical Affairs, the basic question was whether the hospital should align itself with a larger system, as many hospitals have done nationwide. "Although there is a lot of pressure and precedent to become part of a bigger network, we decided to remain an independent community hospital for now," Parker said. "We feel it is most appropriate that healthcare decisions be made locally. We had the financial strength to accomplish a great deal ourselves and felt that we could make better healthcare decisions with our community than individuals in distant metropolitan areas. Once we reached that conclusion, we put together a strategic plan that would support that decision."

In the 1997 Annual Report, Indiana Hospital announced its new mission: "To be the preferred regional health services provider." Unveiling the hospital's strategic plan, Donald D. Sandoval, FACHE, president and CEO of Indiana Hospital and Indiana Healthcare Corporation, assured employees that the hospital would remain independent. "We all concluded that Indiana Hospital can continue to function independently and be successful," citing the "dedicated employees, the high quality medical staff, and the hospital's current financial strength" as the key contributing factors to this decision.

AMBULATORY SURGICAL CENTER

To keep pace with the constantly changing health care industry, the hospital launched an entirely new project in November 1997. "Health care is rapidly changing, and Indiana Hospital is responding," said president and CEO Donald Sandoval. "By expanding the hospital complex to include an ambulatory surgery center and physician office space, we will be able to make a more comprehensive array of services available to our patients in one convenient location." With procedure costs increasing, and the majority of physician offices unable to provide the necessary equipment, the center offered patients another option for surgery.

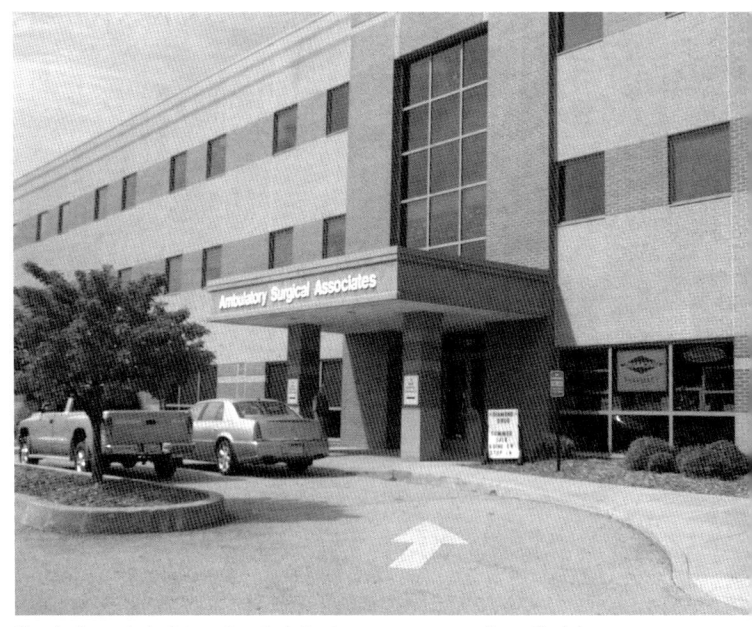

The Indiana Ambulatory Surgical Center was a cooperative effort between Indiana Hospital and Indiana Ambulatory Surgical Associates, LLC, a group of local surgeons and other physicians. Chairman of the Board James Miller echoed Mr. Sandoval's assessment of the wisdom of the project. "We did it because we were convinced it would be an economically viable project. Although the outpatient center sometimes competes with the hospital, the alliance makes sense because of the shared services."

Marshall Erdman and Associates, Inc., who designed and constructed the hospital's Outpatient Services Building in 1992, coordinated the project. The three-story, 48,000-square-foot building cost approximately $6.2 million. Located near the main entrance to the hospital, an enclosed walkway was built to connect the two facilities.

The physicians' group owned the first two floors, which contained three operating rooms, an endoscopy suite, and physician office space. The third floor, owned by Indiana Hospital, was reserved for additional physician offices.

The Indiana Ambulatory Surgical Center was a cooperative effort between Indiana Hospital and Indiana Ambulatory Surgical Associates and opened in 1998.

Before the Center was finished, however, in the April 27, 1998, edition of the *Indiana Gazette*, James Miller announced Don Sandoval's resignation as CEO of Indiana Hospital. "The Indiana County community owes Don Sandoval a debt of gratitude for many of the improvements and accomplishments that have occurred at Indiana Hospital during the past thirteen years." Citing the hospital's high marks from outside agencies that evaluated the hospital's performance, he said, "The health care environment has changed dramatically in recent years, and Indiana Hospital has not escaped the stress of the managed care movement."

Dr. Parker was appointed interim CEO. His current responsibilities for coordinating medical staff activities, assisting medical staff officers and department chairmen, and recruiting new physicians to the area gave him a broad perspective from which to navigate the hospital's future.

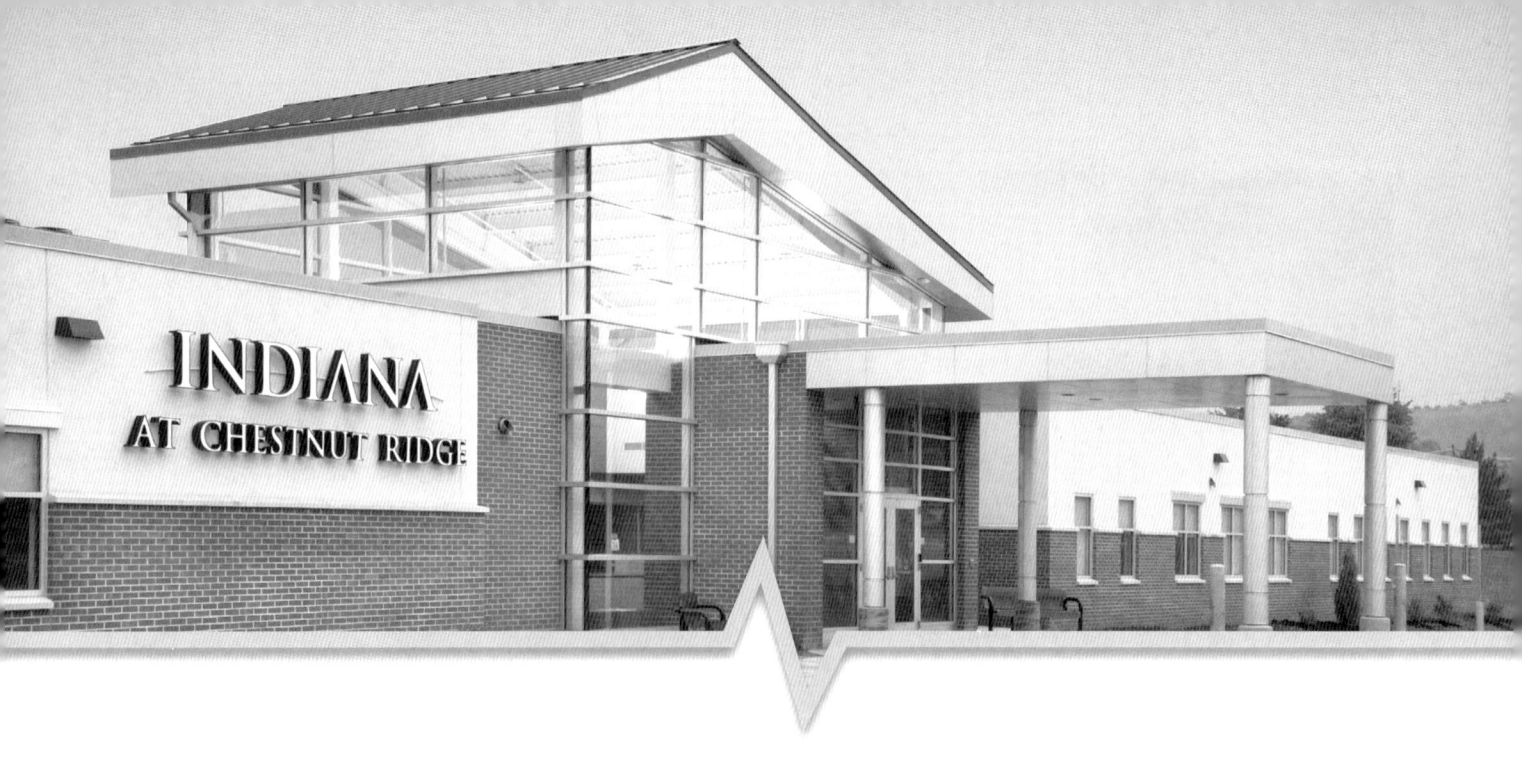

CHAPTER 7
A New Era, A New Commitment, A New Identity

Hospitals across the country continued being squeezed, caught between reductions in Medicare reimbursements and their dedication to providing the best possible care to the communities they served. By necessity, the economics of care was playing an increasingly larger role in their decision-making process. The Balanced Budget Act of 1997, enacted ostensibly to ensure Medicare's fiscal solvency, resulted in further reductions in federal reimbursements. Pennsylvania hospitals were especially hard hit; in percentage of elderly residents, the state ranked second in the nation. On average, Pennsylvania hospitals were losing twenty-three cents on every dollar of care they provided.

That was the state of things when Stephen A. Wolfe became Indiana Hospital's chief executive officer in February 1999. After receiving his master's degree from Pennsylvania State University, Steve spent nine years as director of hospital pharmacies at J. C. Blair in Huntingdon followed by seven years at Clearfield Hospital, four of which he served as CEO. A pharmacist by trade, he regards himself as "a clinician in an administrative office."

Though Clearfield and Indiana Hospitals were very similar, Steve noticed one major difference. "When I first got here, the most memorable reaction I had was when I walked through the halls. Nobody really looked at each other or talked to one another." He soon learned one reason why. His very first meeting was with a labor attorney who warned him that the employees were on the verge of a strike.

The cost containment measures of recent years had taken its toll on all the employees, and the general state of the industry led to fears regarding job security. The nurses did, in fact, vote to join the union, and though by Steve's own account, the contract negotiations were "tough sledding," they did reach an agreement.

As the hospital's new CEO, Steve's approach was unique, preferring to listen rather than speak. He set

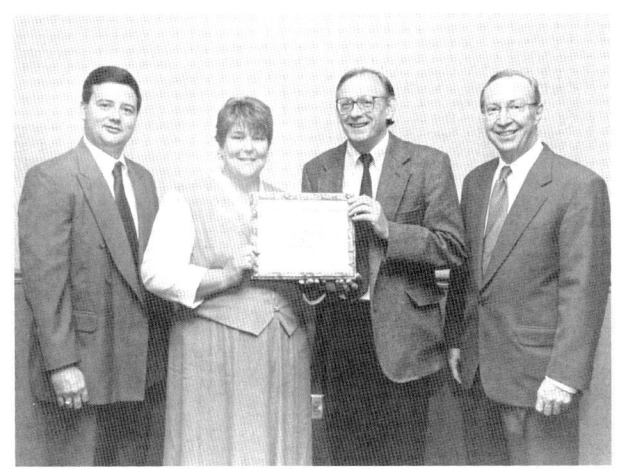

New CEO Steve Wolfe, Sue Majoris, and Dr. Lawrence Pettit with Indiana Hospital's recognition from Postpartum Support International, 1999.

Opposite page: IRMC at Chestnut Ridge was completed in August 2009.

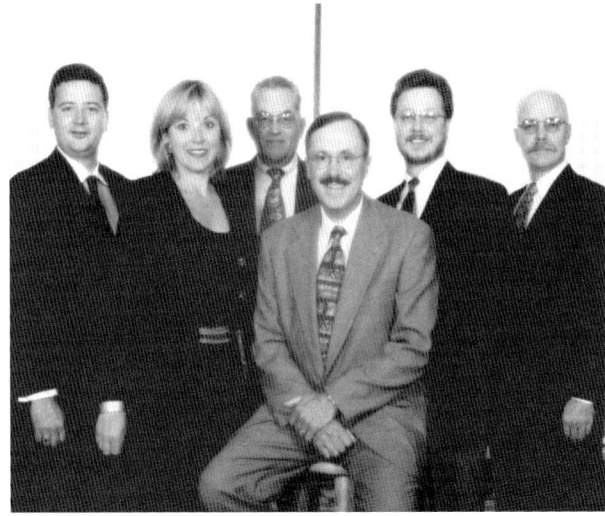

Steve Wolfe with Indiana Hospital's board of directors upon his hire, 1999.

up meetings with board members and key members of the staff and held round table discussions with groups of employees. "They're the ones who know what we really need to do to improve our services and remain viable," he said.

His first order of business was to stabilize and shore up the hospital's finances to protect its autonomy. Describing independents like Indiana Hospital as "an endangered species," the board's determination to remain independently owned had been a major factor in his decision to accept the CEO position. Indiana Hospital's losses for the previous fiscal year

1999

Registered nurses vote for representation by Health Care PSEA.

2000

2002

The First Commonwealth Cardiac Catheterization/Peripheral Angiography Laboratory opens in May.

The Bork Emergency Center opens, having developed an entirely new process for patient care.

The hospital's name is changed to Indiana Regional Medical Center.

2003

The Center for Cardiac and Vascular Care opens on July 16.

The Herbert L. Hanna, MD, Center for Oncology Care opens, located on the first floor of the IRMC Medical Arts Building.

The emergency room implements the "Expert Care in 30 Minutes" initiative.

IRMC receives the People Do Matter award.

2004

Center for Wound Healing opens at 119 Professional Center.

IMRT and radioactive seed therapy are offered at Oncology Center.

2005

IRMC is named #1 large employer among Best Places to Work in Pennsylvania.

M. Dorcas Clark, MD, Women's Imaging Center opens.

Main lobby is renovated; new entranceway is designed.

2006

Dr. James A. Garrettson Physician Excellence Award is created; Dr. Thomas McCoy is the first recipient.

IRMC is named #1 large employer among Best Places to Work in Western Pennsylvania and #3 in the state.

2009

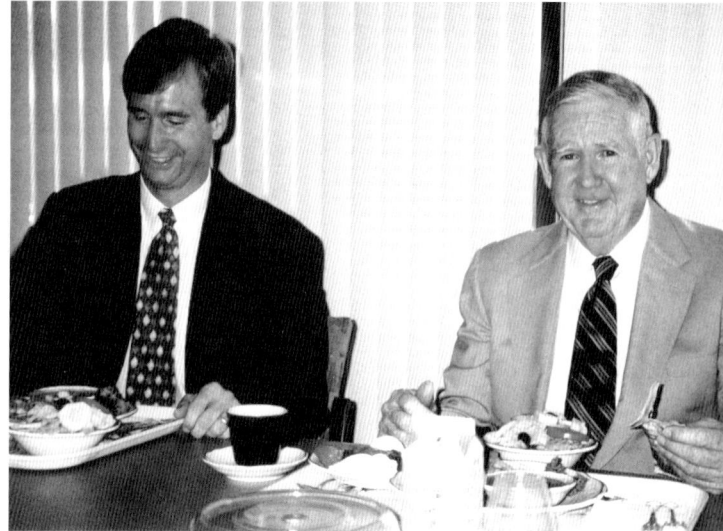

- IRMC at Chestnut Ridge opens.
- Indiana Total Therapy (ITT) is established as a joint venture with COSM.

2011

- New entrance road, IRMC Drive, is formally dedicated.

2012

- IRMC purchases Indiana Ambulatory Surgical Center.
- ST Wellness Center opens on Shelley Drive.
- October 1: Human Motion Institute Building opens.
- October 15: IRMC UrgiCare opens on site.

Mike Donnelly treats John Murtha, US Representative from the Twelfth Congressional District, to lunch at IRMC.

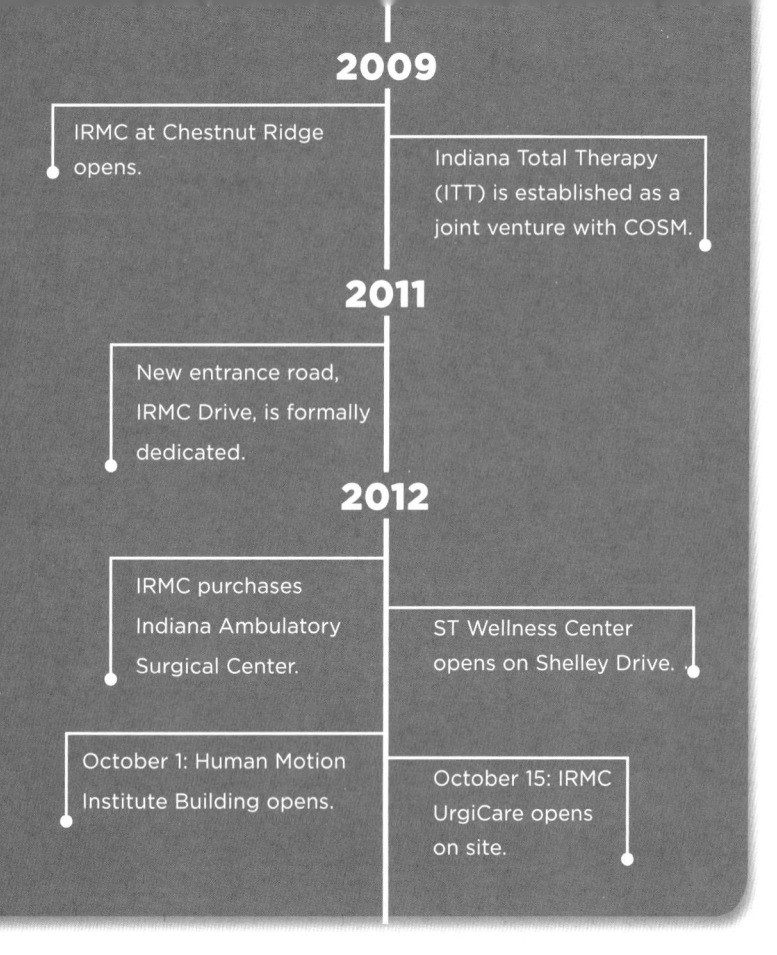

were approximately $997,000, and since provisions of the Balanced Budget Act extended through fiscal year 2004, it was likely the situation would worsen before it improved. Shortly after Mr. Wolfe's arrival, Indiana Hospital played a major role in a national effort to reduce the Medicare cuts provided for in the Balanced Budget Act of 1997. Hospital employees, physicians, volunteers, trustees, and supportive community members sent postcards to Congress and the White House calling for relief legislation. Stephen Wolfe and David Acker, CEO of Charles Cole Memorial Hospital in Coudersport, Pennsylvania, delivered 400 letters with a similar message from rural hospitals nationwide to Congressman John P. Murtha in Washington, DC. As a result, Congress passed relief legislation to restore about $17 billion to Medicare over five years.

In the meantime, medical staff, administrators, and board members evaluated studies and reports from consultants. Their decisions on which programs to keep had to focus on increasing the hospital's visibility within the community while making sure that costs stayed in line with reimbursements. "Community need is the first criterion," Stephen Wolfe said. "If there isn't evidence that a service is sufficiently needed, if projected costs are not in line with projected reimbursements, then the project will probably be discontinued."

One of their primary goals was to increase the hospital's market share. Approximately 50 percent of all county residents hospitalized went to Indiana Hospital, a number Steve regarded as "not good enough," setting a goal to increase market share to 65 percent. Acknowledging that the primary care centers the hospital had established throughout the Indiana County community in recent years were a step in the right direction, he also recognized that future facilities were likely to develop in the form of "synergies rather than brick and mortar."

Beyond the tangibles of finances and services, one of Steve's top priorities since that first day was to change the culture of Indiana Hospital, a task in which the entire staff has participated and excelled. "What I've been trying to impress on the hospital family is we

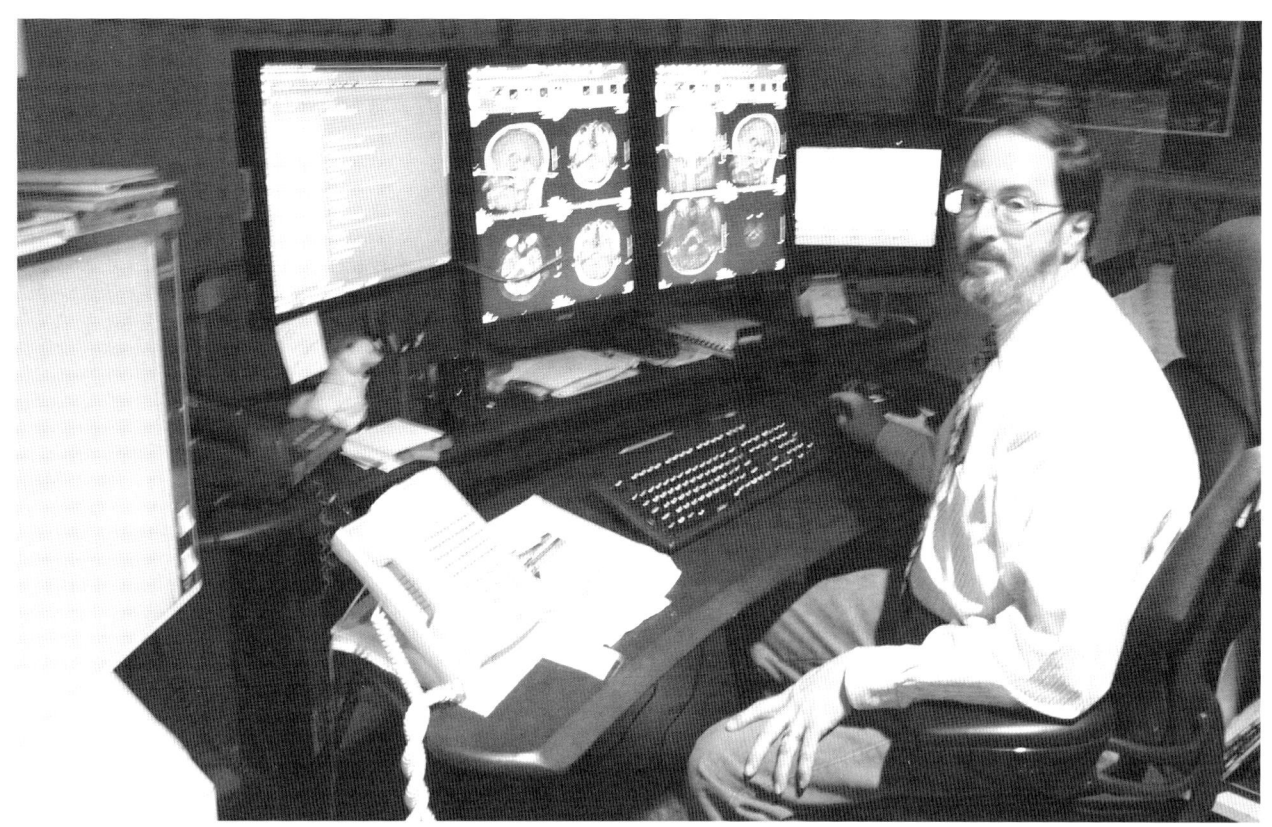

Dr. Frank Simone, director of Diagnostic Imaging Services, sits before the PAC (Picture Archiving and Communication system), by which all radiology images are digitized, eliminating the use of film.

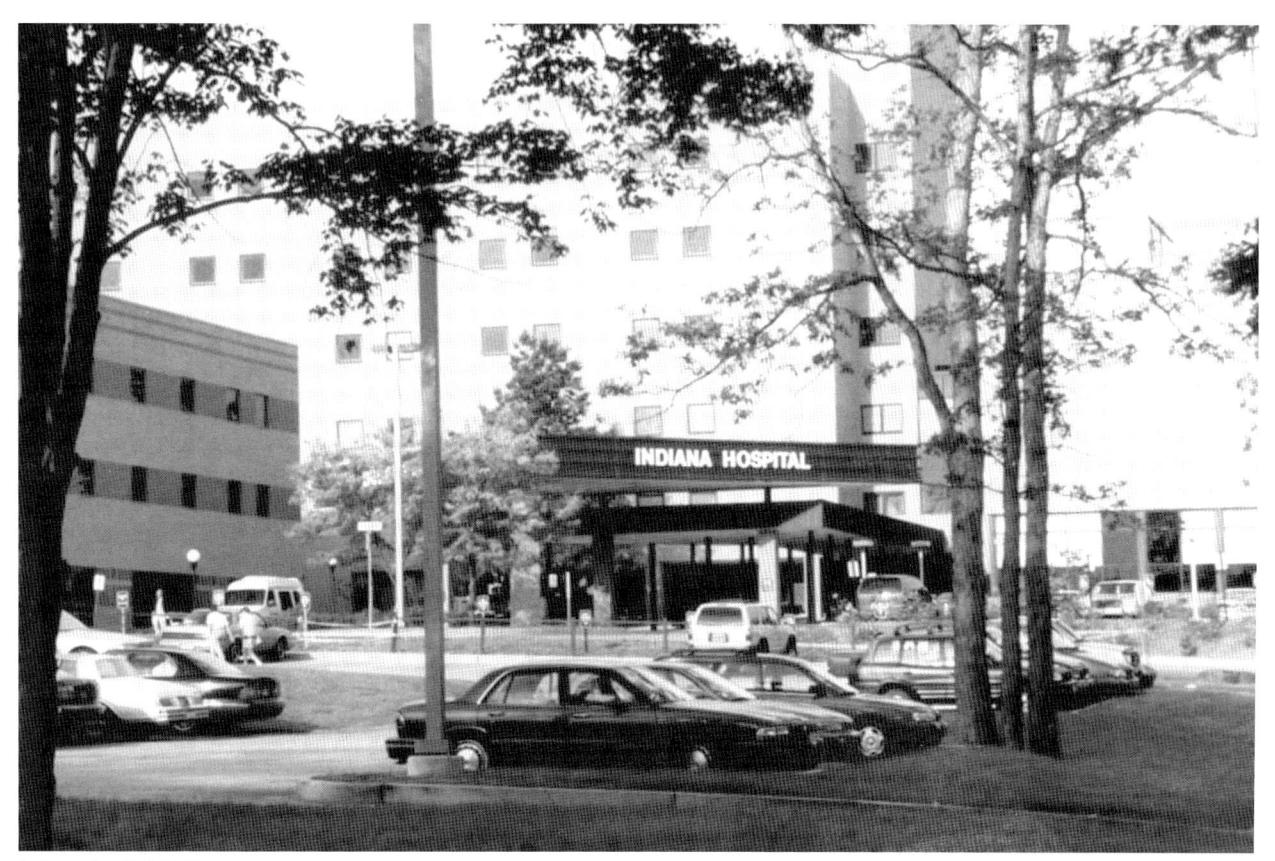

Indiana Hospital, 2000

Chapter 7: A New Era, A New Commitment, A New Identity — 93

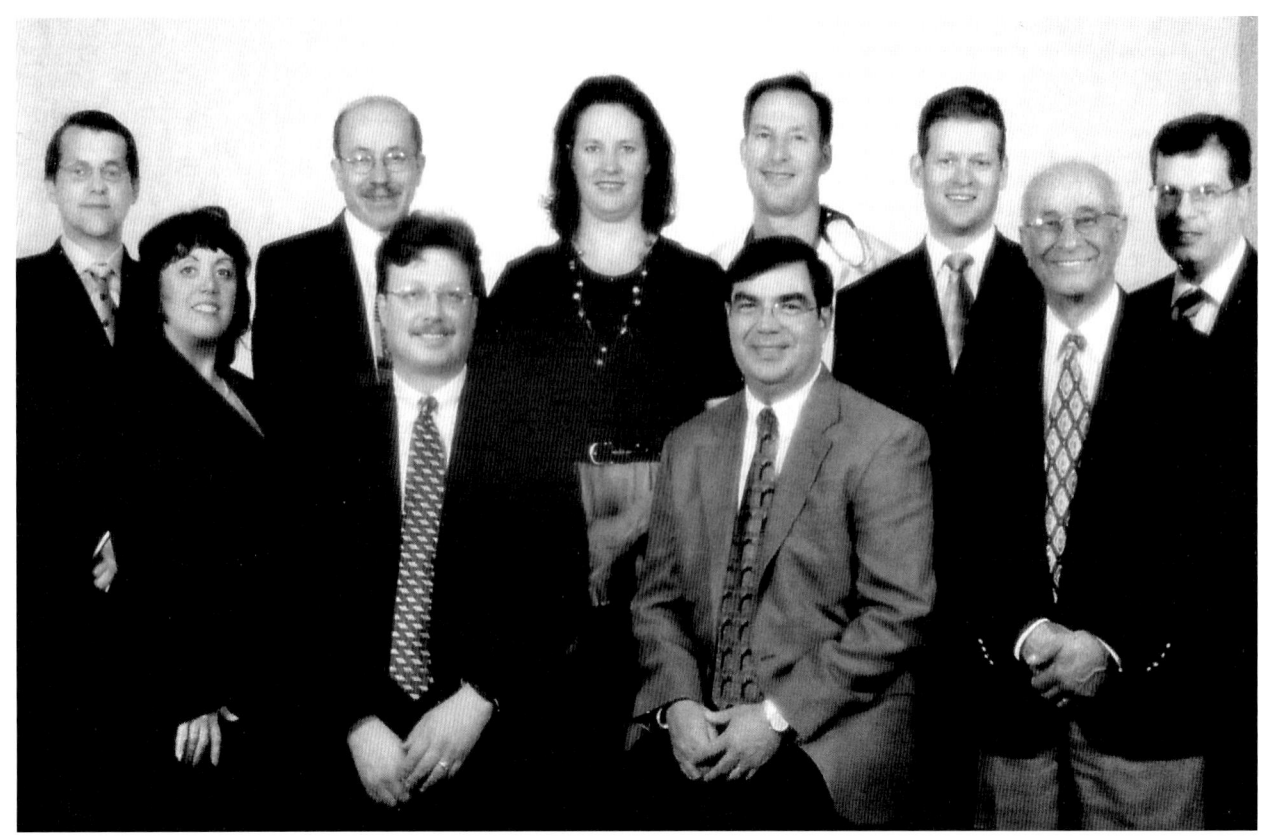

IRMC is understandably proud of its hometown physicians.

have a lot to be thankful for," he said at the time, acknowledging that the pressures put on hospitals by Medicare and insurance companies were causing division between hospital administrations and employees. "If you're divided among yourself, how can you face the challenges externally?" he asked.

In May 2000, through the generosity of First Commonwealth Bank, the First Commonwealth Cardiac Catheterization and Digital Angiography Laboratory became a reality, giving Indiana Hospital the most up-to-date diagnostic and treatment capabilities for its cardiology patients.

Indiana University of Pennsylvania's Small Business Institute completed a six-month-long study of the hospital by the end of 2001. It revealed that Indiana Hospital was perceived as a great place to give birth but lacking in the area of emergency care. The study also revealed that public perception of the hospital was higher among those who had more experience with it. The main problem with the emergency services department, which had not been restructured since it was built in the 1970s, was the long waiting times and the crowded conditions. "Our average door-to-door visit to the Emergency Department is three hours, which is the national average," said Steve Wolfe. "We want to do better. The ED is the front door to the community with 33,000 visits a year."

A capital campaign launched in 2001 raised $10 million from the hospital's very generous and supportive community, and the new Bork Emergency Center opened during the winter of 2002. The $5 million renovation tripled the size of the Emergency Department and increased the number of beds from fourteen to twenty-one, enabling it to treat 42,000 patients a year.

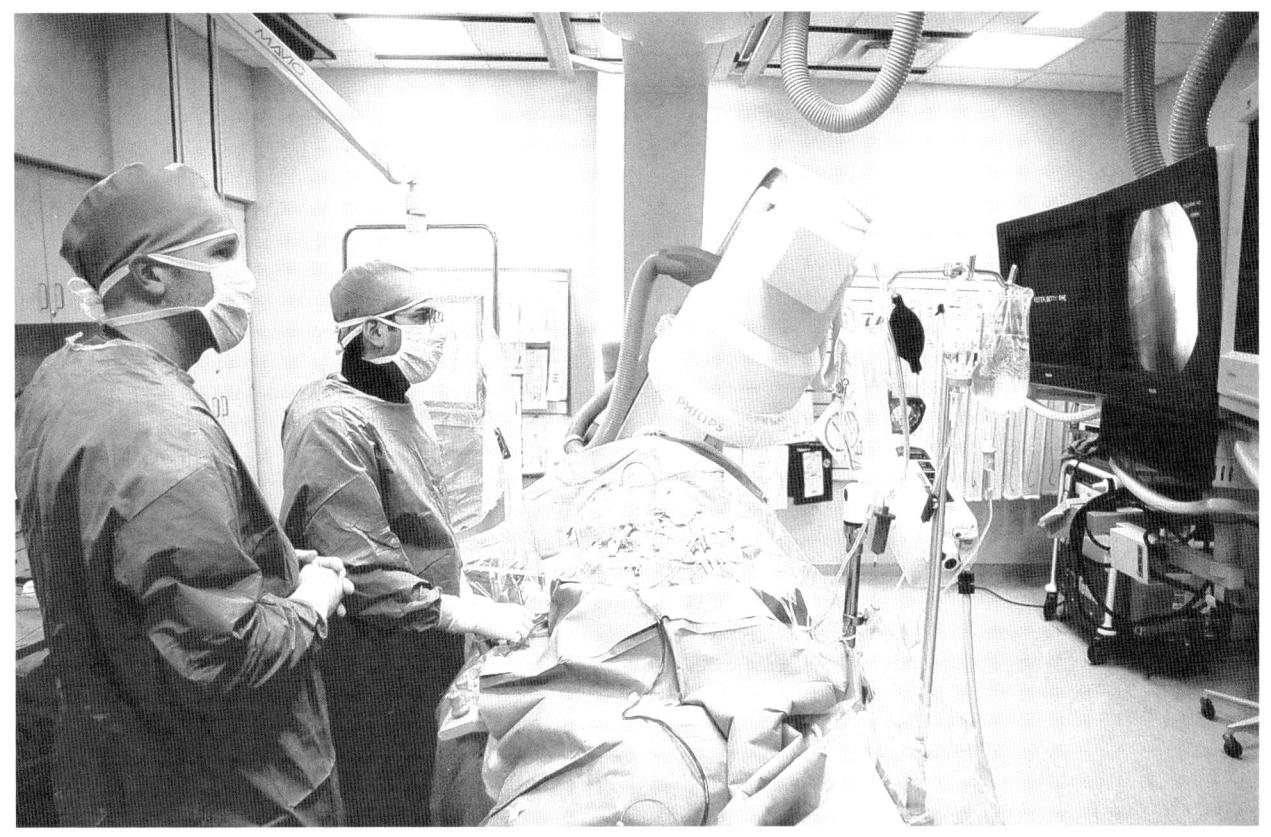

The First Commonwealth Cardiac Catheterization and Digital Angiography Laboratory opened in 2000.

Hundreds of people showed up for the open house; however, the new Center had a surprising result. Expectations throughout the community went way up, but absent changes in the basic processes for handling patients, the Emergency Center's scores actually declined. Brand new procedures for processing patients were initiated. An emergency technician trained to get the patient into the system electronically greeted the patient immediately. A registered nurse then performed a brief triage and escorted the patient to a room. The first available physician then saw the patient to assess their condition. Registration, which used to be the first order of business, was now the final step, taking place in the patient's room. The following quarter, this "patient first" attitude earned the staff of the Bork Emergency Center patient satisfaction scores in the 90th percentile and its highest ever—a 97 out of 100—in the third quarter of 2003.

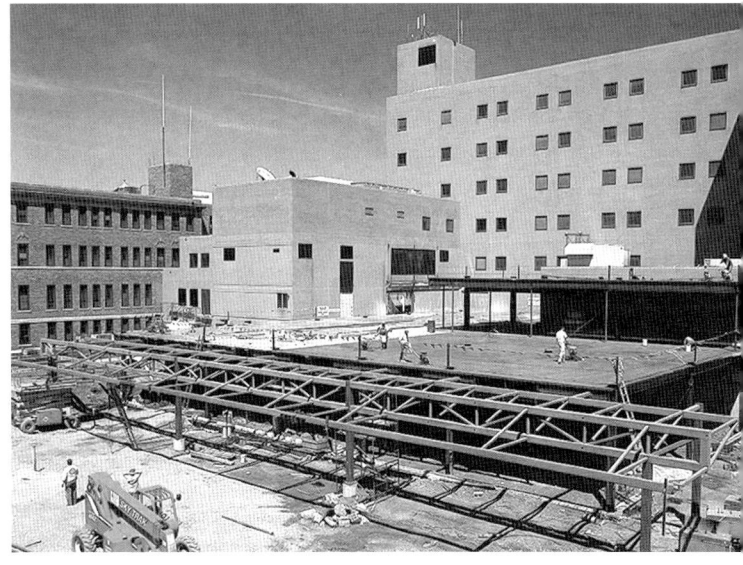

The new emergency center under construction.

In addition to the Bork Emergency Center expansion, the board of directors approved the spending of $5.6 million for a new CT scanner, an MRI scanner, and new imaging and monitoring devices for the cardiac catheterization lab.

When the Bork Emergency Center opened during the winter of 2002, people from the community were welcomed to the open house.

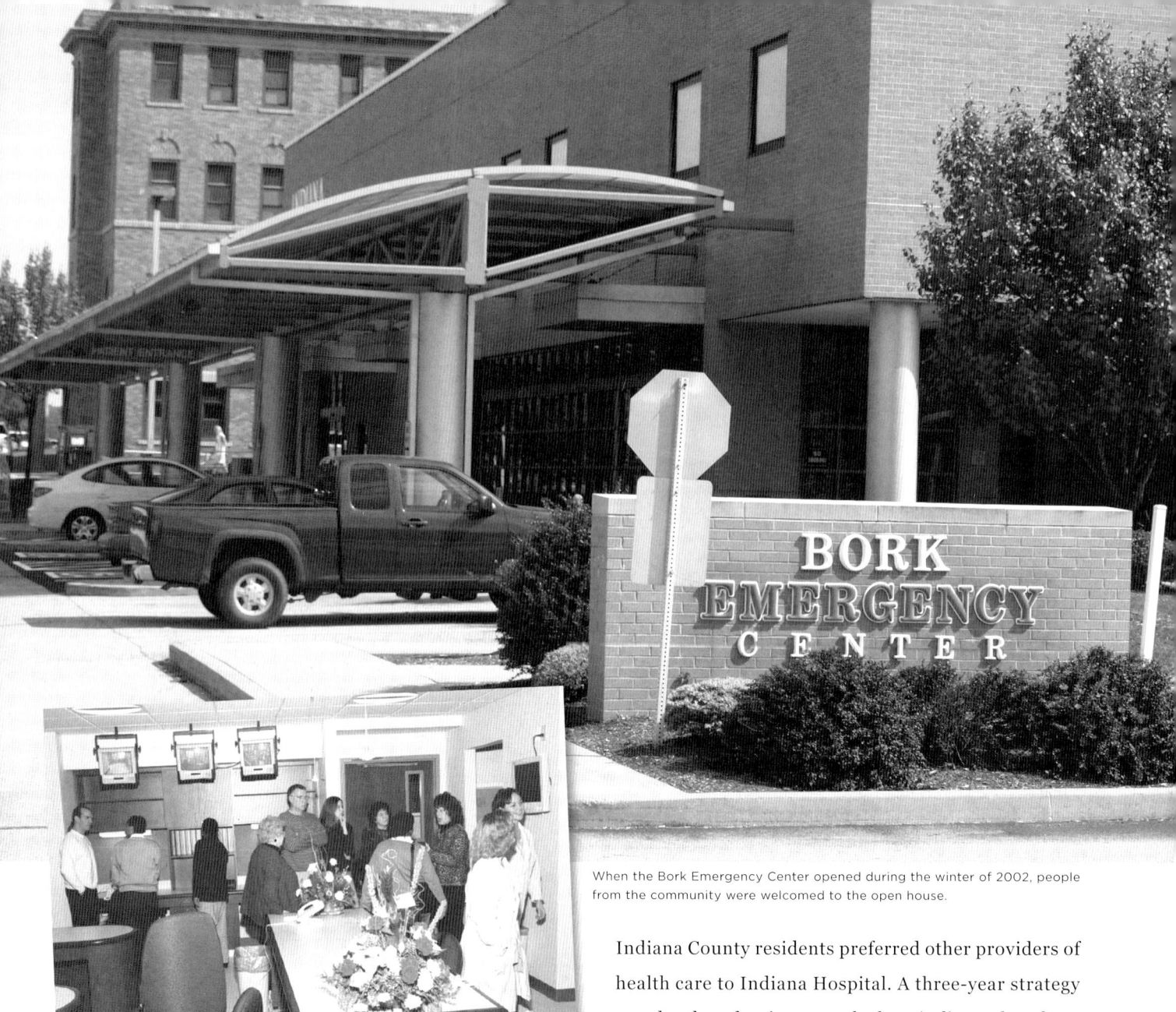

By May 2002, Indiana Hospital over the previous four years had added a cardiac digital angiography lab, a stationary MRI, a new CT scanner, a dialysis center, an ambulatory surgical center, and an expanded Emergency Department; in addition, twenty-nine new physicians had been recruited. Still, only 41 percent of the hospital's revenues were coming from inpatient services. Public perceptions are difficult and slow to change, and another survey showed that 48 percent of Indiana County residents preferred other providers of health care to Indiana Hospital. A three-year strategy was developed to increase the hospital's market share to 66 percent.

Based on survey information, Indiana Hospital developed a brand new theme: Take a Closer Look. They also announced the adoption of a new name, designed to shed the old image and more accurately reflect the broader geographic reach of the hospital. Indiana Hospital would now be known as Indiana Regional Medical Center. "Our new name reflects the new nature and capabilities of our facilities and the recommitment of our people to satisfy every patient, every day," said CEO Steve Wolfe. "Just as our theme—Take a Closer Look—asks members of the public to evaluate our services based on their treatments today, so does our new name: Indiana Regional Medical Center."

By 2003, Pennsylvania was one of twelve states in the union facing a medical liability insurance crisis. According to the Pennsylvania Medical Society, rising premiums and a shrinking number of insurance companies offering coverage was causing the state's physicians to eliminate risky procedures, move out of state, or simply retire early.

Chairman of the board of directors Joe O'Dell considered the hospital to be at a pre-crisis state, "with clear handwriting on the wall." After all, physicians generate revenue for hospitals, and the situation was making it difficult for IRMC to retain and recruit physicians. The loss of two or three specialists could put the hospital's entire future in jeopardy.

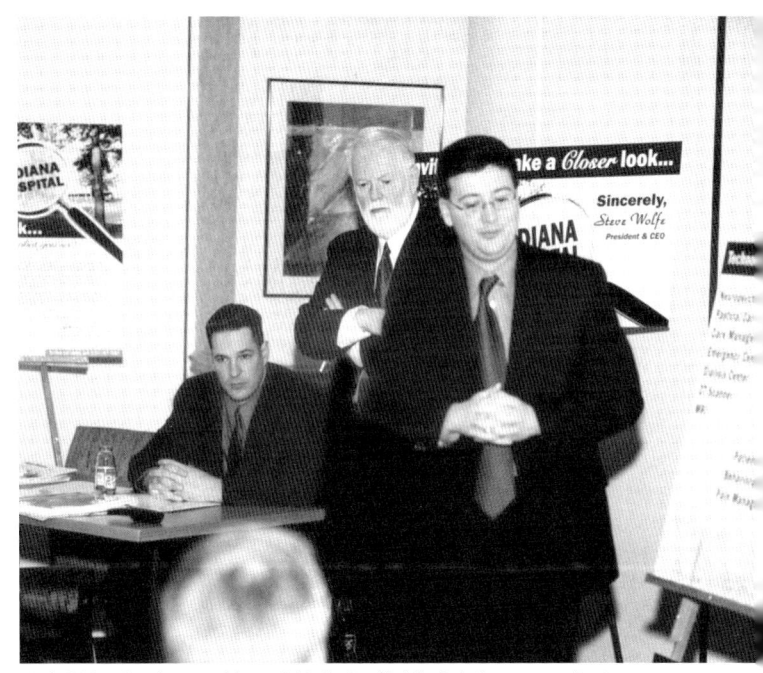

IRMC employees put on their best holiday smiles while working on Christmas Day 2001.

Mark Richards, vice president of Marketing/Public Relations; consultant Frank Ryan; and CEO Stephen Wolfe share information with staff on the name change to Indiana Regional Medical Center, 2002.

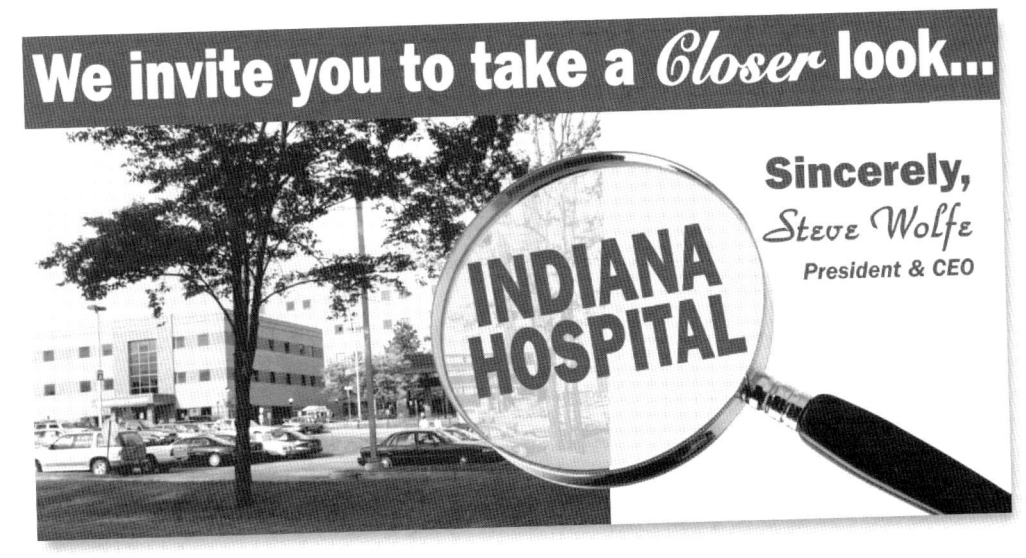

A billboard invited area residents to "take a *Closer* look" at the hospital.

Chapter 7: A New Era, A New Commitment, A New Identity —⌁— 97

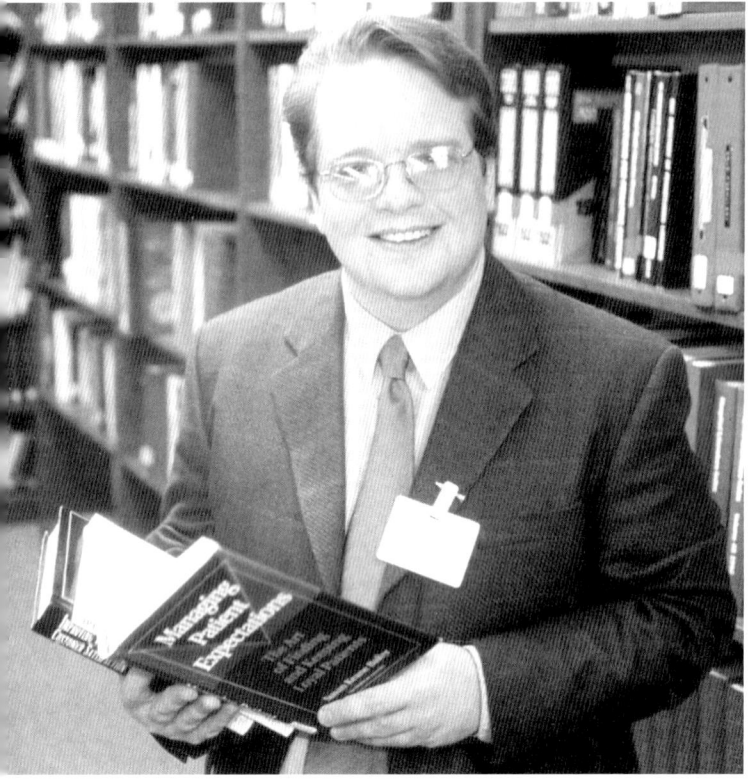

Jim Kinneer, vice president of People Development.

The crisis could not have come at a worse time. IRMC lost $1.6 million in 2002 and was projected to lose $500,000 during the 2003 fiscal year. To avoid the overhead costs of a big insurance company, IRMC joined with thirty-one other Pennsylvania community hospitals to create a Risk Retention Group to act as the medical liability carrier for the hospitals. By doing so, IRMC avoided an anticipated 90 percent increase in its own medical liability premium from the hospital's commercial insurer. Instead, it jumped only 10 percent to nearly $2 million for 2004.

The Transitional Care Center, originally developed in 1994, was renamed the Rehabilitation Care Center. The revised treatment program was designed to help patients recovering from stroke, spinal cord injuries, amputation, brain injuries, congenital deformities, and burns restore their life skills.

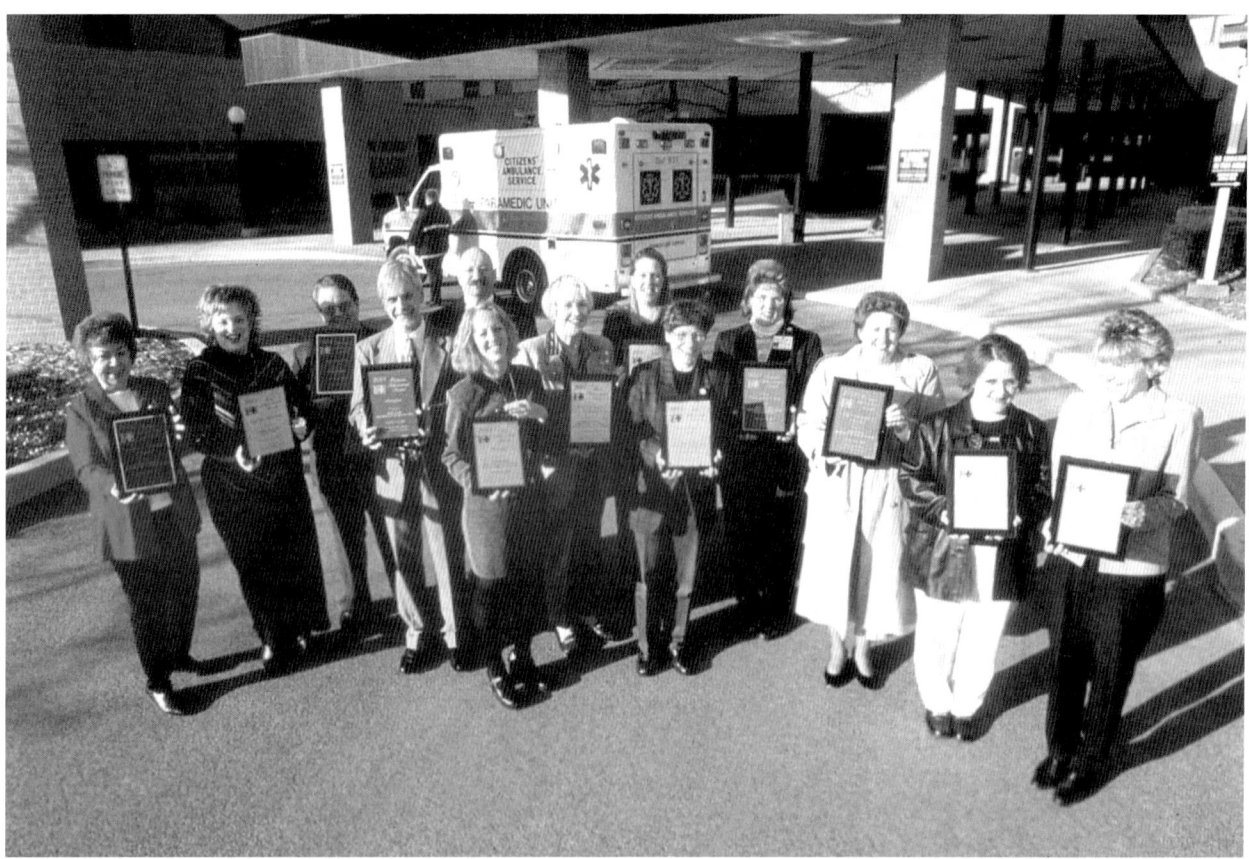

Patient Satisfaction Award winners.

Indiana Regional Medical Center

The Visiting Nurses Association also moved back to the IRMC campus in the Medical Arts Building in 2003. The proximity to the hospital enhanced their role in the patient's health care continuum. The VNA now offered the full range of services for the entire family—home care, hospice and palliative care, and extended private duty care.

In 2002, with cancer care being the second largest part of the health-care need after cardiology, Indiana Hospital moved to "the front lines in the battle against cancer," according to Stephen Wolfe. The hospital purchased the cancer center that was located in the Overlook Building. With that commitment, Indiana Hospital began construction on a $4.4 million, 10,000-square-foot building known as the Medical Arts Building where Indiana Hospital would take oncology care to a new level. Indiana Hospital opened on September 15, 2003, the newly constructed Herbert L. Hanna, MD, Center for Oncology Care. Dr. Hanna, a family physician and IRMC board member, died of lung cancer in October 2002. This center, funded through the hospital's capital campaign, included a Varian Linear Accelerator, considered the best by radiation experts, which used high-intensity computer-guided x-ray beams to pinpoint cancer cells and eliminate unnecessary exposure to radiation dosages that could damage surrounding healthy tissue. In addition, the PA Hematology Oncology Group relocated chemotherapy services to this center creating a full-service cancer center for community patients. Another treatment option, brachytherapy, was also offered. By inserting radioactive seeds directly into the tumor, brachytherapy could in some cases reduce the length of treatment from six to eight weeks of ra-

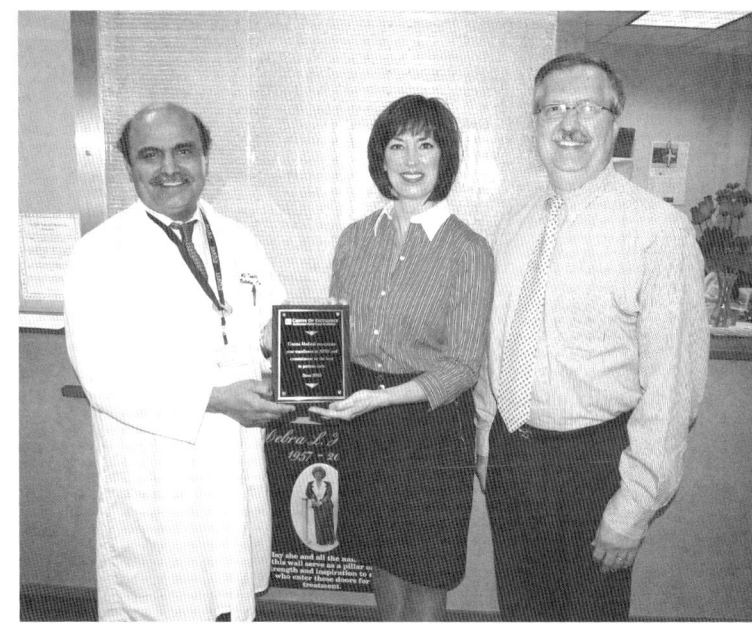

The Herbert L. Hanna, MD, Center for Oncology Care won the award for Excellence, 2005.

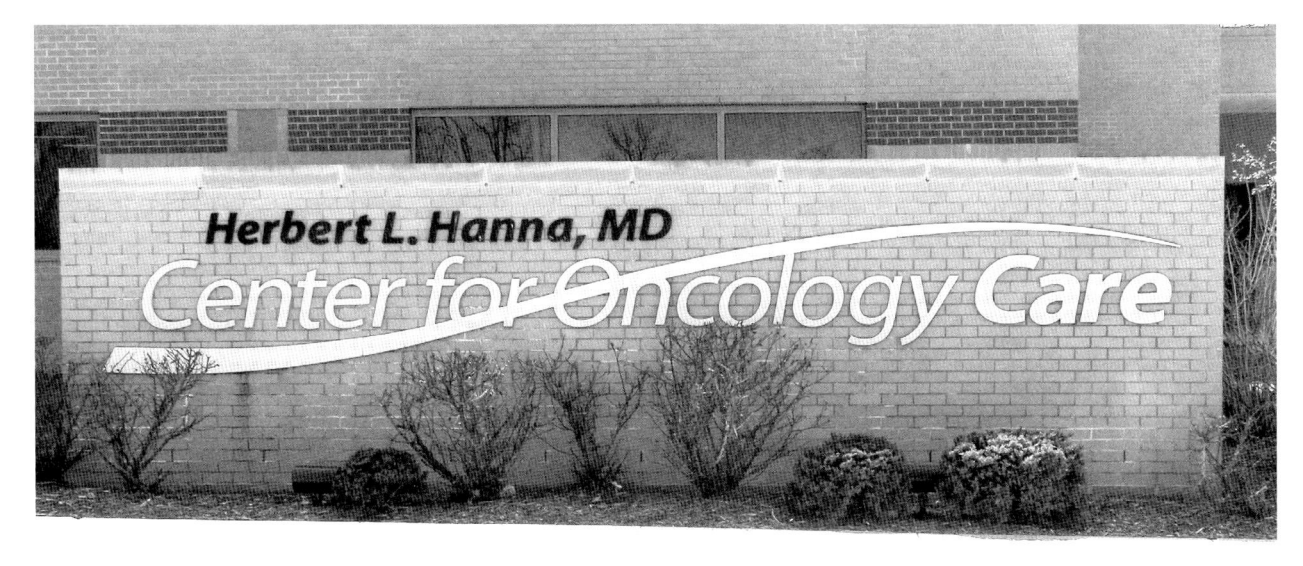

Opened in 2003, the Herbert L. Hanna, MD, Center for Oncology Care was named for one of Indiana Hospital's most respected physicians.

diation down to only one. In addition, the new Oncology Center offered inpatient transportation from the hospital, social service assistance, nutritional counseling, cosmetic and prosthetic consultation and supplies, and pain management to provide comprehensive care for cancer patients and their families. Dr. Hanna's widow Merle Hanna, knowing how happy her husband would have been to see the level of patient care the new Center provided, commented, "I think Herb would be so proud of what this has to offer to the community."

In the fall of 2004, IRMC became the only regional hospital to offer a dedicated Center for Wound Healing to help heal chronic wounds as well as hyperbaric oxygen therapy for nonhealing wounds. This new outpatient program was located in the 119 Professional Center in Indiana.

RECOGNIZING PROGRESS

The management team at IRMC understood that there is a direct link between patient satisfaction scores and staff members' workplace satisfaction. "We're people caring for people," said Dominic Paccapaniccia, who has been the hospital's chief operating officer since 2004. "If we're angry or stressed people caring for people, some of that undoubtedly translates directly to the patient and their family."

In 2003, the hospital was recognized for its culture change efforts through gathering employee feedback with an internal survey process and for implementing incentive plans and benefits to enhance employee satisfaction. In recognition of its commitment to best people practices, IRMC was awarded a People Do Matter Award.

The next year the hospital took things another step further and began benchmarking itself against other hospitals. They changed consultants and began working with Press Ganey, a leading patient-care consulting firm. With more than 1,200 hospitals in their database, the patient satisfaction survey would now make it possible for departments to check themselves against similar departments in other hospitals. "We had some key areas that were scoring very poorly," Steve Wolfe said. "There were some emotional reactions but we finally resolved that something had to happen." As an example, Outpatient Services scored originally in the 30th to 50th percentile. With their ability to benchmark themselves against other hospitals, they quickly moved into the 90th percentile.

Patient satisfaction scores continued to improve. In 2004, the hospital scored above the 80th percentile in three of the four global indicators for hospitals—Emergency Services, Outpatient Services, Inpatient Services, and Ambulatory Care. IRMC's x-ray department scored in the 99th percentile. Other departments now scoring above the 90th percentile included Ultrasound, CT scan, OB/GYN, the Bork Emergency Center, and Inpatient Discharge. For the second year in a row, IRMC was selected as a finalist for the People Do Matter Award.

During the fall of 2004, IRMC was chosen as one of the best places to work in the region by *Pittsburgh Business Times* and recognized at an awards program at the Omni William Penn in Pittsburgh. In the first list of the Top 30 Places to Work, IRMC was ranked tenth overall—eighth among large employers—and was the number one ranked hospital on the list. Employing over 1,100, IRMC was the second-largest employer in Indiana County. Steve Wolfe credits the award as a turning point in the culture at IRMC primarily because the honor is based on the employees' opinions. "I think that's when it sunk in," he said.

Once again, the IUP Small Business Institute conducted a community perception survey, and this time public perception of the medical center improved significantly over the 2001 study. Based on 2,500 random phone calls and 1,600 mailed surveys, IRMC received an overall perception score of 4.1 on a scale of 1 to 5. Individually, all twelve departments or services mentioned in the survey saw their scores increase as well. "This survey is important because I believe it's a validation of the hard work that's going on here at IRMC," Steve Wolfe said. "Our mission is to serve this region, and today we can say with confidence that the image and perception of IRMC is at an all-time high."

The *Pittsburgh Business Times* named Indiana Regional Medical Center 2005's #1 Large Employer in Western Pennsylvania, and less than a month later, the hospital was recognized as the number one large employer in the entire state. The Best Place to Work in Pennsylvania award program was created in 2000 and was one of the first of its kind in the country to be offered by a state. The program is a public/private partnership of the Pennsylvania Department of Community and Economic Development, Team Pennsylvania Foundation, *Central Penn Business Journal*, Best Companies Group, and the Pennsylvania Chamber of Business and Industry. In 2006, IRMC achieved the number three spot among Best Places to Work across Pennsylvania and took the number one spot in Western Pennsylvania.

Indiana Regional Medical Center was also spotlighted in the April 2005 edition of *Healthcare Executive*, a magazine for hospital professionals published by the American College of Healthcare Executives. The article recognized IRMC as "one of the fastest growing hospitals in the United States," having doubled in size over the past eight years. In 2007, the magazine ran a repeat feature on the hospital, focusing on its success at sustaining its outstanding performance.

Obviously, the hospital's initiatives regarding both patient and employee satisfaction were reaping rewards. The financial status of the hospital was improving, in part because of cost containment measures and because its market share had increased by 25 percent over the previous six years. Revenue increased from $54 million in 2000 to $88 million in 2005, an increase of almost 63 percent, which CEO Steve Wolfe remarked at the time could take many hospitals more than fifteen years to achieve.

The interdependent relationship between the hospital and the community at large reaped dividends for both. The success of the 2001 capital campaign helped to build the Bork Emergency Center and a cardiac catheter lab, and aided with the recruiting of a total of fifty-four new physicians in recent years. Beyond the improved health care the community received in return, the nearly $90 million a year it cost to operate the hospital was nearly all recycled back into the community, most of it in the form of wages and benefits.

When clinics in Bolivar, New Florence, and Seward, which were previously run by UPMC, were closed during the summer of 2005, IRMC made the bold decision to reopen them. The *Johnstown Tribune-Democrat* compared it to "a knight on a white horse." Steve Wolfe, president and CEO of IRMC, humbly considered it "doing our part."

Also during the summer of 2005, the M. Dorcas Clark, MD, Women's Imaging Center opened at IRMC adjacent to the Bork Emergency Center. Named for Dr. M. Dorcas Clark, who began her career at Indiana Regional Medical Center in January 1980, the center offered an integrated interdisciplinary team approach to mammography. The center included three mammography units, one stereotactic mammography unit, one bone density measurement unit, and one breast ultrasound. Adjacent to the imaging center is the upgraded MRI unit, allowing for breast magnetic resonance.

By the end of 2005, approximately 15,000 of the 203,000 annual outpatient visits were by people who lived outside Indiana County. The emergency room was now treating more than 38,000 patients per year, up from 24,000 in 1999. The Herbert L. Hanna, MD, Center for Oncology Care almost doubled its number of patients served since opening in September 2003, and the hospital's Center for Wound Healing in the 119 Professional Center was on track to meet its predicted eighteen-month investment payback since opening in May 2004. The hospital's net revenue was $90 million in fiscal 2005, up from $54.5 million in 1998.

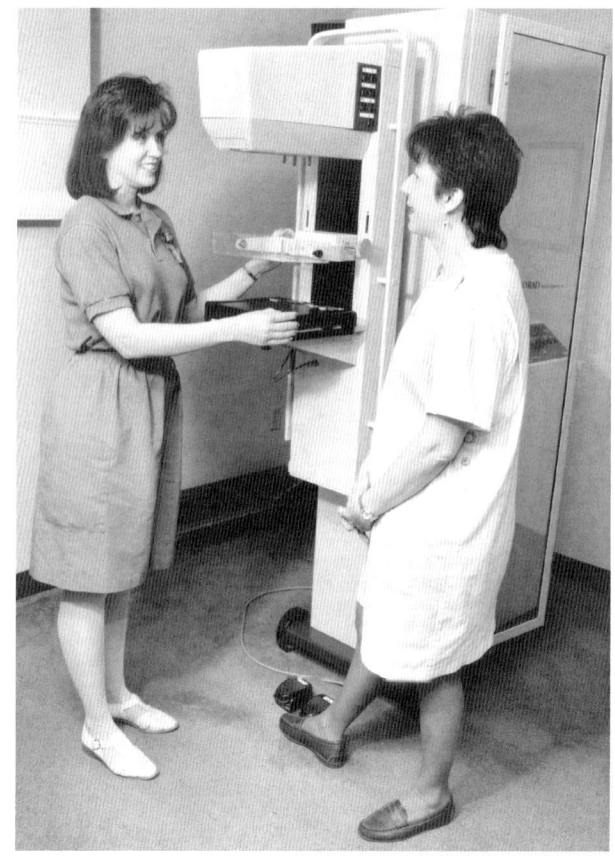

Tracey Ross reassures a patient in the M. Dorcas Clark, MD, Women's Imaging Center.

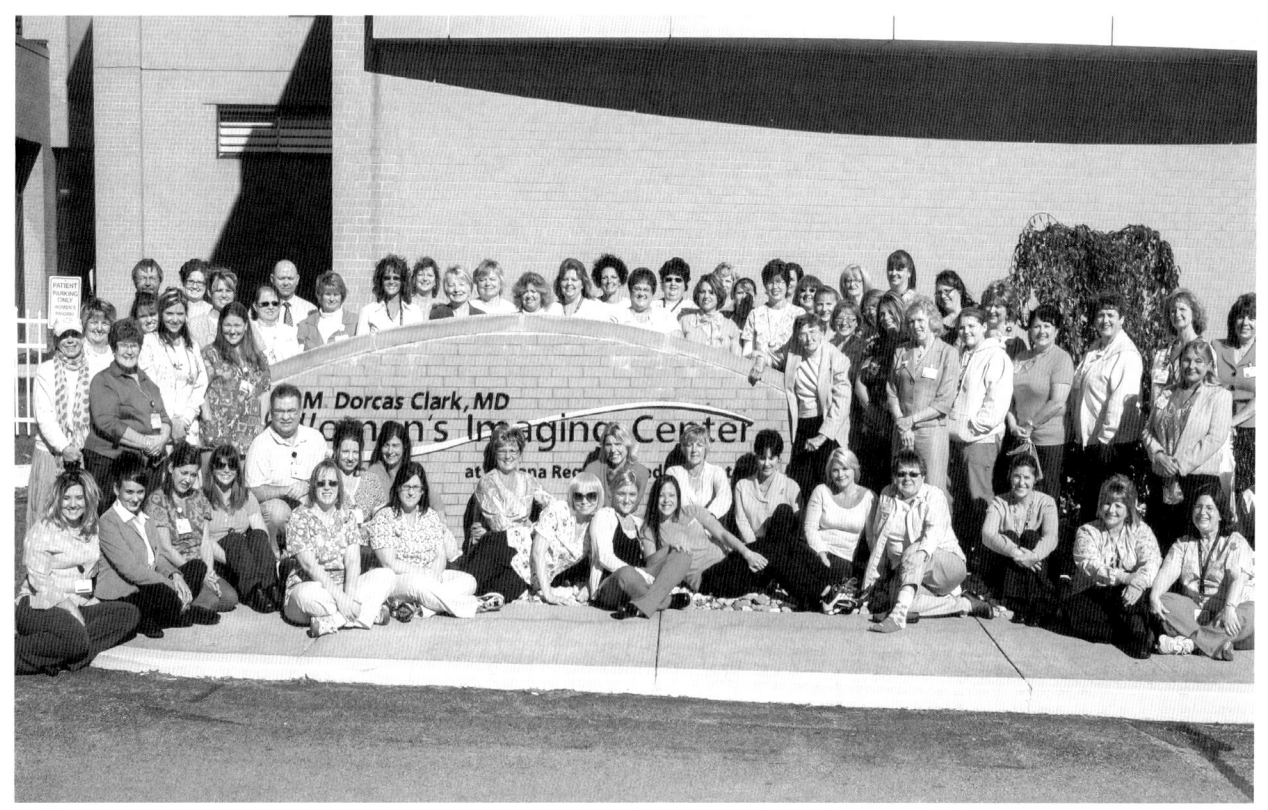

The M. Dorcas Clark, MD, Women's Imaging Center opened in 2005 and was quickly awash in pink.

In 2006, IRMC established the Dr. James A. Garrettson Jr. Physician Excellence Award to honor physicians who demonstrate the highest standards of professionalism in patient care, in their interaction with their peers and other staff, and in their community service. All physicians and members of the IRMC staff can nominate potential recipients, which are then evaluated by a selection committee. Dr. Thomas McCoy was the first to receive the award in 2006. In succeeding years, the award has been given to Dr. Shafic Twal, Dr. Alex Juhasz, Dr. Russell Drozdiak, Dr. Donna Balewick, Dr. Stella Boron, and Dr. Mark Boykiw.

During the first quarter of 2007, four areas of Indiana Regional Medical Center achieved a 90th percentile for patient satisfaction from Press Ganey's surveys, putting them among twenty national semifinalists for Press Ganey's Turnaround award. When IRMC was notified in September that it was once again one of

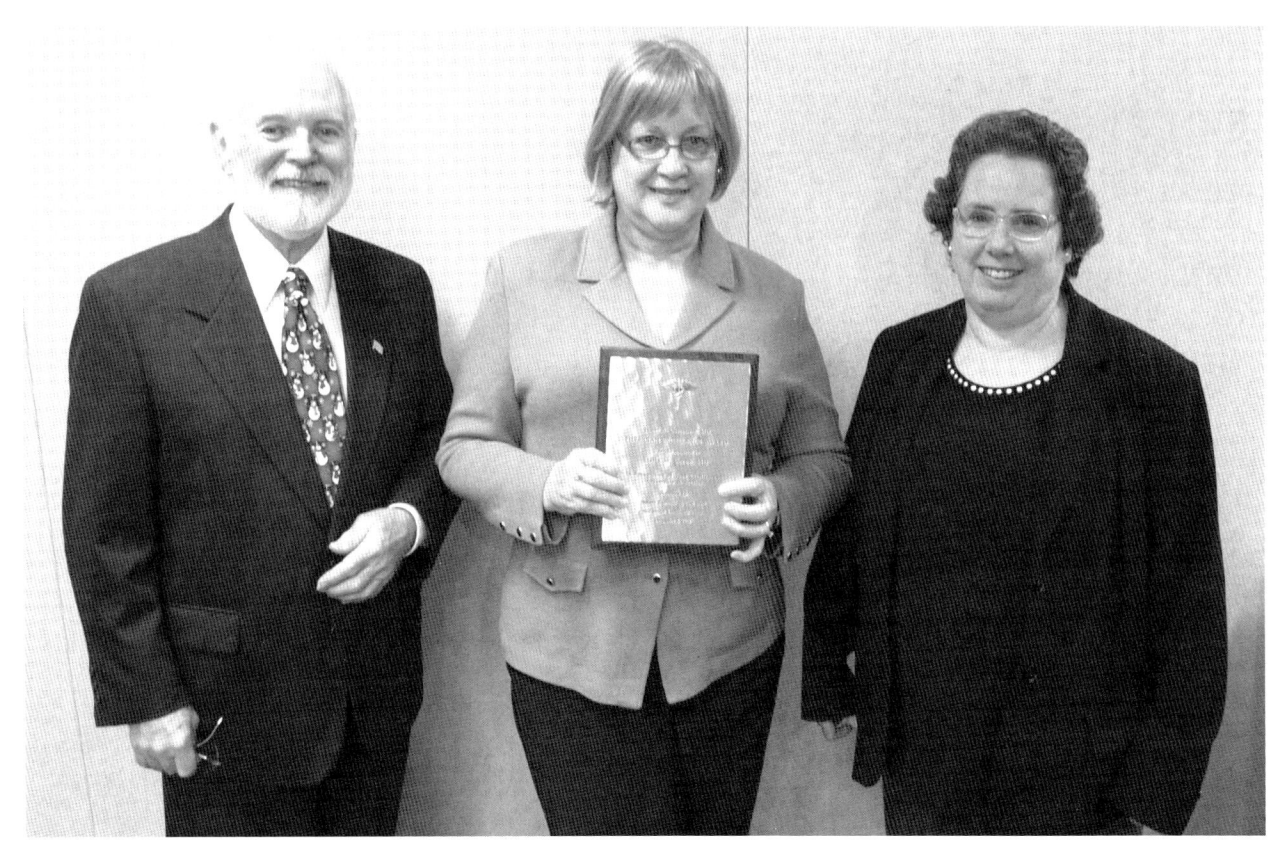

Dr. Shafic Twal, pediatrician, examines a toddler, 2000.

Dr. Stella Boron, center, received the Physician Excellence Award in 2011, named for Dr. James Garrettson, left.

Chapter 7: A New Era, A New Commitment, A New Identity — 103

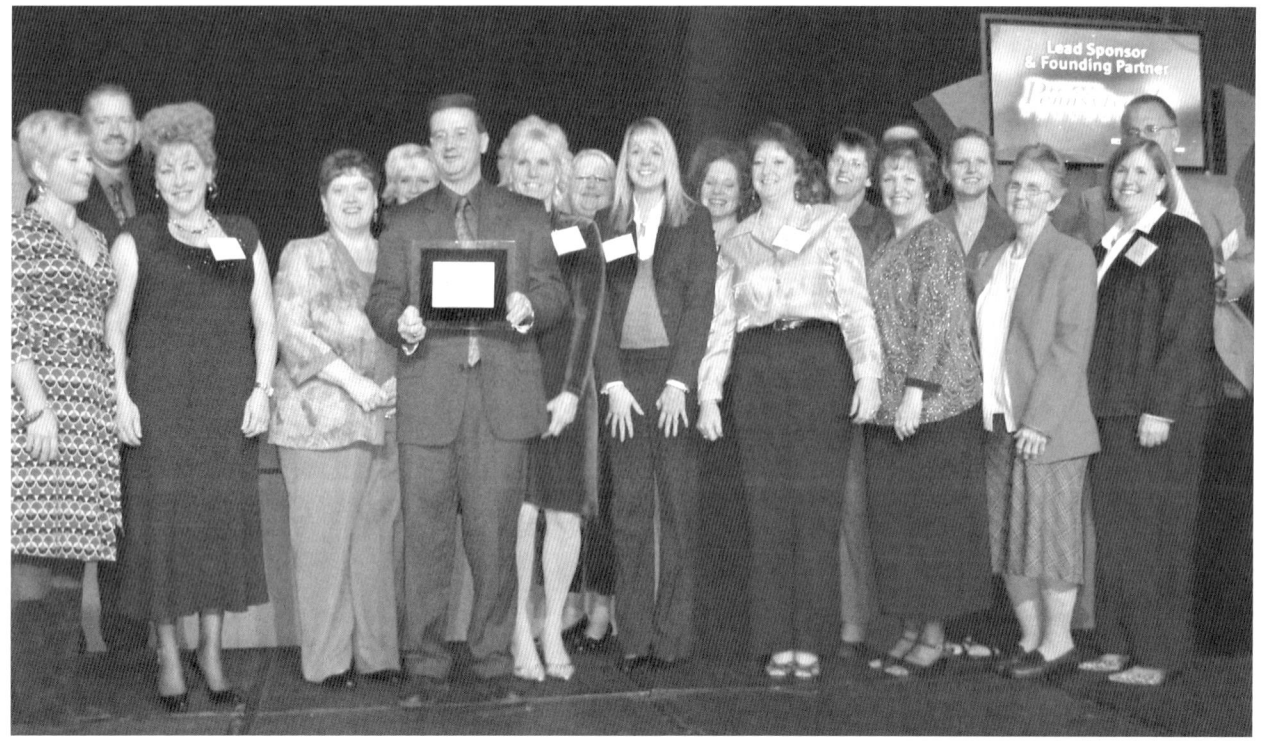

Staff members surround Steve Wolfe as the hospital is awarded the "Best Places to Work" Award in 2007.

the top fifty large employers eligible for the Best Place to Work in Pennsylvania award, President and CEO Steve Wolfe decided to hold a random drawing to select several frontline employees to attend the event where the winner was to be announced. In the glamorous but suspense-filled ballroom of the Hershey Lodge in Hershey, Pennsylvania, those very lucky and very proud employees waited as the winners were counted down. More than 1,000 attendees applauded IRMC employees who assembled behind the podium along with President and CEO Steve Wolfe and Board Chairman Bob Rout when it was announced that IRMC was again ranked #1 Best Place to Work in Pennsylvania in 2007. IRMC was the only organization in the history of the program to repeat recognition as the top-ranked employer. A house-wide celebration of the honor was held in early December with a catered event that served all shifts of employees. "We wanted to celebrate this award with all our employees," Steve explained, "because it is through their efforts that we are able to sustain a winning workplace culture."

IN FLIGHT—ON TIME

Anyone who has spent a day waiting while a loved one underwent surgery knows how agonizing the hours can be, particularly since the average person does not have a full grasp of the process. To help ease that anxiety, the surgical services department launched a new patient tracking system in 2008. A new software system and big screen monitors positioned throughout the hospital made it possible for surgeons, physicians, nurses, and family members to track a surgical patient's trip through the operating room "from departure to landing." The patient's family was given a patient identifier, a code used on the waiting room board in place of the patient's name to protect privacy. The boards are updated every few seconds to help the families follow their loved one through the process. The patient's clinical information is displayed on boards seen only by medical personnel. This "flight board" style of tracking made the entire surgical process smoother and is part of the reason why patient satisfaction scores at IRMC continued to rise.

THE MARTIN AND BARBARA BEARER CENTER FOR HEALTH

Recognizing that the bulk of Indiana County's growth was occurring in the southern part of the county evidenced by the growing number of admissions from that area, IRMC established IRMC at Chestnut Ridge, a new comprehensive ambulatory care facility on the grounds of Blairsville's Chestnut Ridge Golf Resort and Conference Center. Named in honor of Chestnut Ridge developer Martin Bearer and his wife Barbara, the 31,000-square-foot facility costing approximately $10 million opened in August 2009.

The center represented IRMC's largest investment since the patient tower was built in 1979. The internal medicine practice of Drs. Matthew Klain, Matthew Nettleton, and Eric Heasley, long-established medical care providers in the area, anchored the facility. In addition to making a wide range of specialists available to area residents, IRMC at Chestnut Ridge provides dialysis, outpatient imaging services, laboratory services, and rehabilitative therapies through Indiana Total Therapy (ITT). Chestnut Ridge is just one of four locations where ITT provides services through a joint venture with IRMC.

Of primary importance to area residents, however, is the UrgiCare center at Chestnut Ridge. Open seven days a week, it puts medical care for common illnesses within easy reach.

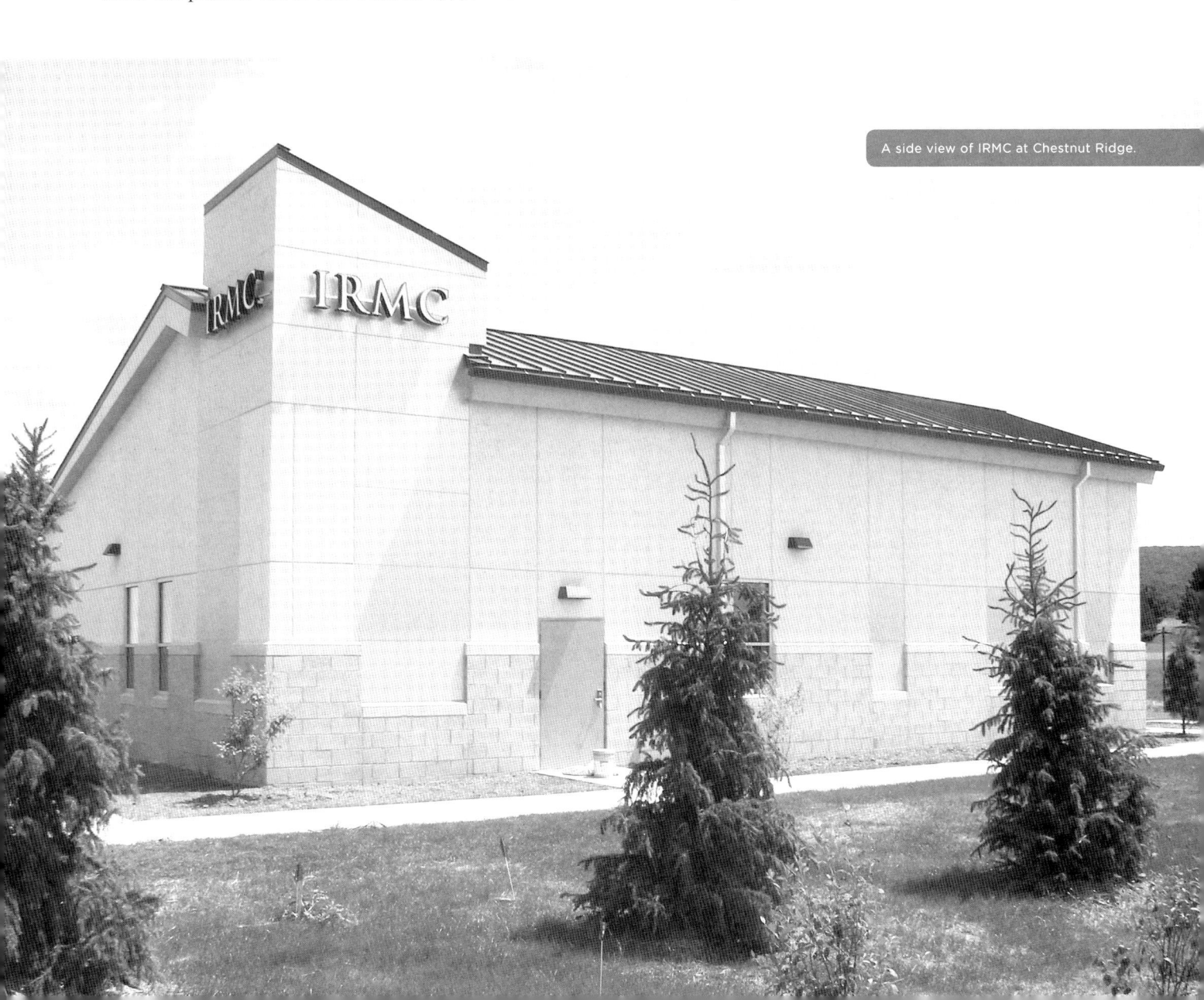

A side view of IRMC at Chestnut Ridge.

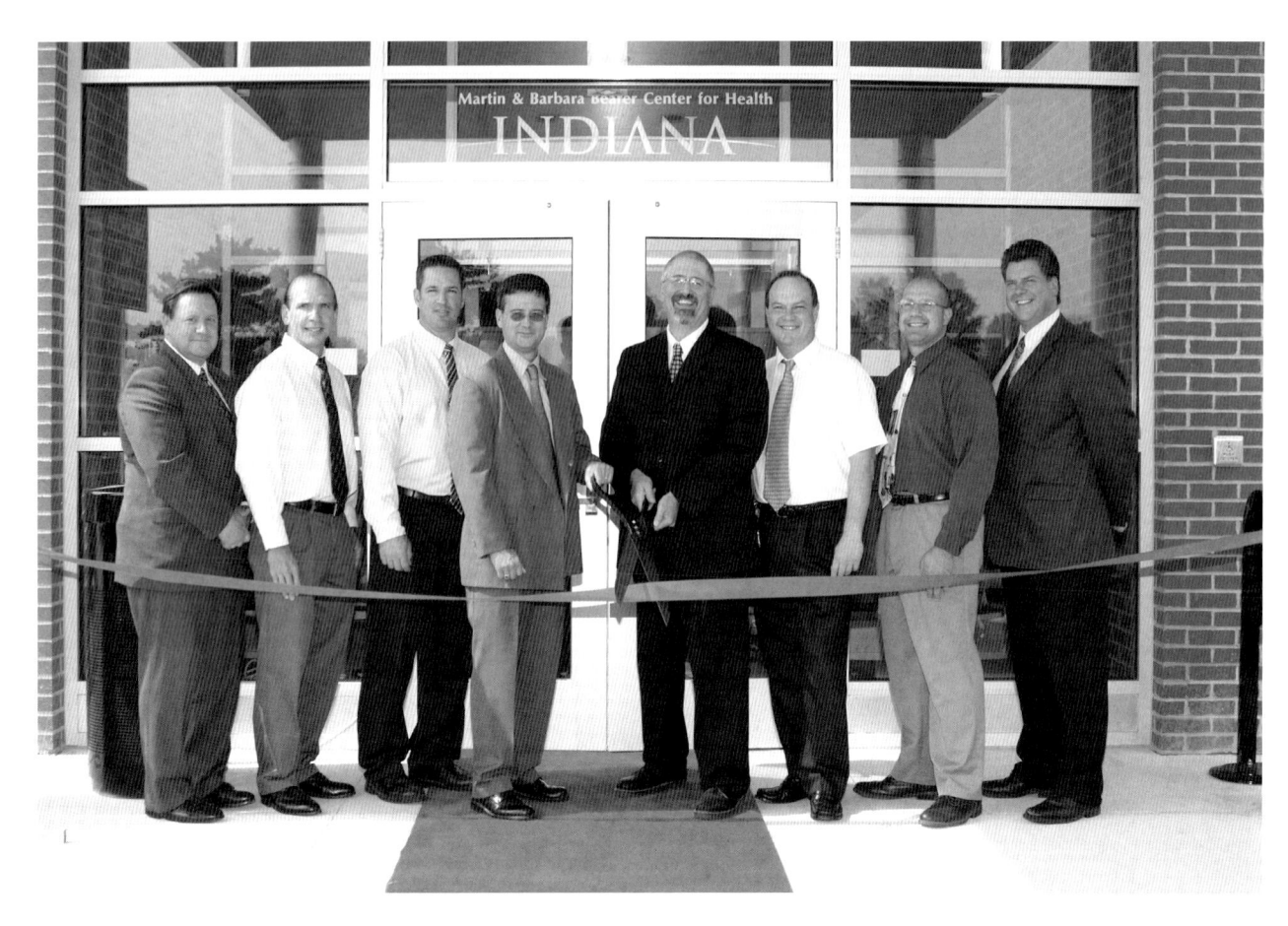

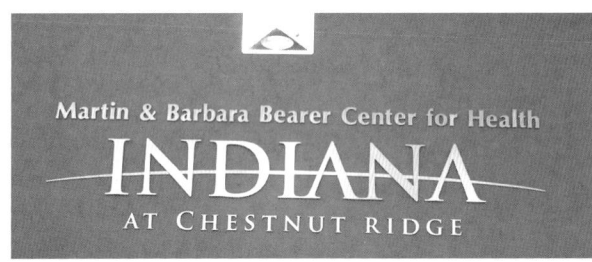

The new facility was named in honor of Chestnut Ridge developer Martin Bearer and his wife Barbara.

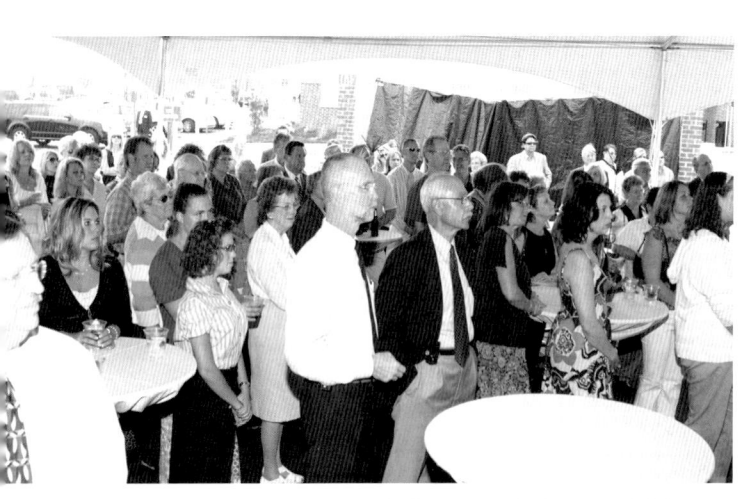

Hundreds of residents, grateful for the new facility, attended the open house.

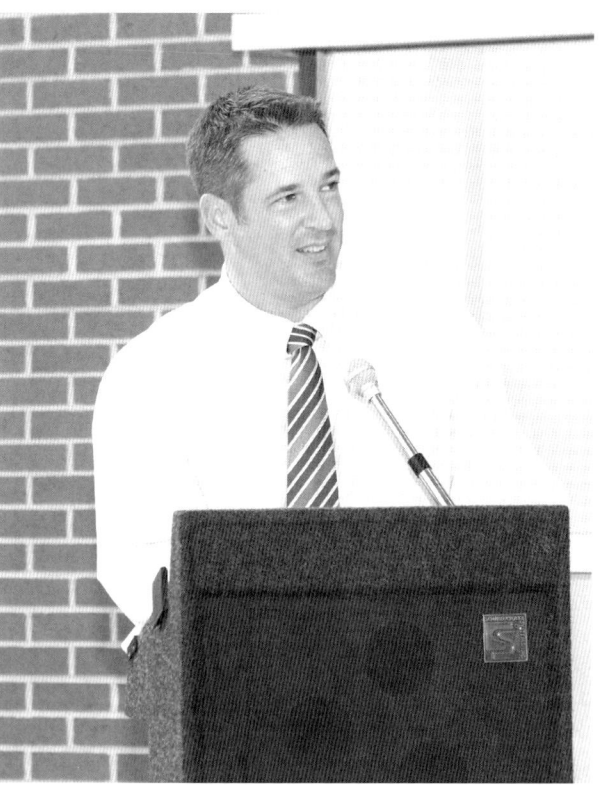

Mark Richards welcomes the crowd, and IRMC CEO Steve Wolfe and Dr. Matthew Klain cut the ribbon on the new Chestnut Ridge facility on August 27, 2009.

SETTING THEIR SIGHTS HIGH

With numerous awards to their credit, Indiana Regional Medical Center set its sights on winning the coveted Baldrige award, a national quality award program managed by the US Commerce Department's National Institute of Standards and Technology (NIST). Congress established the award, given by the President of the United States, in 1987. The success IRMC enjoyed over the last few years could have created the temptation to "rest on our laurels," Steve Wolfe said. "Instead, we decided that we've come a long way, but we're going to go a lot further."

The process began with a detailed fifty-page application designed as a self-assessment tool to help organizations identify strengths and opportunities for improvement by comparing themselves to high-ranking organizations in their category. While winning the award was a goal in itself, the real prize they

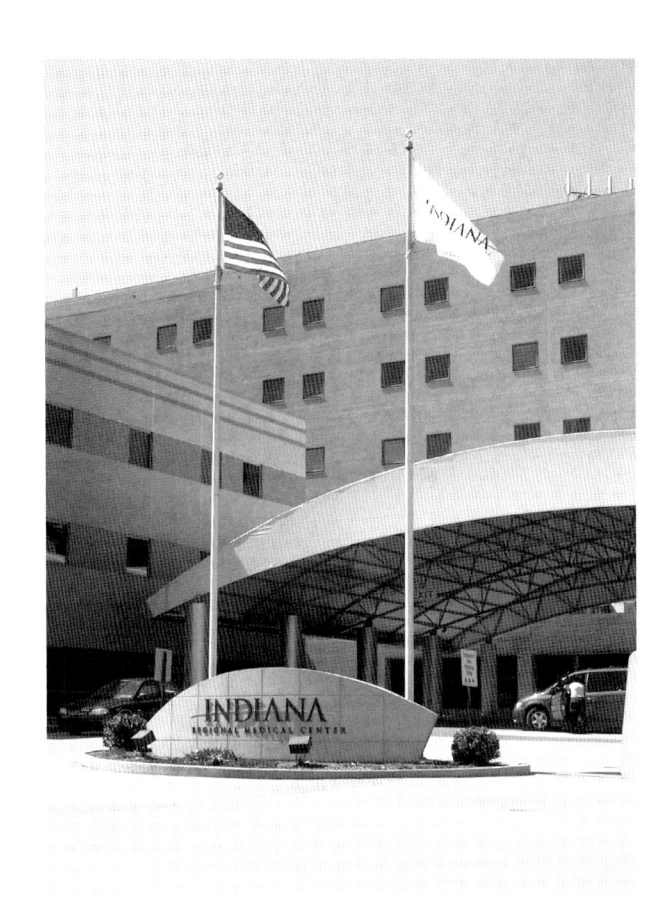

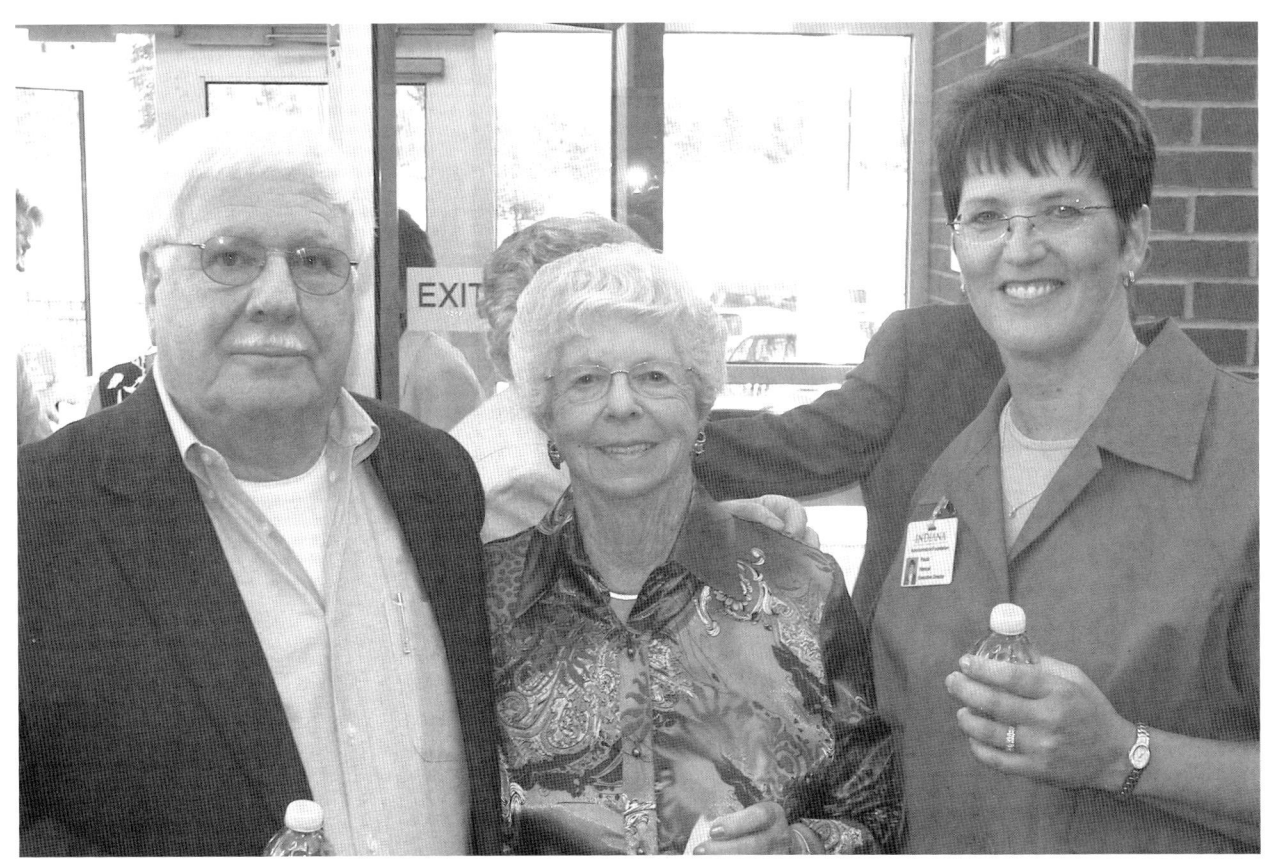

In 2005, the main lobby was renovated and the front entrance redesigned. Mr. Kovalchick, Mrs. Bearer, and Paula Hencel visit at the open house.

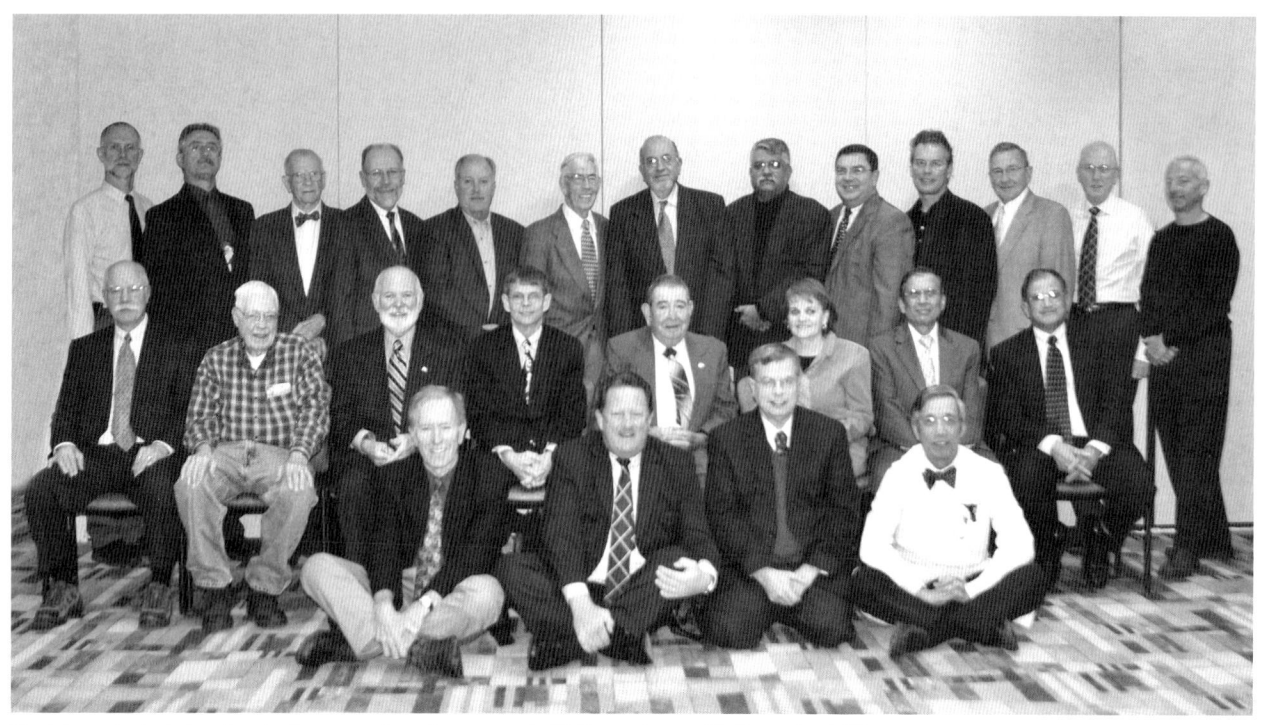

Physicians who had given twenty-five years of service or more to IRMC were honored in December 2010.

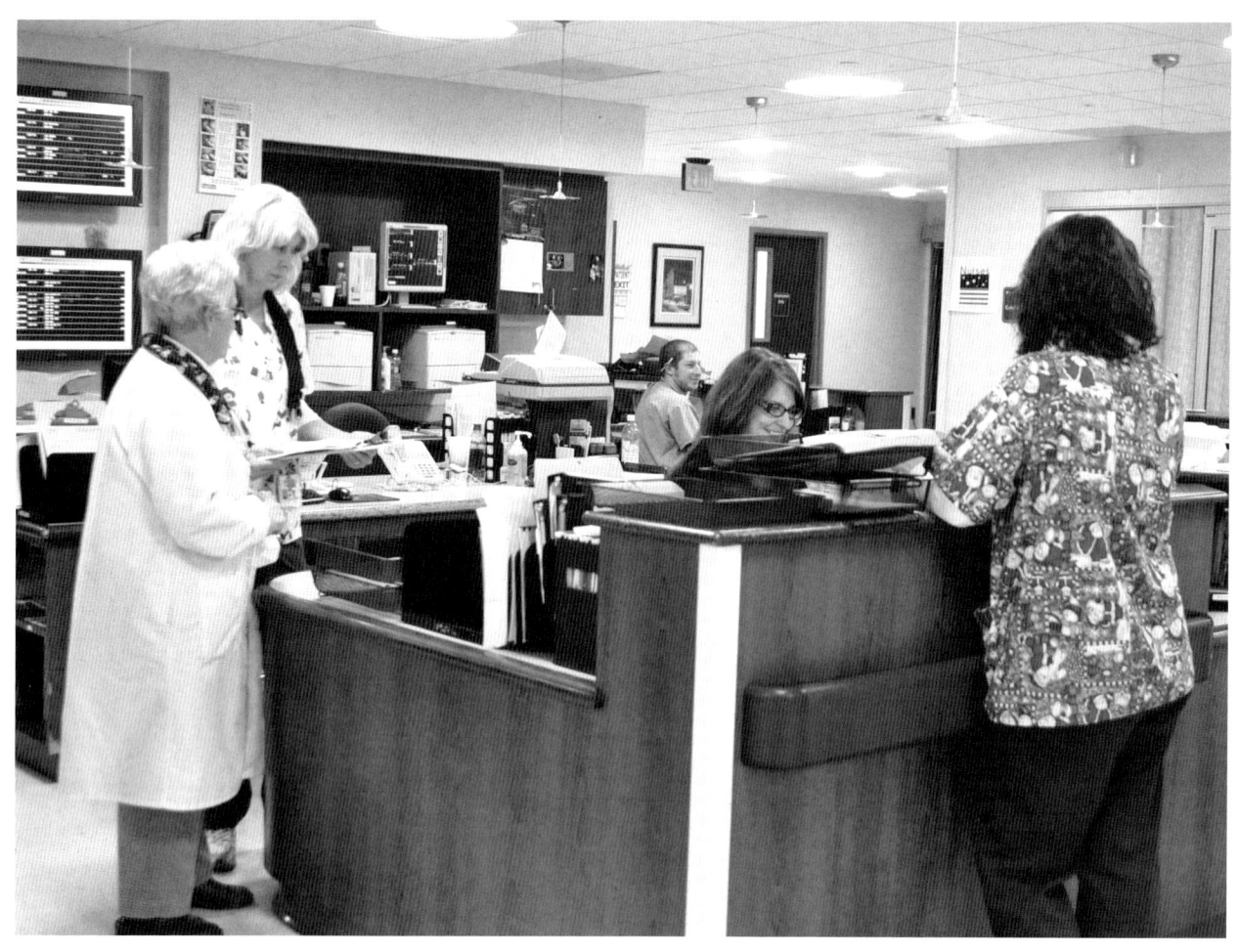

The staff of Bork Emergency Center, Christmas 2010.

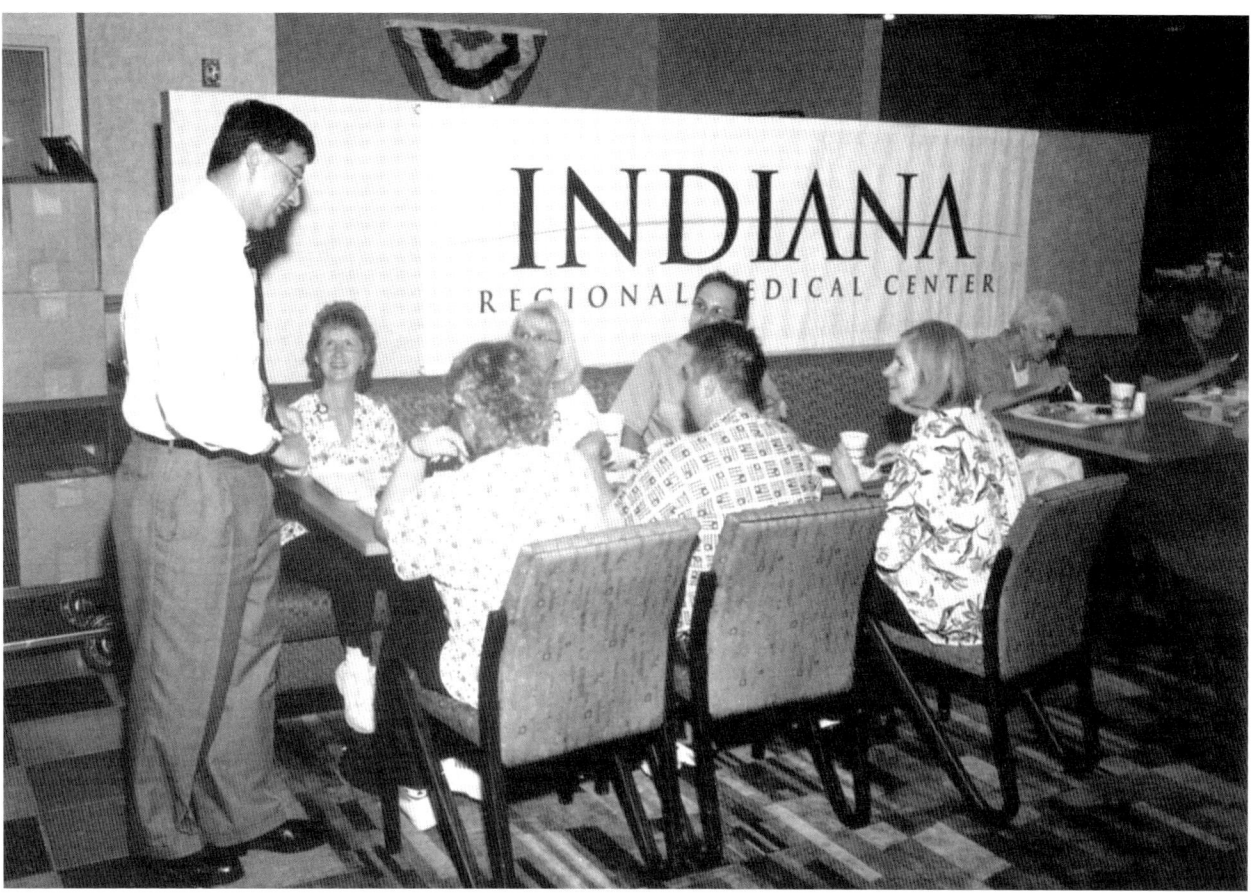

CEO Stephen Wolfe visits with Environmental Services Staff, 2002.

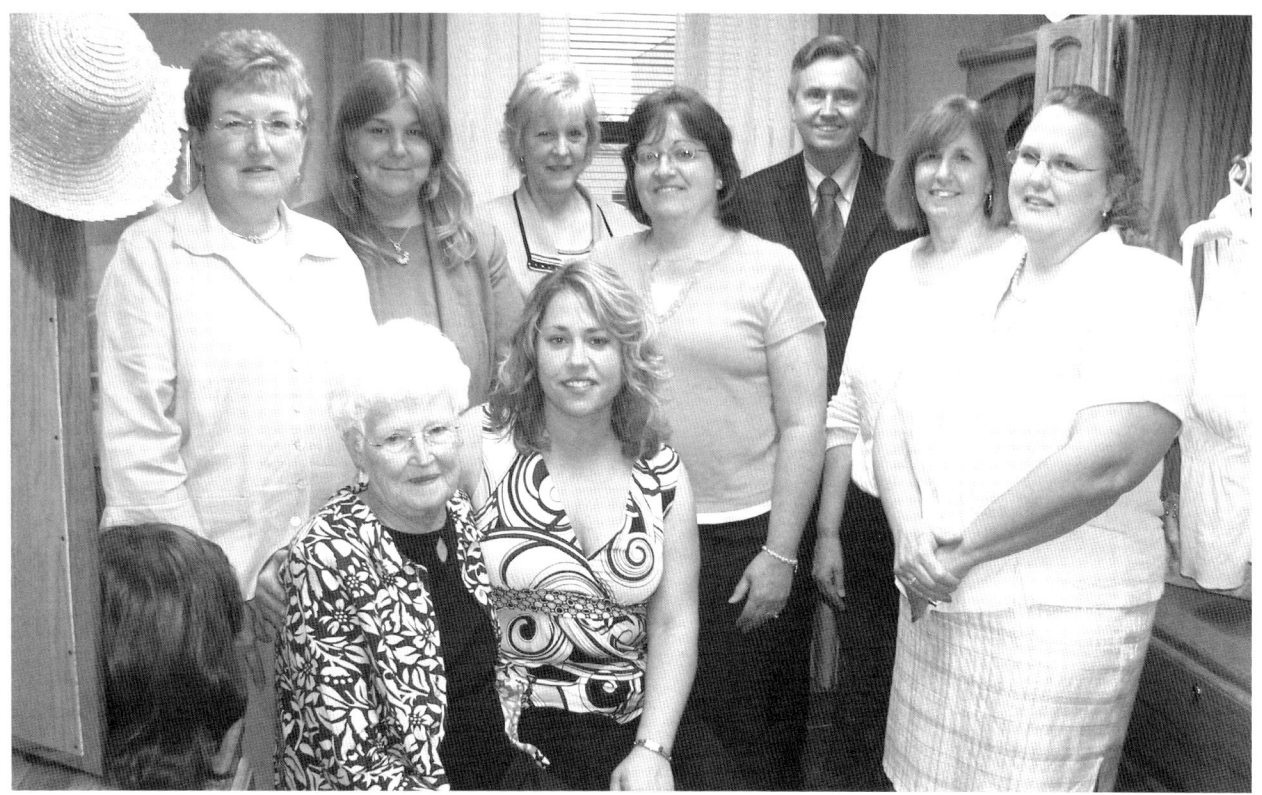

Birdie's Closet, devoted to helping cancer survivors, was dedicated in June 2008.

Chapter 7: A New Era, A New Commitment, A New Identity — 109

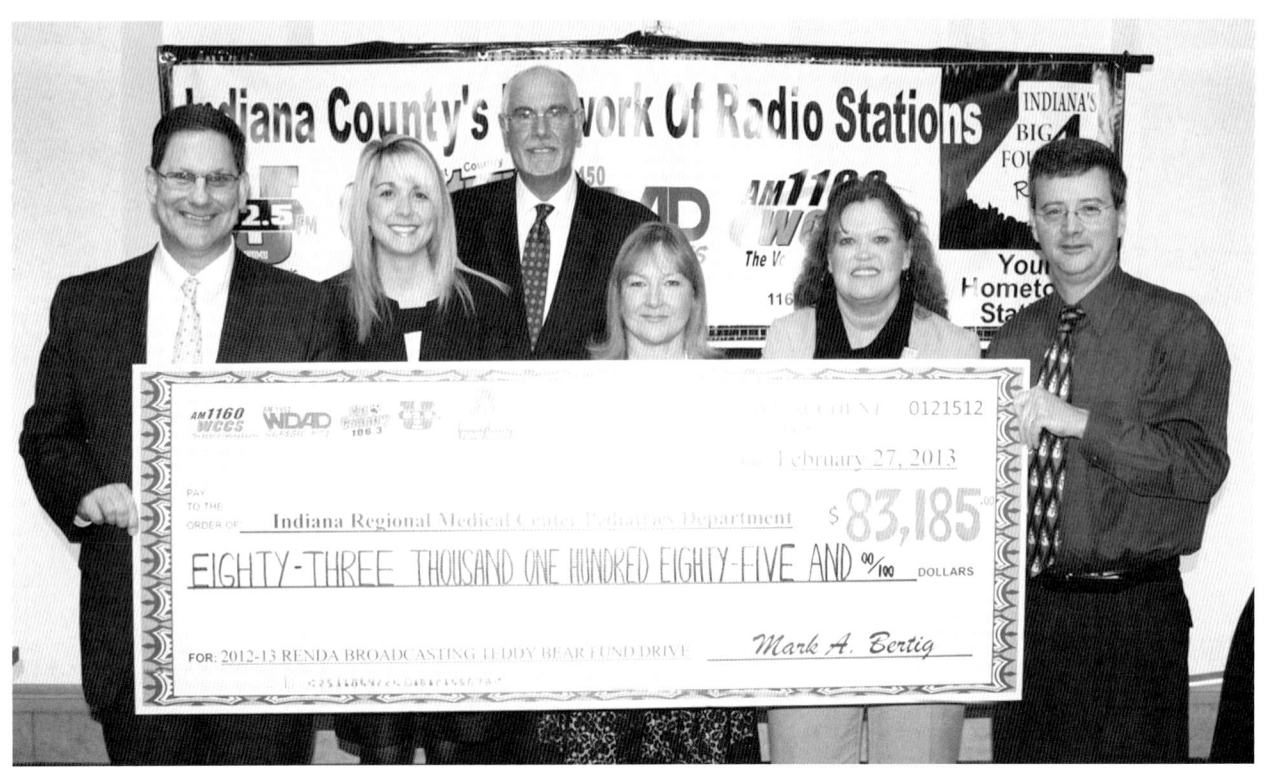

Renda Broadcasting's Teddy Bear Fund Drive raised more than $83,000 in 2013 in support of OB and Pediatric Services.

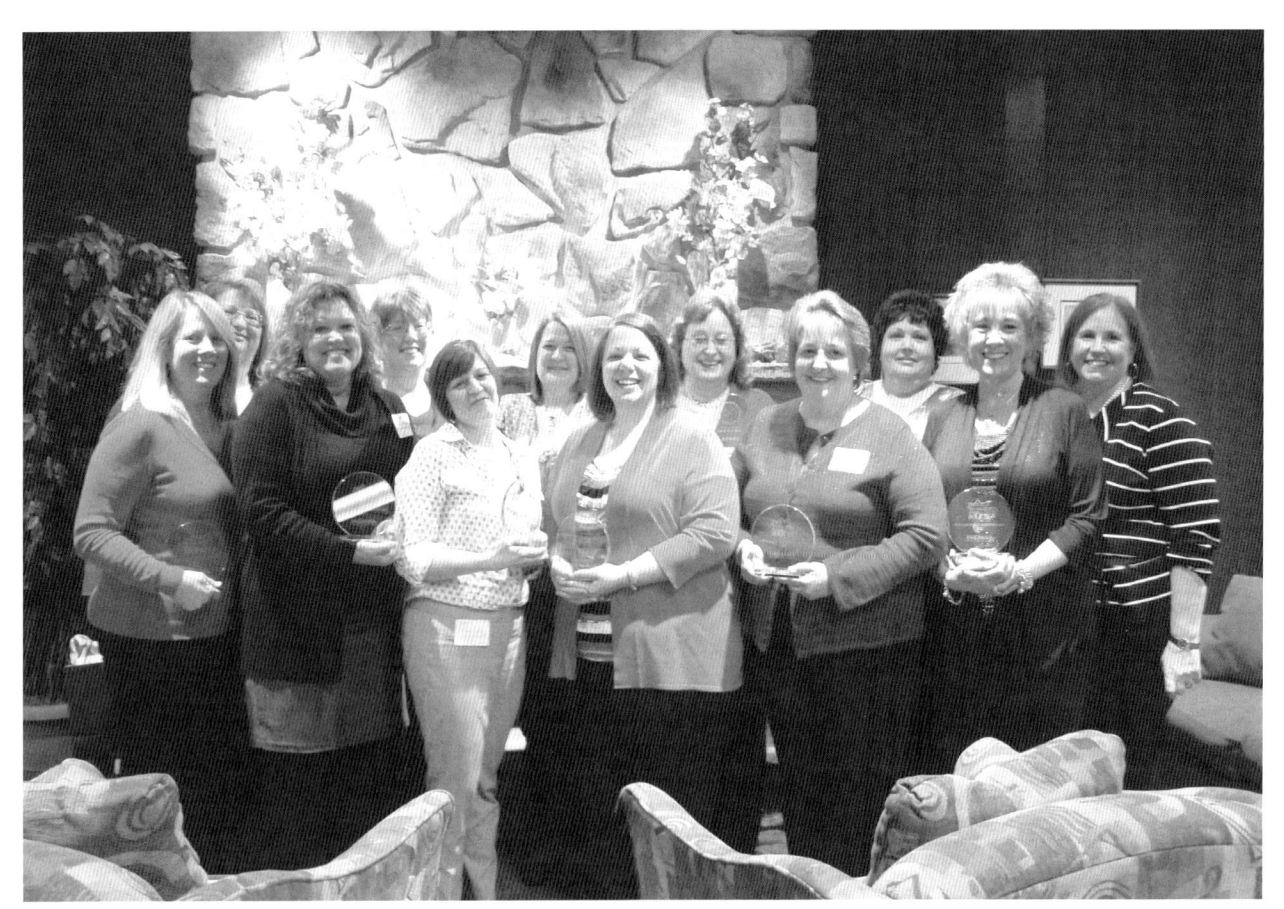

The 2013 Compass Award winners celebrate together.

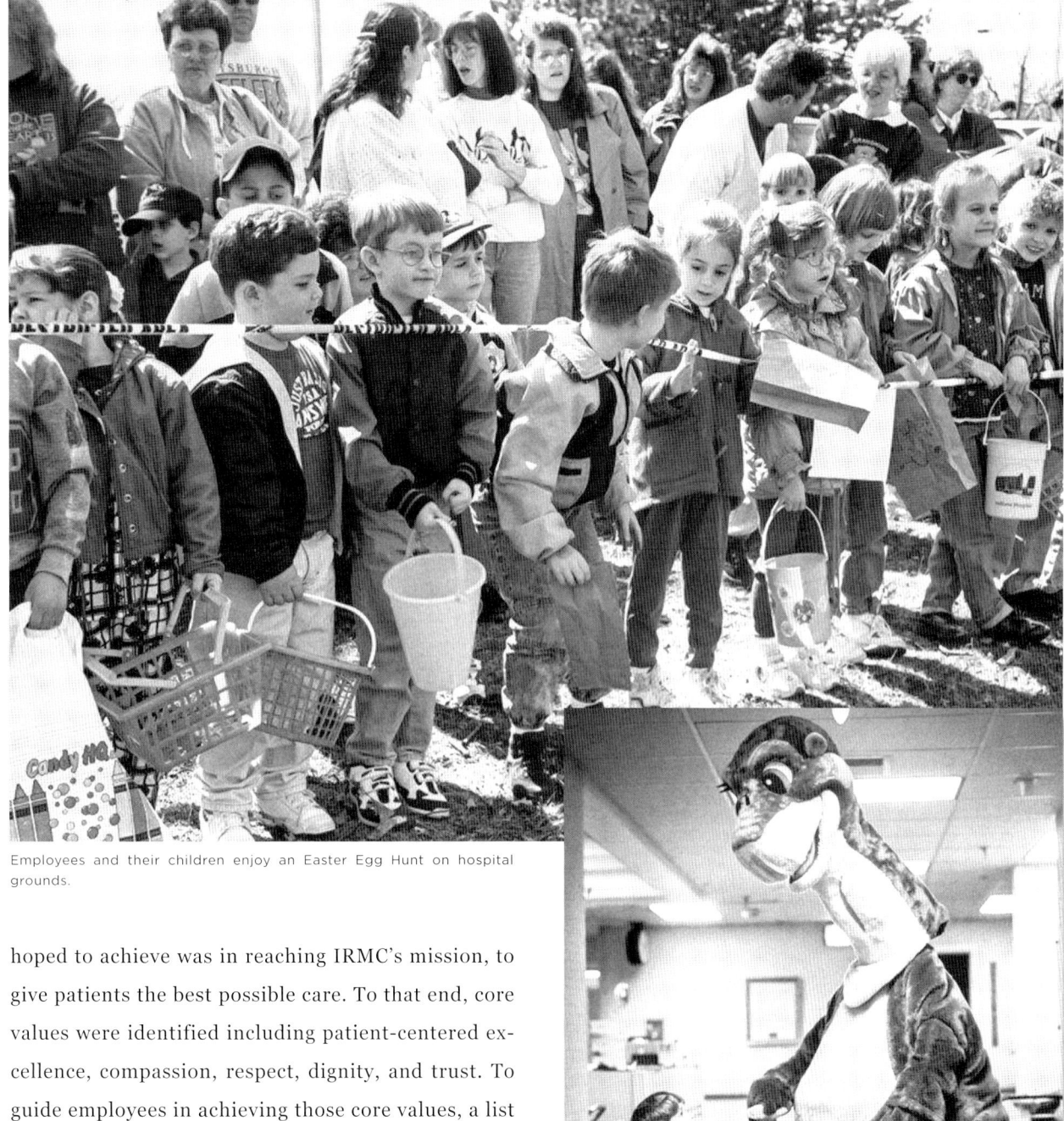

Employees and their children enjoy an Easter Egg Hunt on hospital grounds.

hoped to achieve was in reaching IRMC's mission, to give patients the best possible care. To that end, core values were identified including patient-centered excellence, compassion, respect, dignity, and trust. To guide employees in achieving those core values, a list of Compass Commitments was developed. They included Courtesy, Acknowledgement, Confidentiality, Safety, Innovation, Teamwork, Empowerment, Professionalism, Responsibility, Attitude, Communication, and Pride in Work—key behaviors that support the core values. In 2008, IRMC established the Compass Award to recognize employees, volunteers, and physicians who demonstrate IRMC values in action and exemplify the mission.

A costumed character visits a child in the pediatric ward.

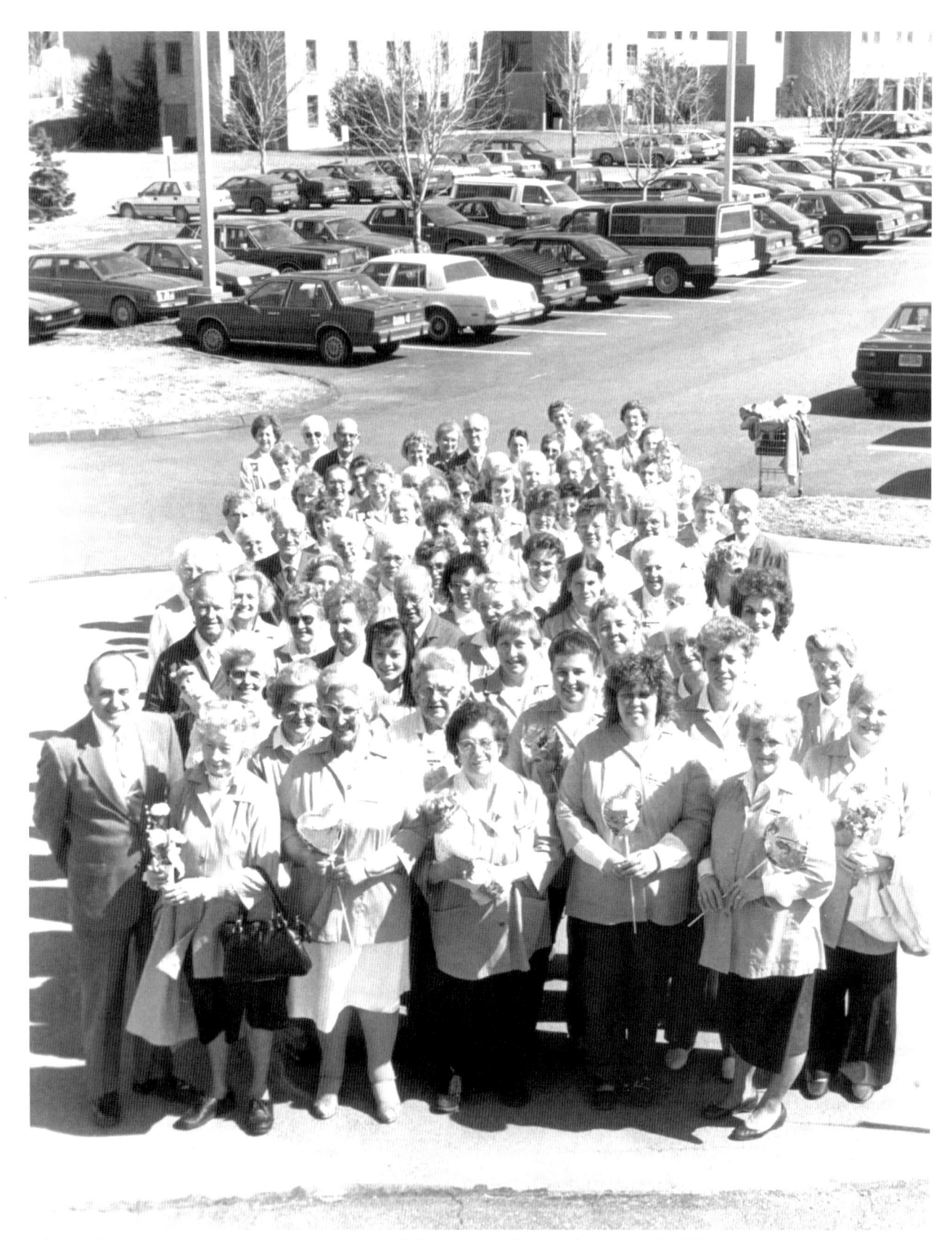

Volunteers have been an integral part of the care provided at IRMC since the Auxiliary was first organized in 1916.

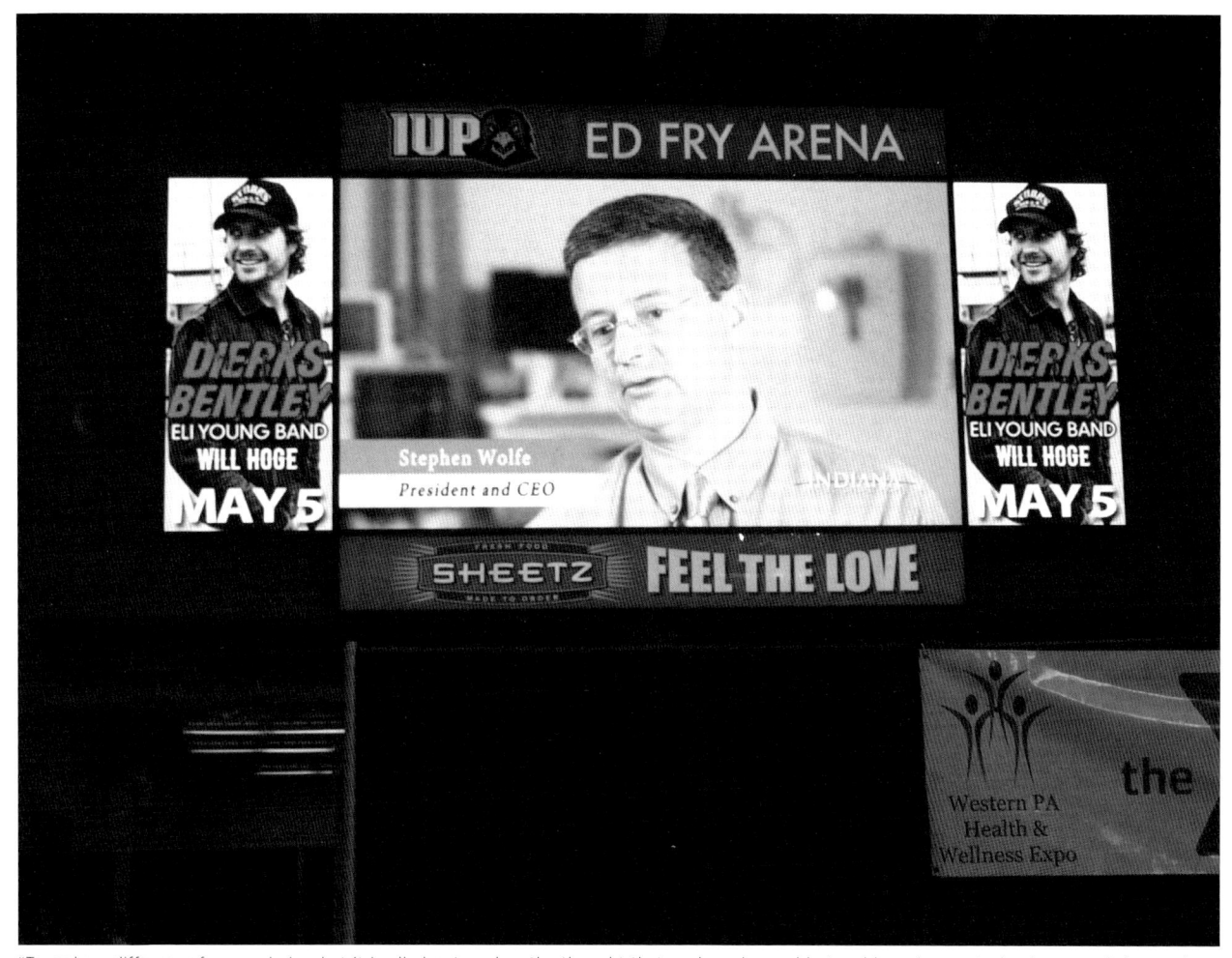

"To make a difference for people is what it is all about, and so the thought that we have been able to add services or technology or whatever where we can really care for people in a very high quality way and hopefully in a setting where they are closer to their family and have all of those other supports—I mean—that's what it is all about."

Seeking to improve in ways that most of us never think about, IRMC also received the Unison Gold Star Provider award in 2009, which included a $50,000 grant, for reducing the number of hospital-acquired infections. The award was based on data gathered by the Pennsylvania Health Care Cost Containment Council, data showing that IRMC reduced the rate of infection by 25.12 percent compared to the statewide average of 7.8 percent for the same two-year period.

Chapter 7: A New Era, A New Commitment, A New Identity —⋀— 113

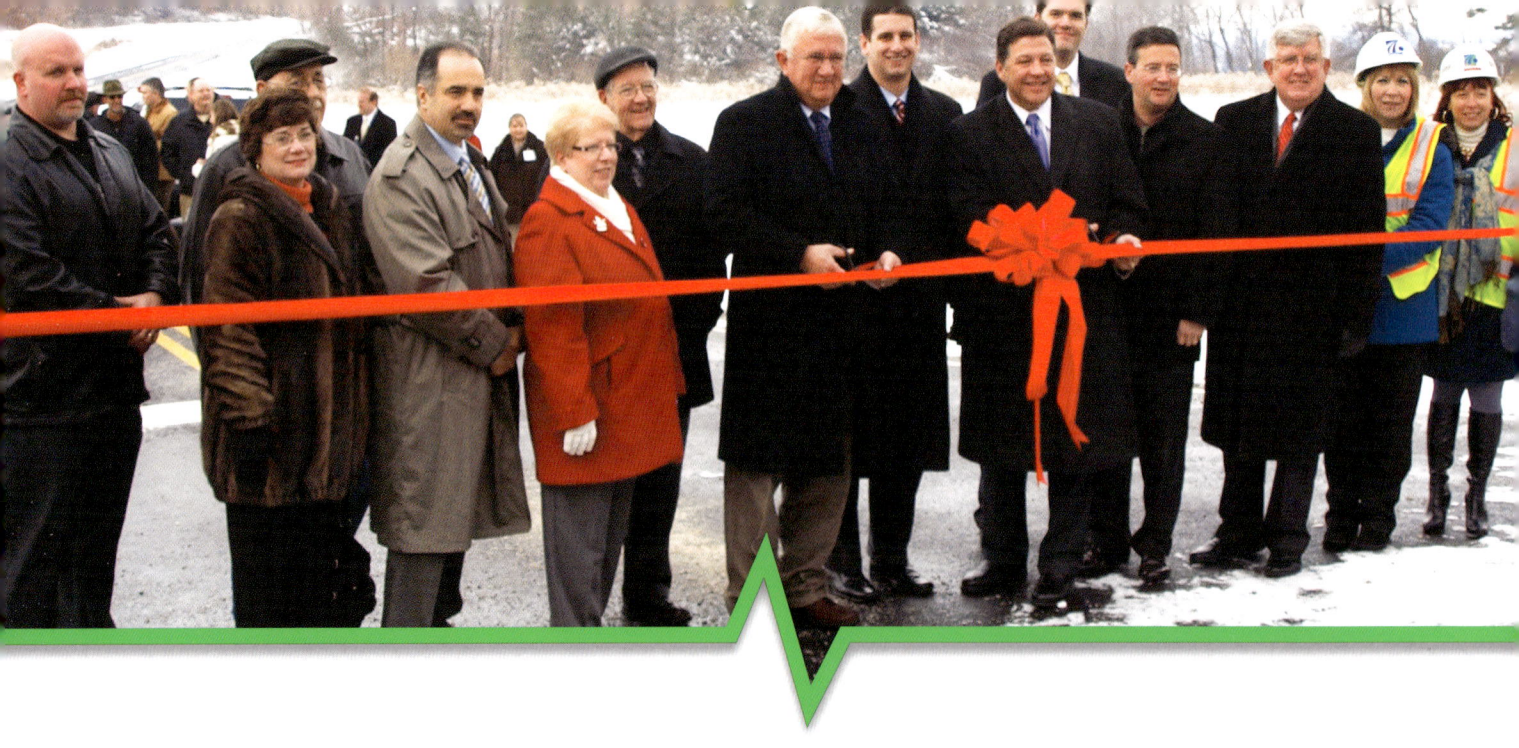

CHAPTER 8
Honoring Our Past, Embracing Our Future

As Indiana Regional Medical Center prepares to celebrate its centennial year, the sharp contrasts between the practice of medicine in 1914 and now in 2014 will loom large. Virtually nothing about the hospital's day-to-day operations has been unchanged. And yet, the door that originally opened in 1914 is still there, as is the Mack Wing portico where decades of nursing graduates posed for their class photo. Millions of dollars have been spent expanding and upgrading the hospital, and yet its history remains intact. In an age when our "bricks and mortar" history is too often turned to rubble to make way for steel and glass, the original structure of Indiana Hospital remains at the heart of Indiana Regional Medical Center. What has also remained constant, in the midst of growth, financial challenges, and stunning technological advances, is the commitment to compassionate patient care. "I think, of all the vocations you can choose," Stephen Wolfe reflected, "wanting to care for people, making them better, keeping them healthy, and even in the worst case scenarios helping them pass on with dignity and compassion . . . I don't know that there is a greater calling on all the planet. I'm really proud of our people and the hard work, sacrifice, and dedication they all give to provide that for our patients."

A CONSTANT AMID CHANGE

It is difficult to imagine anyone who more aptly personifies the core values at Indiana Regional Medical Center than Marge Scheeren, director of volunteers since 1975, and the 150 volunteers who fall under her charge. Volunteers help staff the hospital every day including holidays in twelve-hour shifts. They help in the Pantry and the gift shop, take the hospitality cart through the hospital, sort and deliver the mail, and, of course, staff the information desk where they are the first people to greet visitors when they enter the hospital. Marge is herself a volunteer; her life can be defined by one word—service. Beneath her gentle, ladylike demeanor is a strict level of professionalism that she also requires from her volunteers.

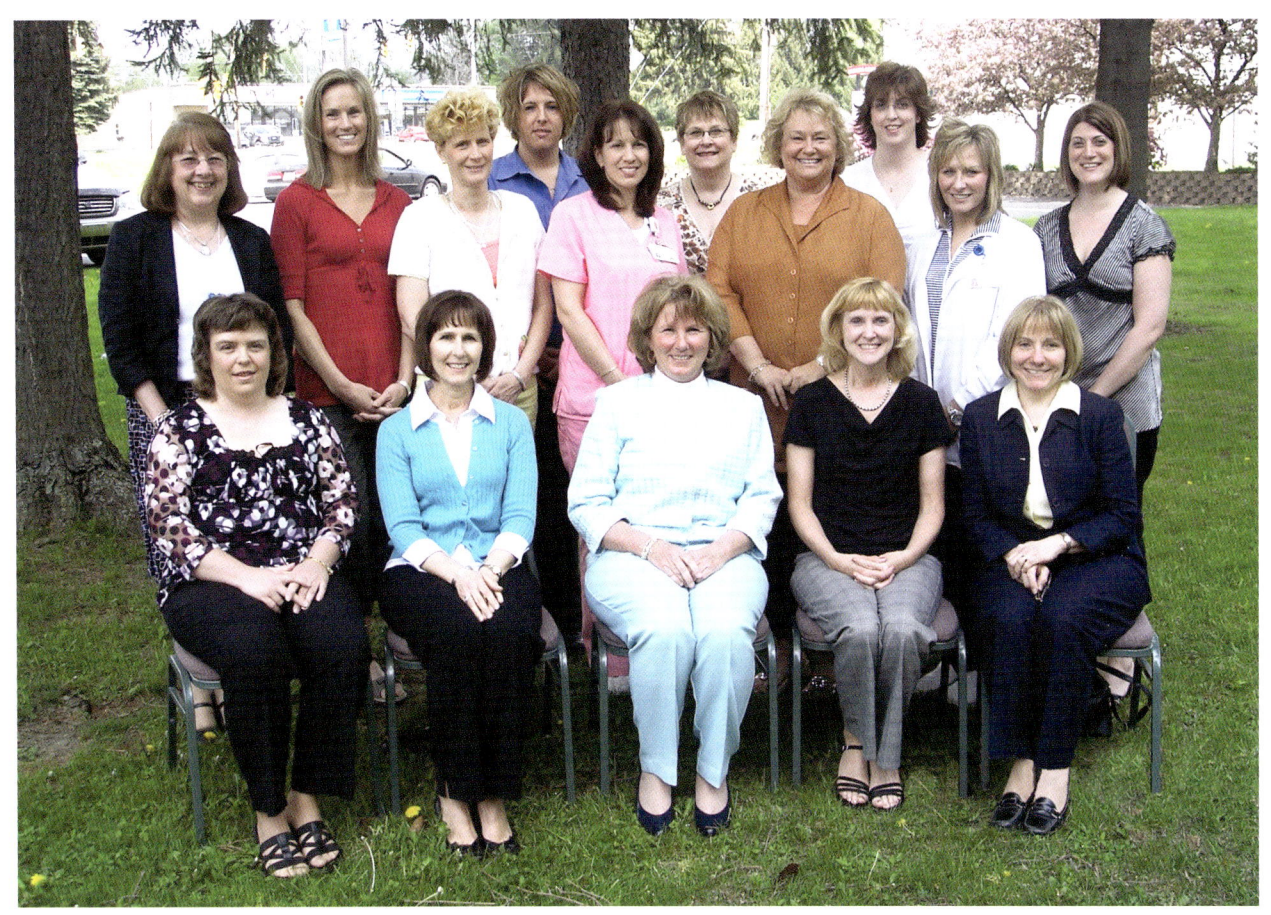

IRMC's nominees for the Cameos of Caring award created by the University of Pittsburgh School of Nursing in 1999 to honor nurses who demonstrate exceptional levels of skill and care.

Opposite page: From the beginning, Indiana Hospital and now IRMC have illustrated what can be accomplished when the people of a community pool their time, talent, and treasure.

The Indiana Regional Medical Center Auxiliary is the parent organization overseeing the volunteers, and Marge is understandably proud of the long list of donations for which the Auxiliary has been responsible over the years. While the list includes some of the hospital's primary equipment, what touches Marge's heart the most are the little gestures that have undoubtedly made a tremendous difference to patients over the years. "Long ago we started a program to supply tiny little gold rings when a mom loses a baby," she said. "On the door of any room where there has been a baby lost, there is a little card with a leaf on it and a dew drop. So everybody knows when they see that card that a baby has not survived." Every year on Christmas Day, patients receive small bags filled with

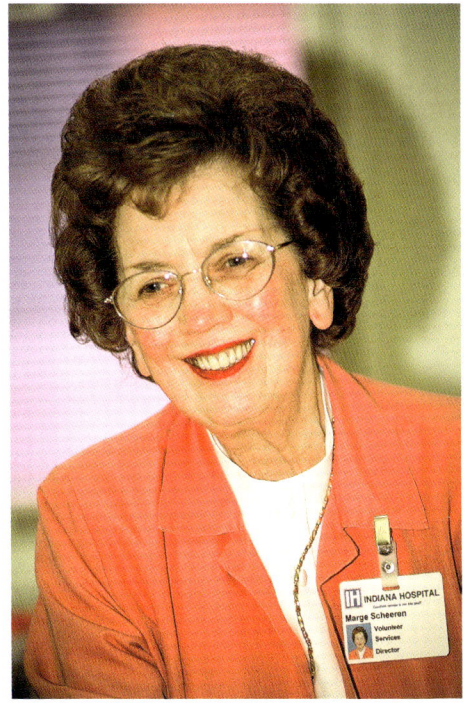

Marge Scheeren has been director of volunteers since 1975.

Chapter 8: Honoring Our Past, Embracing Our Future —⋏— 115

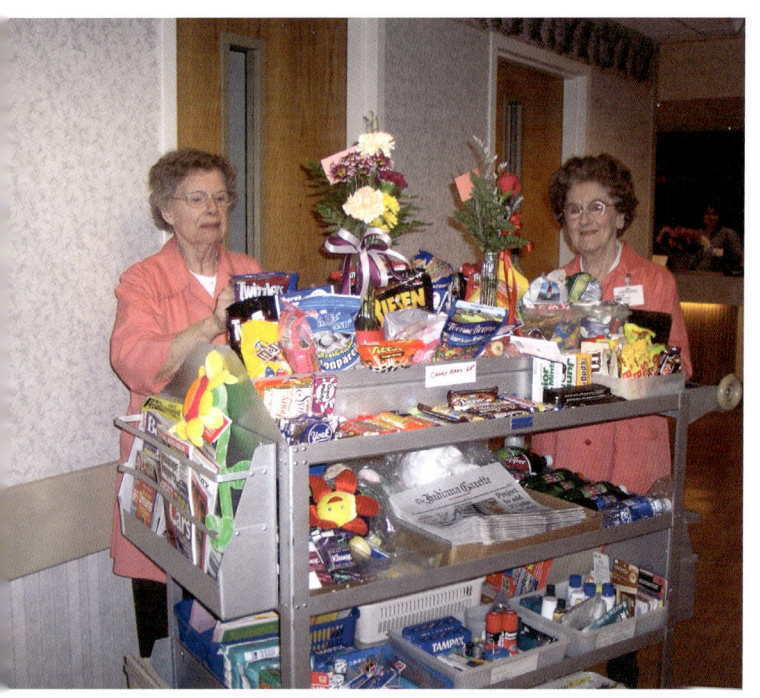

The hospitality cart offers patients and their families items of comfort and convenience but most importantly a drop-in visit and a smile.

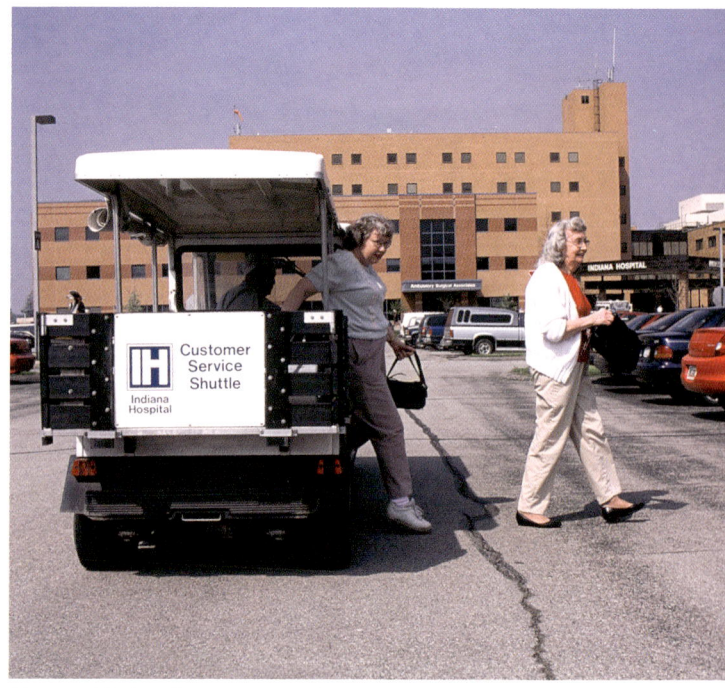

Above and below: For many years the hospital provided a shuttle service. The Auxiliary now provides visitors even more ease and comfort by supporting the courtesy van.

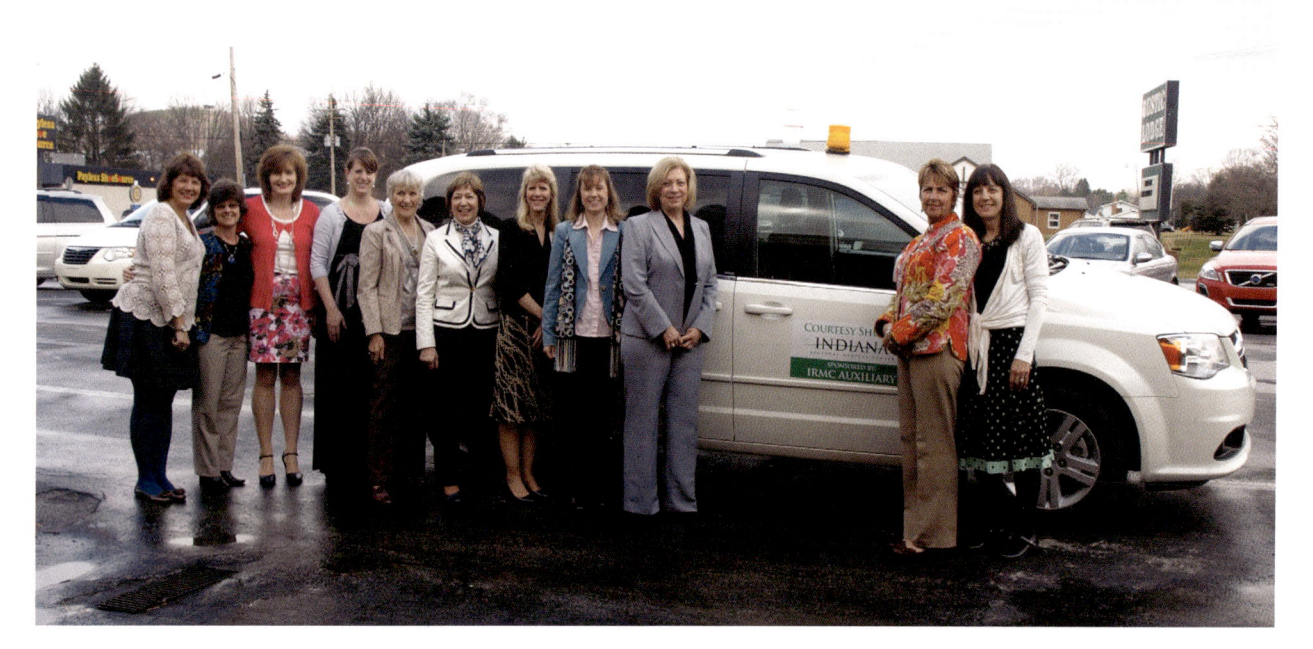

individually wrapped items of everyday usefulness. "Many times we have found," she said, "that little bag is their only Christmas."

For nearly forty years, the Auxiliary was the major supporter of the Lifeline program but recently shifted its support to the hospital's shuttle service, a courtesy that the hospital opted to discontinue as a cost-cutting measure. Instead of the previous golf cart, the Auxiliary will sponsor all costs related to the minivan shuttle, providing a higher level of passenger comfort, particularly during inclement weather.

THE NURSES

There is a striking contrast between the nurses' starched white caps and white stockings of years ago and the colorful and unarguably more comfortable nurses' uniforms of today. From the modern viewpoint, it might be easy to assume that those starched uniforms represented greater discipline among the nursing staff, but to assume that they represented better patient care would be an error.

In truth, the visible changes in nurses are rooted in two factors: the women's movement, which sought to erase our rigid expectations about how women should look and act, and the entrance of men into the nursing profession. White stockings, shoes, and caps no longer suited the new gender-neutral profession.

Education and training has changed over the years, and according to Cindy Virgil, vice president of Nursing Services, it is more common in recent years for nurses to have bachelor degrees. Approximately 73 percent of the patient care staff are registered nurses. Licensed practical nurses, nursing assistants, transporters, and clinical secretaries make up the remaining 27 percent. While some nurses with master's degrees opt to go into education or leadership positions, "at IRMC," Cindy commented, "we have nurses with master's degrees who choose to stay right at the bedside." That commitment to patient care is often the result of personal experience. Nancy Smith, director of the Institute for Healthy Living, made the decision to go into nursing her senior year of high school. "I had a simple appendectomy," she recalled, "but the care I received was so good that I decided that was what I wanted to do." She began working at the hospital in 1974 making $5,000 per year. The nurse who inspired her career path was Indiana Hospital's own Diane Petras.

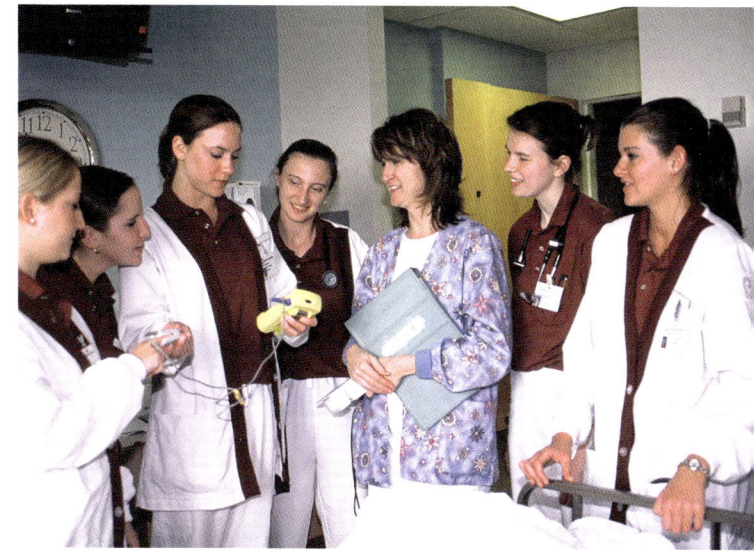

Besides the classroom, student nurses learn from the best source of all—the experienced and dedicated nurses of IRMC.

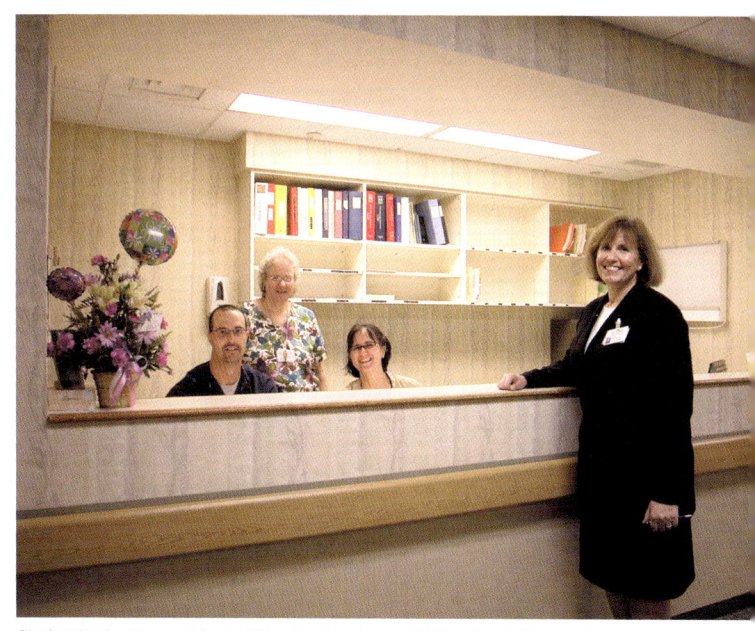

Cindy Virgil, vice president of Nursing Services, with the fourth floor staff.

When asked about the hospital's current strengths, retired surgeon Dr. Alex Juhasz immediately identified the nursing staff and their enhanced role within the hospital. "In 1977 [when he joined the staff], the nurses couldn't really say anything, couldn't suggest anything for improvements. That has vastly changed." Now, nurses are involved with establishing policies, procedures, and practices, and selecting equipment and vendors. Like all other depart-

Chapter 8: Honoring Our Past, Embracing Our Future

ments at IRMC, the nursing staff is also involved in the LEAN performance improvement initiative based on the renowned Toyota production system. As part of the hospital's goal of achieving the Baldrige award, the program provides a structured framework for determining best practices. As the front line of patient care, the physicians, surgeons, and hospital administration now rely heavily on the nurses' input.

Perhaps more than anywhere else, IRMC's role as a sole community provider of health care is illustrated through its staff of nurses. "Our staff is very committed, extremely compassionate, and knowledgeable," said Cindy Virgil. "Our nurses are taking care of friends, neighbors, people from their place of worship, people who take care of them in restaurants and grocery stores. So there is a level of commitment and compassion that comes from that. To me, that's palpable in this organization. It's real."

THE PHYSICIANS

"Nothing happens at Indiana Regional Medical Center until a physician signs an order," Stephen Wolfe is often heard saying, acknowledging the foundational role of IRMC's dedicated physicians. "We're incredibly blessed to have been able to attract and retain an outstanding medical staff," he said. "Certainly our current staff is as good as any you'll find in a community hospital anywhere in the United States." Though house calls are not nearly as much a part of the doctors' daily routine as they once were, some physicians at IRMC still make home visits, particularly in the more rural areas. And though their services are no longer bartered with homemade treasures, according to Dr. Edward McDowell, the doctors provide as much charity care as ever.

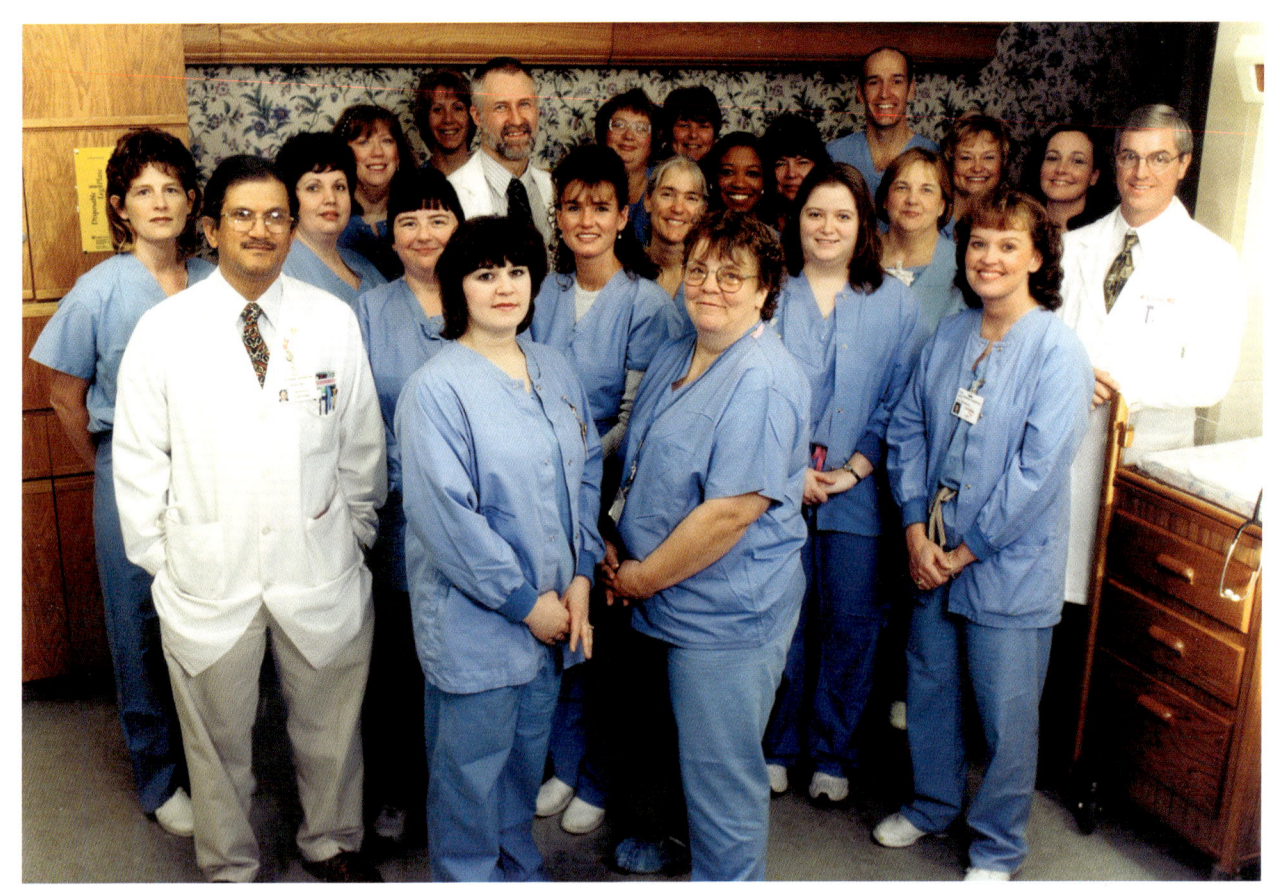

IRMC's obstetrics physicians, nurses, and staff.

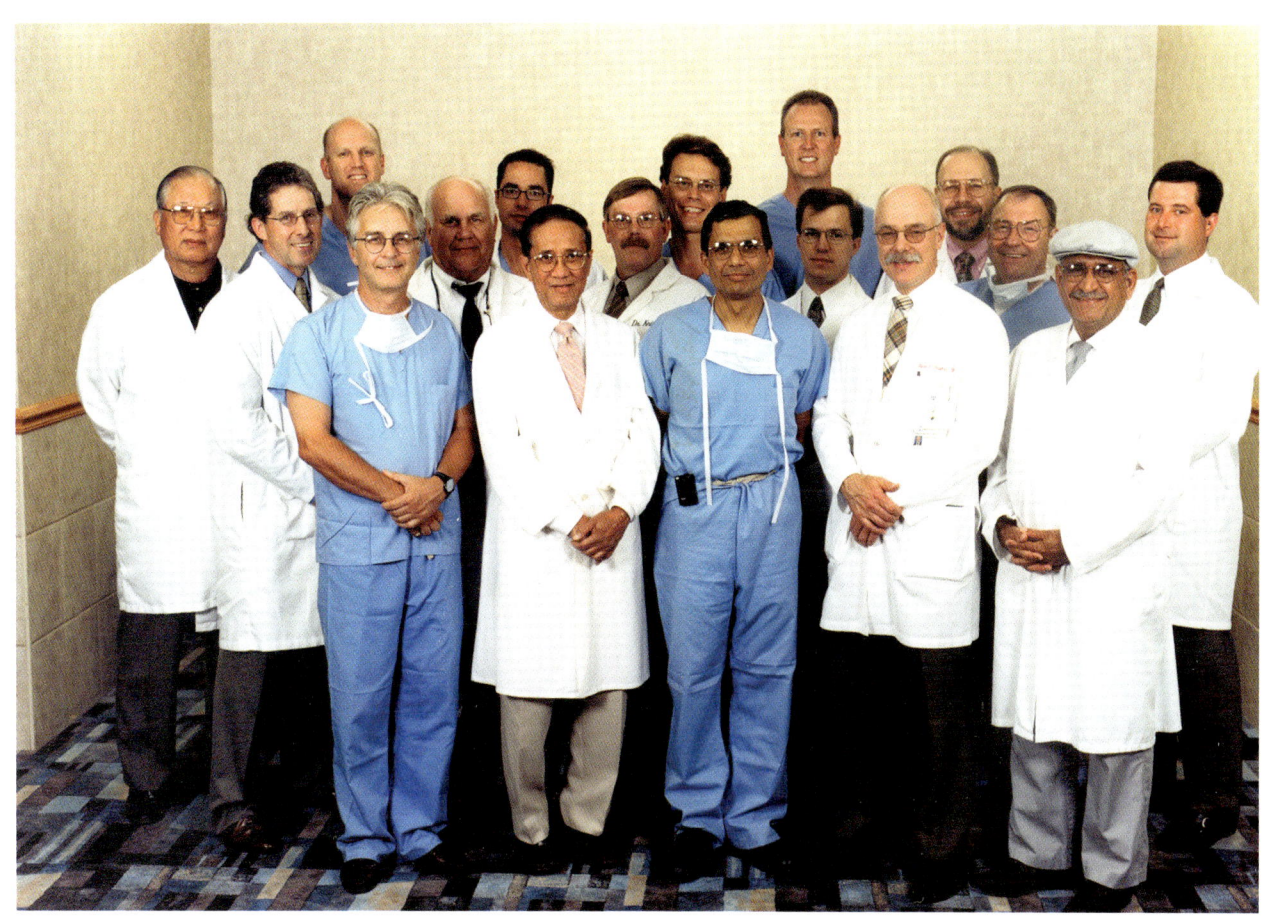

IRMC's surgical physicians stay abreast of the rapid advances in surgical equipment and procedures.

Having come to Indiana Hospital in 1982 following his training at Allegheny General, Dr. McDowell became medical director of IHPS in April 2012. Still a practicing cardiologist, he has seen numerous changes in both medicine in general and the physicians over the past thirty years. "It's just astounding to me when I look back—the procedures, the medications, the things that we have to help people now that we didn't have thirty years ago," he said. "Every day, I see how it makes a difference in the patient's quality of life." Unlike years ago when physicians offered cradle-to-grave care, today IRMC has a highly specialized staff of physicians, an inevitable result of those medical advances, along with the advanced services the hospital now offers.

The other major change Dr. McDowell and others have observed is the growing difficulties of private

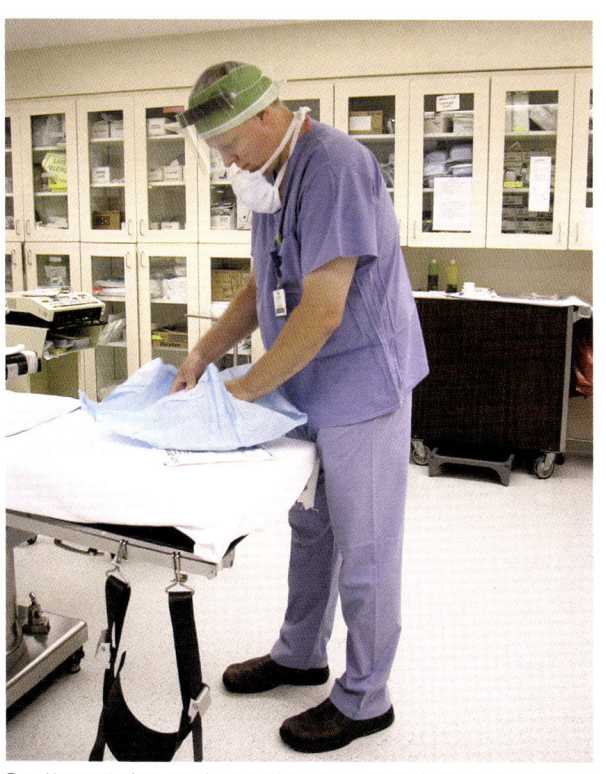

Ron Homer makes certain everything is ready for both the patient and the surgeon.

Chapter 8: Honoring Our Past, Embracing Our Future — 119

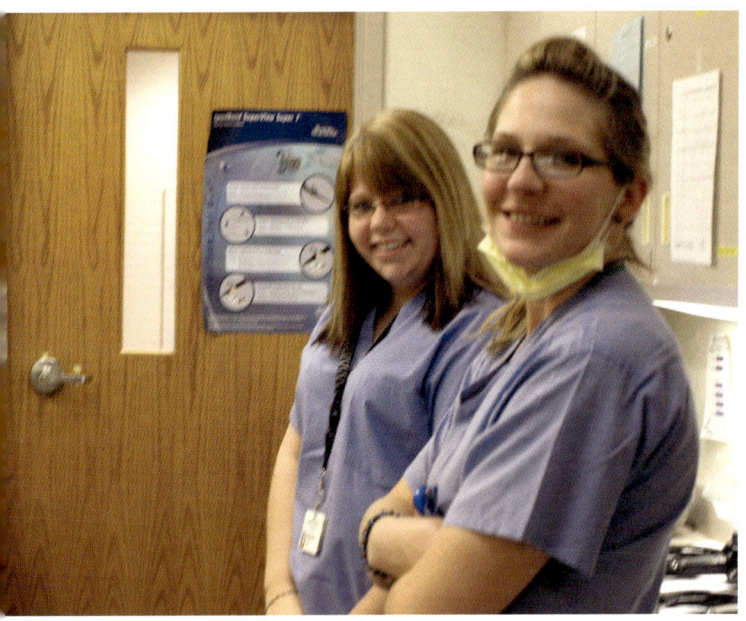

IRMC's greatest asset is its people, who provide quality care and service with a smile.

practice. The increased regulations and the red tape that comes with them pose tremendous challenges for the individual practitioner. Electronic medical records, despite their eventual advantages, come at great expense in both money and time for the solo physician. In contrast to the days when the emergency room doctors were the only physicians employed by the hospital, 20–30 percent of the physicians are now employees. "If Indiana follows the rest of the country, that will probably be much higher in another ten years," he predicted.

Today nearly 20 percent of IRMC's physicians are women, and they, as well as the men, are changing the very nature of the practice of medicine. Instead of the frequent sixteen-hour days of years ago, many of the younger doctors are seeking a better quality of life for themselves as well as their families. "Many of our physicians don't want to be absentee dads," Dr. McDowell commented. Toward that end, many rely on physician extenders in the form of physician assistants and nurse practitioners, who make it possible for the doctor to see more patients in the course of a day and provide personal attention to those who require it.

Despite the challenges and uncertainties surrounding the Affordable Health Care Act, Dr. McDowell remains optimistic about the future. "It's still a good time to be a physician," he said. "To be able to serve people . . . it's a privilege, and I think most of the people at IRMC feel the same way."

IRMC TODAY

Since its early days, IRMC's "front door to the hospital," the emergency department, has continued to provide EMS medical control through a variety of methods, including pre-established care protocols, radio and telephone communications, and medical review and continuing education for EMS providers. Today, IRMC's Center for EMS/Prehospital Medicine, in concert with the Bork Emergency Center, coordinates eighteen specially trained Medical Command Physicians who continue to provide EMS personnel with access to EMS medical direction. Dr. John Cawley, director of the Bork Emergency Center and the

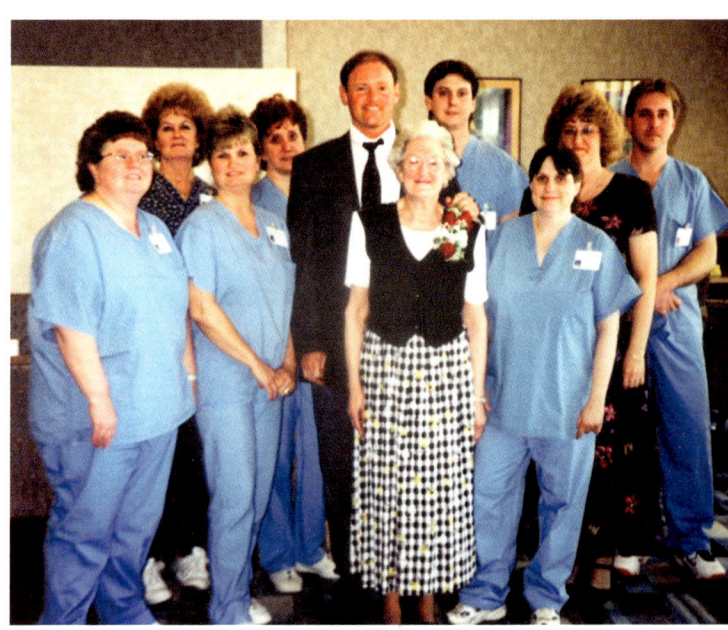

Bob Jeffrey and the Laundry and Linen staff congratulate long-term employee Barb Lockard (center) at her retirement party.

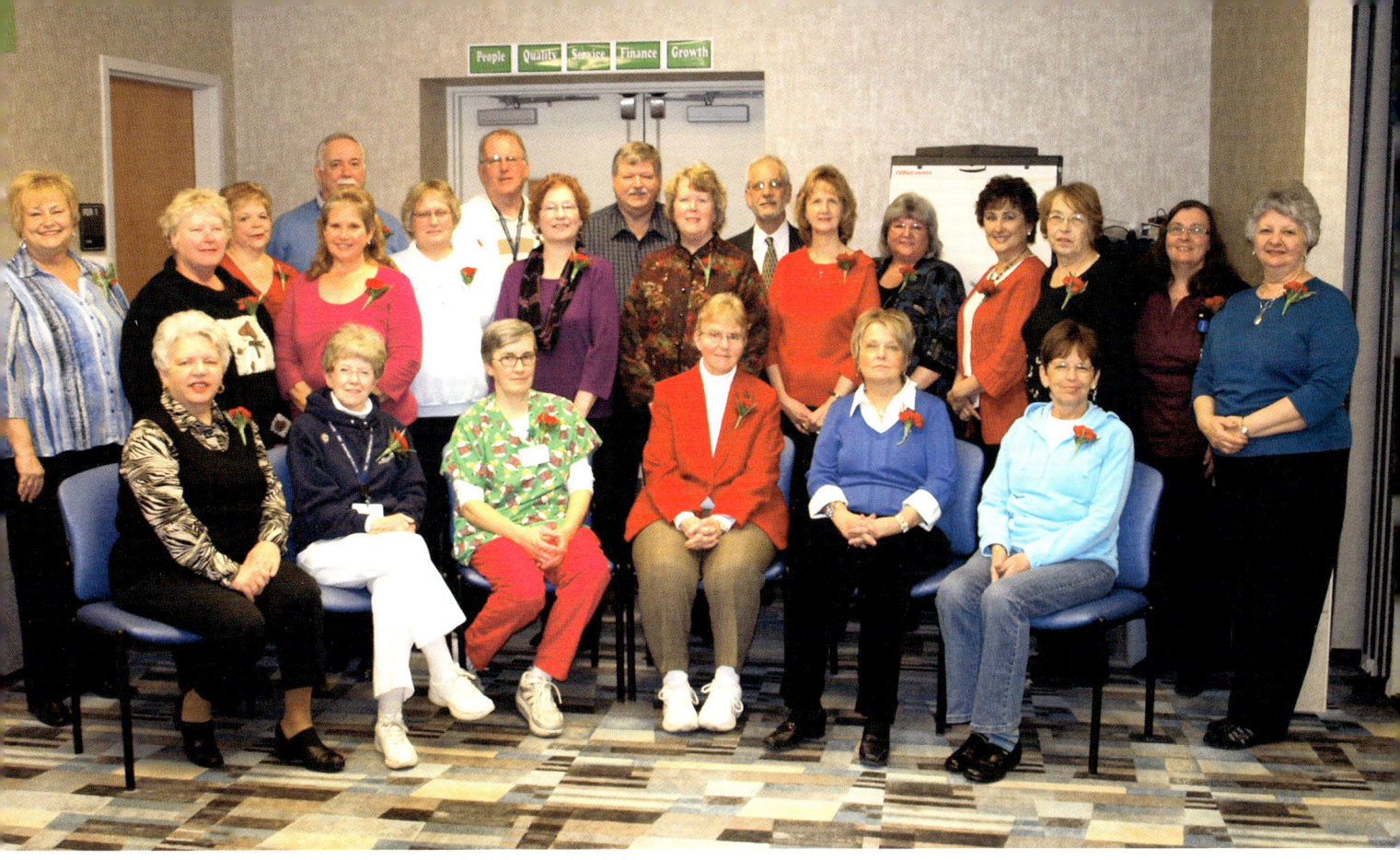

Even after retirement, IRMC employees come back for occasional visits.

Center for EMS/Prehospital Medicine stated, "The EMS crew is the physician's eyes and ears in the pre-hospital setting. Through the medical command system, the interaction between physicians and the paramedics permits emergent therapeutic modalities to be skillfully and rapidly initiated in the field, with the goal of achieving the best patient care possible."

IRMC offers the full range of services required from a sole community provider. The services within the hospital's walls include the Behavioral Health Unit, Center for Cardiac and Vascular Services, the Diabetes Education Center, the It's a Wonderful New Life Maternity Center, Occupational Health, Bork Emergency Center, Rehab Care Center, Sleep Disorder Center, Center for Spine and Pain Management, Palliative Care, and the M. Dorcas Clark, MD, Women's Imaging Center. Within each of these units, there are numerous services available to make the delivery of health care services easier and more efficient for the patients and their families.

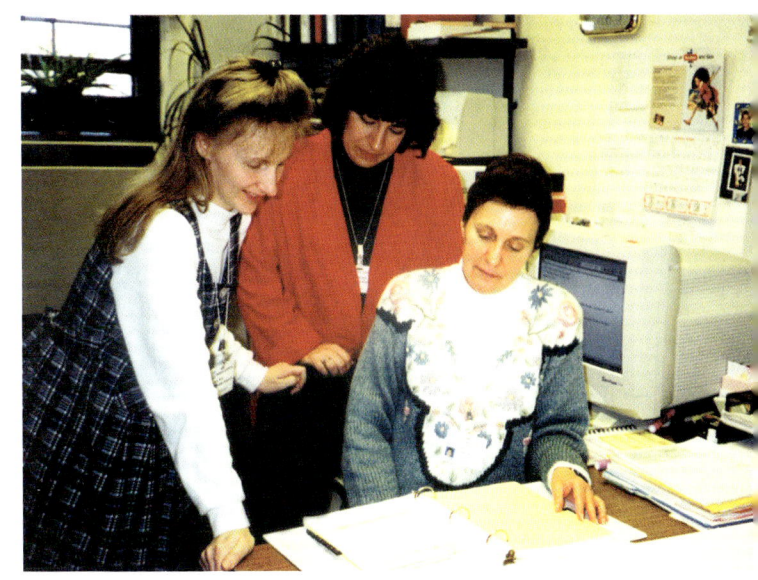

Human Resources staff members Michele Neese, Stacey Hrubochak, and Jean Williams.

Outside the hospital's walls but on the main campus, the Herbert L. Hanna, MD, Center for Oncology Care treats thousands of patients every year with state-of-the-art equipment and methodology. The Ambulatory Surgery Center and Outpatient Services Center flank the hospital.

Chapter 8: Honoring Our Past, Embracing Our Future — 121

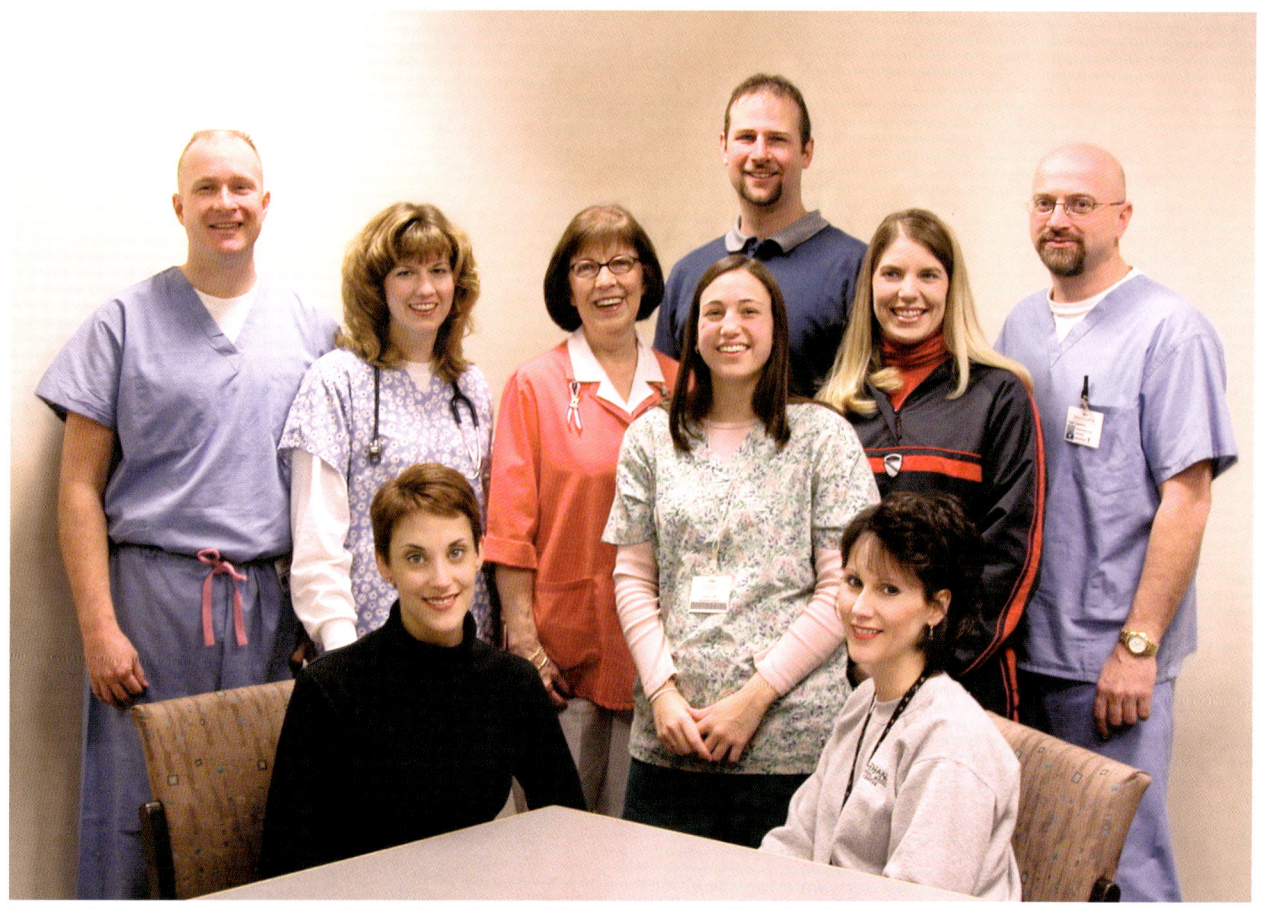

These staff members are representative of those who perform the full range of services offered by IRMC.

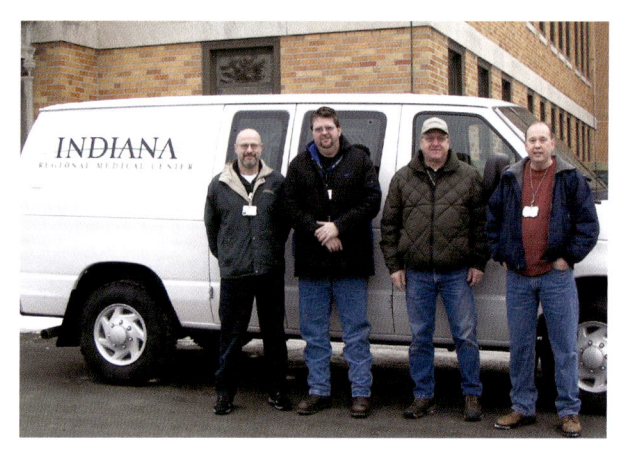

In a rural area like Indiana County, the couriers play an important role between the various satellite locations.

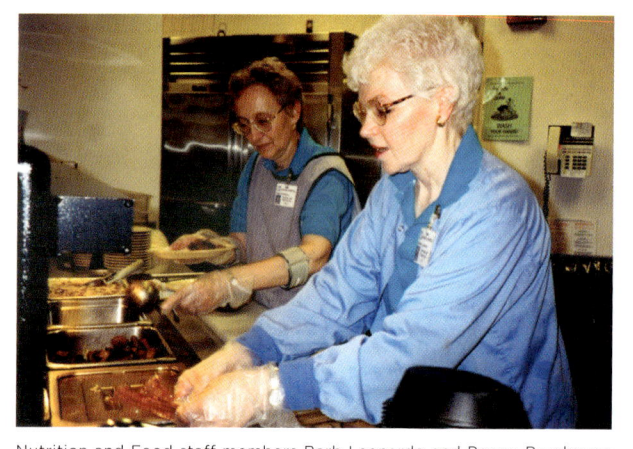

Nutrition and Food staff members Barb Leonardo and Peggy Barnhouse make sure everyone is well and safely fed.

IRMC has two UrgiCare Centers, one at the Main Campus and the other at IRMC at Chestnut Ridge in Blairsville. Other satellite facilities include IRMC at 119 Professional Center in Indiana where the Center for Wound Healing is located, IRMC at Marion Center, IRMC at Northern Cambria, and IRMC at Seward, all of which offer a full line of laboratory and routine x-ray services.

In October 2012, the Human Motion Institute opened its doors at 120 IRMC Drive. The 40,000-square-foot, $15 million center was designed to provide everything under one roof related to muscles and skeletons. IRMC partnered with COSM, the Center for Orthopaedics and Sports Medicine, to create "a comprehensive, leading edge approach to the pre-

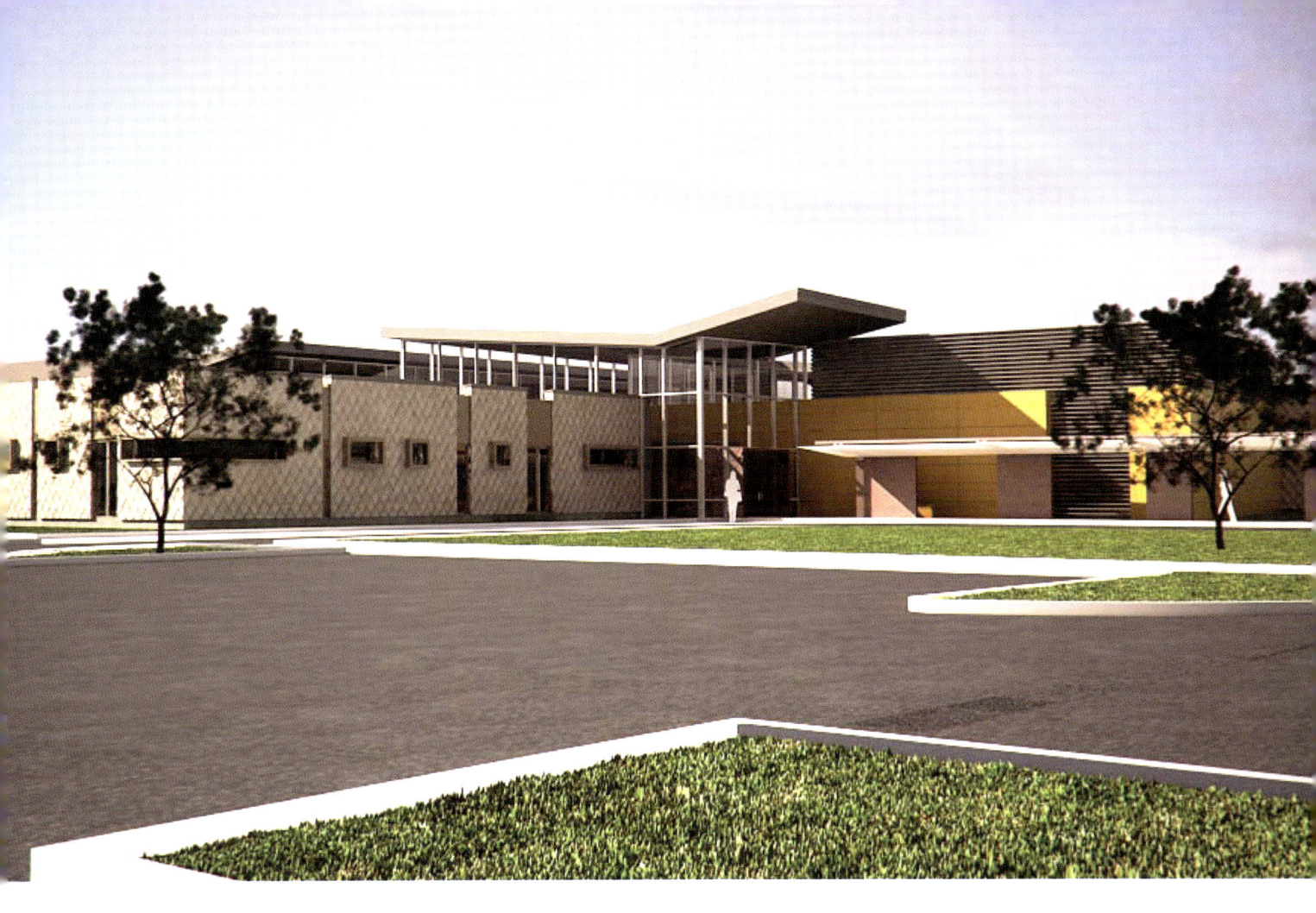

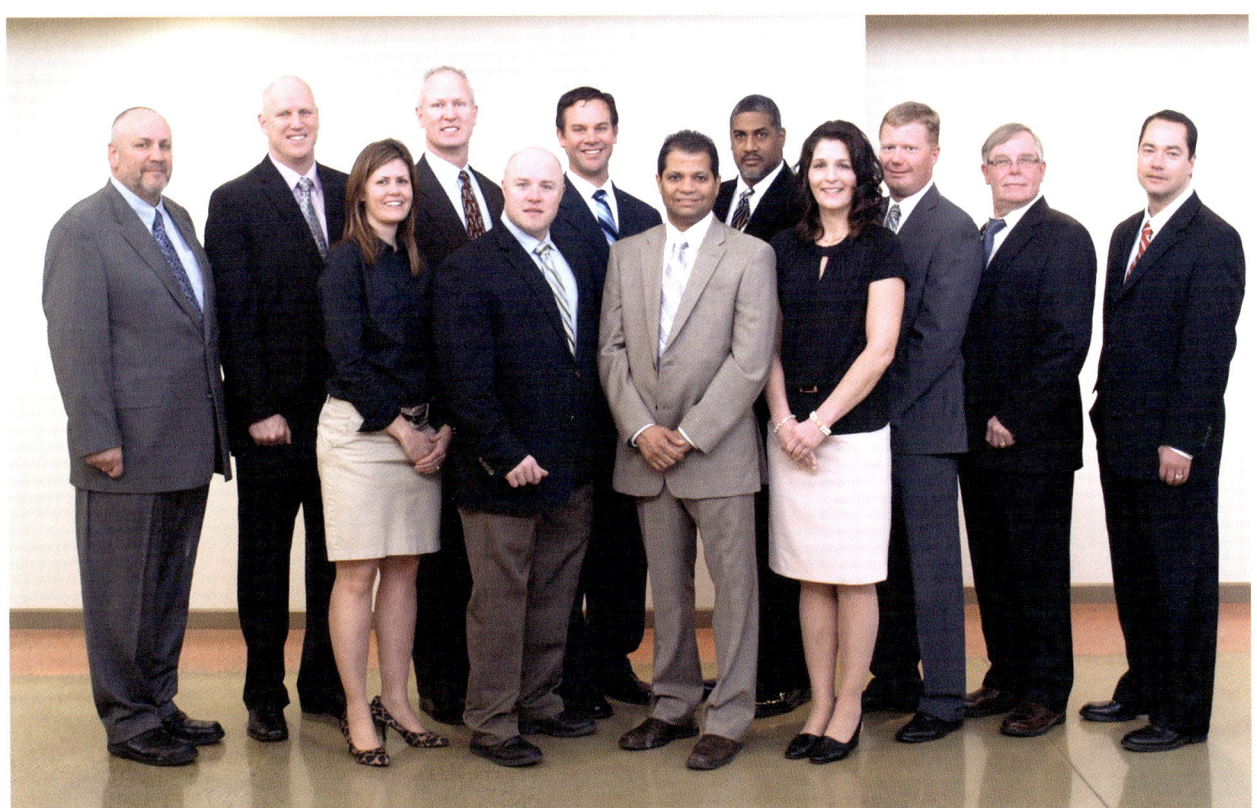

The Human Motion Institute, which opened in 2012, and its staff represent yet another joint venture formed to bring the best possible medical care to the people of Indiana County.

Chapter 8: Honoring Our Past, Embracing Our Future

vention, assessment, treatment, and rehabilitation of musculoskeletal injuries."

A MAJOR CHANGE

Without question, the overwhelming majority of people will tell you that, beyond the technology that has developed in recent decades, the most notable change at Indiana Regional Medical Center is its culture. Nancy Smith, director of the Institute for Healthy Living and a nurse at IRMC for more than thirty-five years, has experienced the culture change firsthand and seen its impact on the community's perception. "The environment now at the hospital is the best that I've worked under—the focus on customer service, the focus on patient satisfaction and employee satisfaction—it's just a much better working environment."

In fact, the culture at IRMC is Steve Wolfe's proudest achievement for the time he has spent here. "We've

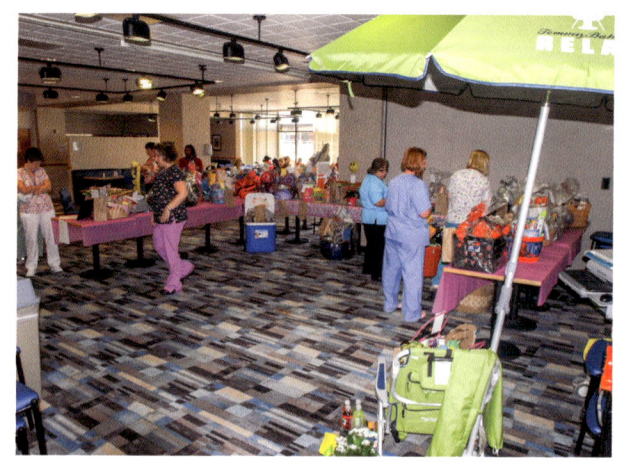

Baskets of goodies are raffled, and employees help fellow employees in need.

created a culture that believes in itself," he said. "Our core competency now is our culture of people."

At the root of the culture is the open communication that is the first vital step to creating sustainable change. "We try hard to communicate. We have an open door policy, and a lot of people take me up on

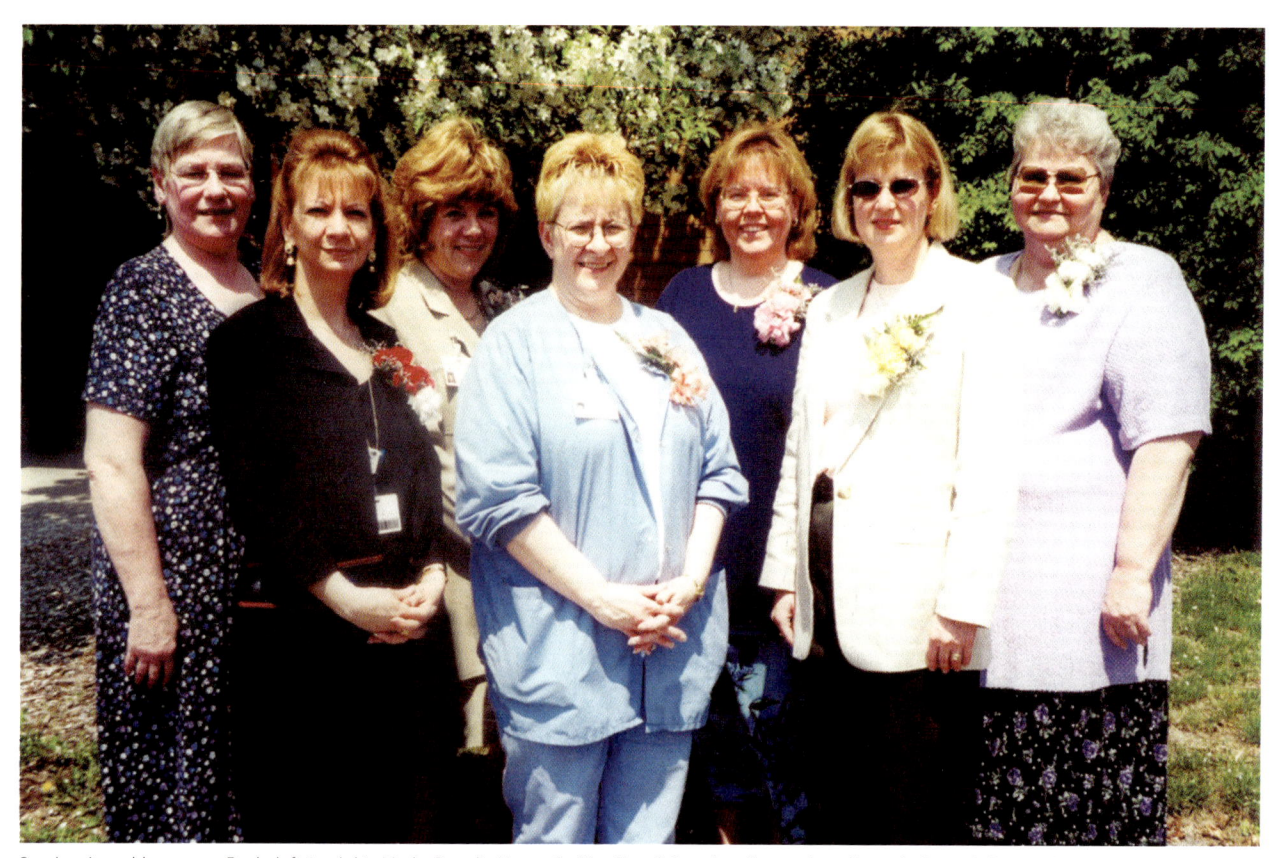

Service Award honorees. Back, left to right: Linda Oswalt, Nancy Smith, Cheryl Gromley, Nancy Jean Hannak. Front, left to right: Debbie Knapic, Annie Plowman, Karen Budris.

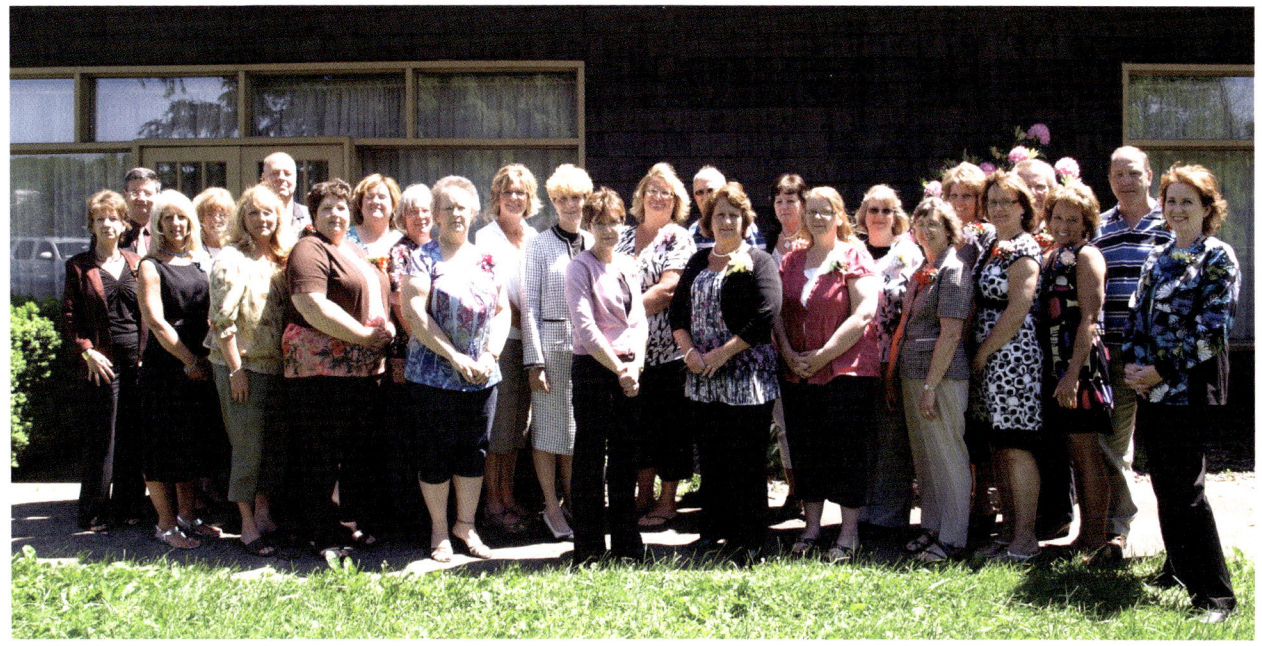

Service Award recipients for 2011.

that," Steve says with a smile. In an unheard-of measure of commitment, his cell phone is published in the patient handbook, making it possible for anyone who is frustrated with some aspect of his or her care to call him personally.

Dominic Paccapaniccia, IRMC's chief operating officer, sees the culture change and the resulting benefits to the employees, the patients, and the hospital itself. "We have five key 'vitals,' which are critical success factors and the number one is people. We try, no matter what we do, to keep that in mind," he said. "In eight years we doubled the size of our revenue. When you put people first, good things happen."

IRMC employees enjoy an excellent benefit package that, besides health care, includes avenues for professional advancement, annual wellness screenings, recreational activities, and even discounts for local restaurants, movies, and shops. The benefit package is just one reason why so many of IRMC's employees are long-term. Of the hospital's 1,316 employees, a whopping 24 percent have worked there for twenty-plus years.

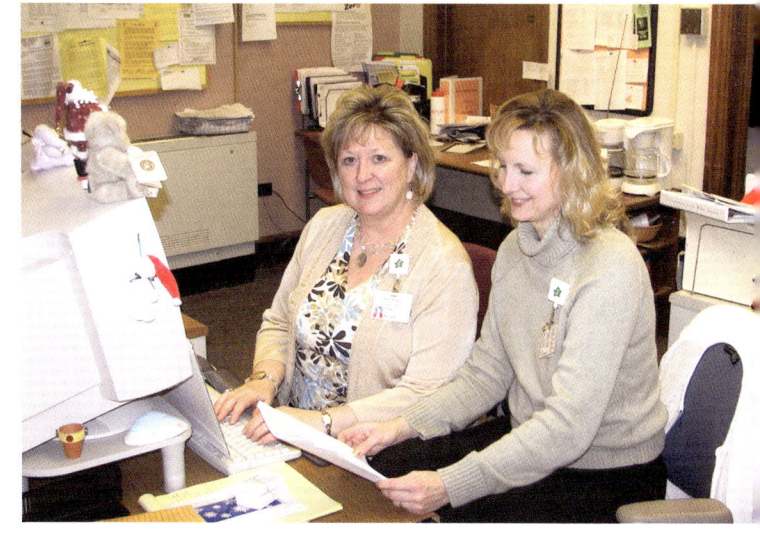

Dawn Zoldak and Annette Cusimano in the Case Management Department.

In 2010, IRMC was once again named among the Best Places to Work in Pennsylvania, Best Places to Work in Health Care by *Modern Healthcare* magazine, and *Fortune* magazine's 100 Best Companies to Work For. Upon receiving the news, Steve Wolfe commented, "For us, the *Fortune* designation was the biggest goal we could set among the best places to work. The Fortune 100 was always the biggest, so we were excited about it." Again in 2012, IRMC was named one of the top five places to work in Pennsylvania by the Best

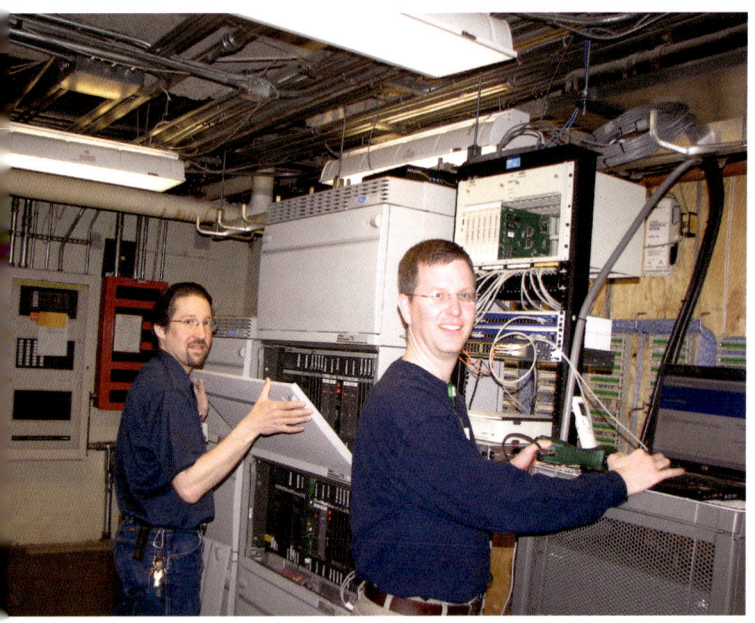

Communication is key! Allen Gray and P. J. McDermott in the Facilities Department keep the telephone service in order.

Places to Work in Pennsylvania program for the fifth year in a row.

Beyond the satisfaction of receiving the award itself, the impact on the hospital and the region is measured in the boost it provides in recruiting physicians and other employees, as well as economic development for the entire county.

There are challenges ahead, to be sure, for IRMC and the entire industry. The primary challenge for the immediate future lies in the provisions contained in the

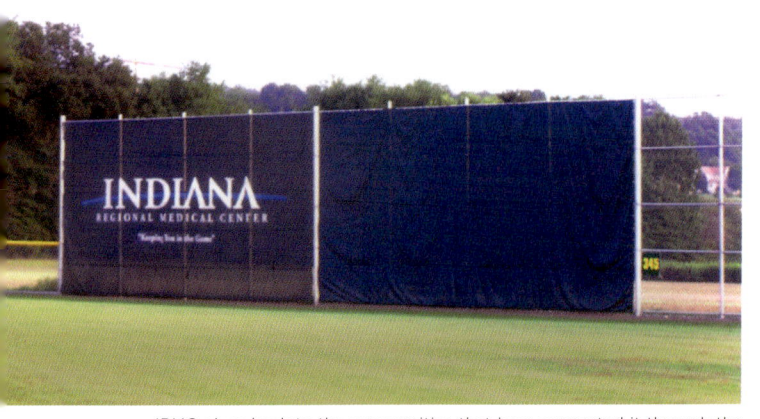

IRMC gives back to the communities that have supported it through the years in numerous ways, including support for Homer City's baseball field.

Patient Protection and Affordable Care Act of 2009. The landmark legislation of the administration of President Barack Obama, its implementation has to date created more uncertainties than solutions. Of particular concern is the creation of mandates and federal subsidies the law includes and contradictory opinions, even within the federal government itself, regarding their funding. "The magnitude of change that's going to occur," said Stephen Wolfe, "will probably be the biggest changes since the advent of Medicare and Medicaid back in the early 1960s."

Whatever payment system ultimately arises as a result of health care reform, there is little question that patients will see their portion of the bill increase. To ease that burden, IRMC is embracing the change by exploring a variety of options to keep costs down and still provide quality care.

Driving IRMC toward its quest for excellence, the steps taken toward the Baldrige award help every department in the hospital to continually refine its processes. For the third year in a row, IRMC has won the Mastery Award, the second highest level in the state, and though the Baldrige sets a very high bar, they are getting there.

Beyond the initiatives driven by Baldrige, the hospital's number one priority as it celebrates its centennial is moving toward a system of physician-driven governance. Identified as a "best practice," physician-driven governance creates a team of designated physicians who play a primary role in administrative decisions. Second only to the goal of physician integration is assuring the hospital's financial viability. Given the current economic and legislative environment, the hospital may be facing a 5–8 percent reduction in its margin, which amounts to approximately $6–10 million. Along with setting a vision for growth that would take the hospital to a 70 percent market share, "We've got to watch the expense side," Steve Wolfe said, "so we're launching a LEAN initiative now." Published reports consistently indicate that 20–40 percent of medical care is waste, and IRMC has set a goal to find out where that waste might be occurring within its system in order to eliminate or minimize it.

Continuing patient satisfaction is the third, albeit continuous, area of focus for IRMC.

Indiana Regional Medical Center is a community asset, a 501(c)3 corporation governed by a twelve-member board of directors, all of whom are volunteers. Unlike hospitals that are accountable to shareholders, every decision the directors make is driven by their concern for the welfare of the community. Their tradition of fiscal conservancy has put IRMC in the top 5 percent of hospitals across the country for financial indicators.

At a time when many other hospitals are being forced to merge, IRMC has renewed its commitment to retaining its independence in order to continue making

The Auxiliary Takes a Stand

Indiana Hospital Auxiliary's minutes from 1949 read, "a resolution was introduced and passed that the Indiana Hospital is opposed to any form of socialized medicine and will do all in its power to defeat such legislation." Unfortunately, we have no way of knowing what event inspired the Auxiliary to pass the resolution. There is no doubt, however, where they stood on the issue.

healthcare decisions that put the community's needs first. As the hospital attains new levels of excellence, providing comprehensive services, economic growth for the region is enhanced. "We're very blessed," Steve Wolfe said, "to have a robust business community with whom we've had a tradition of partnering." The people of IRMC are understandably proud of their role as the community's sole healthcare provider. As the second largest employer, IRMC is the heartbeat of the communities it serves. And the people they care for are not just patients—they are friends, they are family, and they are neighbors.

"To think that in 1914 when the founders established this community," Steve Wolfe reflected, "this coalescing of people who wanted to take care of others . . . they were volunteering or making very little money. To see that continue to evolve after one hundred years is exciting." Despite the challenges and the uncertainties that lie ahead, Indiana Regional Medical Center is in a strong position for the future. "We've earned the right to remain independent, at least for the next three to four years," Mr. Wolfe said. "To go beyond that depends on all of us and our ability to stay focused like a laser on the things we can control—great quality and great service."

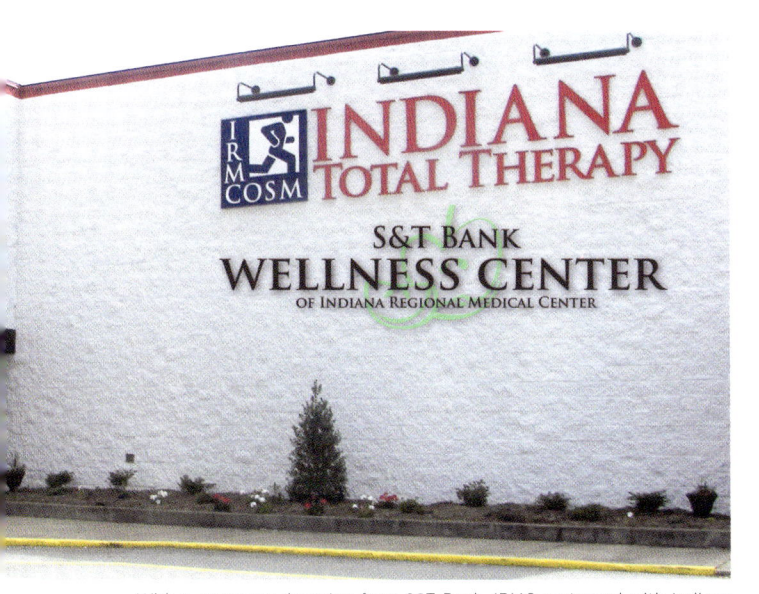

With a generous donation from S&T Bank, IRMC partnered with Indiana Total Therapy (ITT) in 2012 to create the S&T Wellness Center at the ITT West location on Shelly Drive in Indiana. The Center specializes in medically based fitness, giving patients a safe, medically supervised environment for the exercise that is so vital to recovery and overall quality of life.

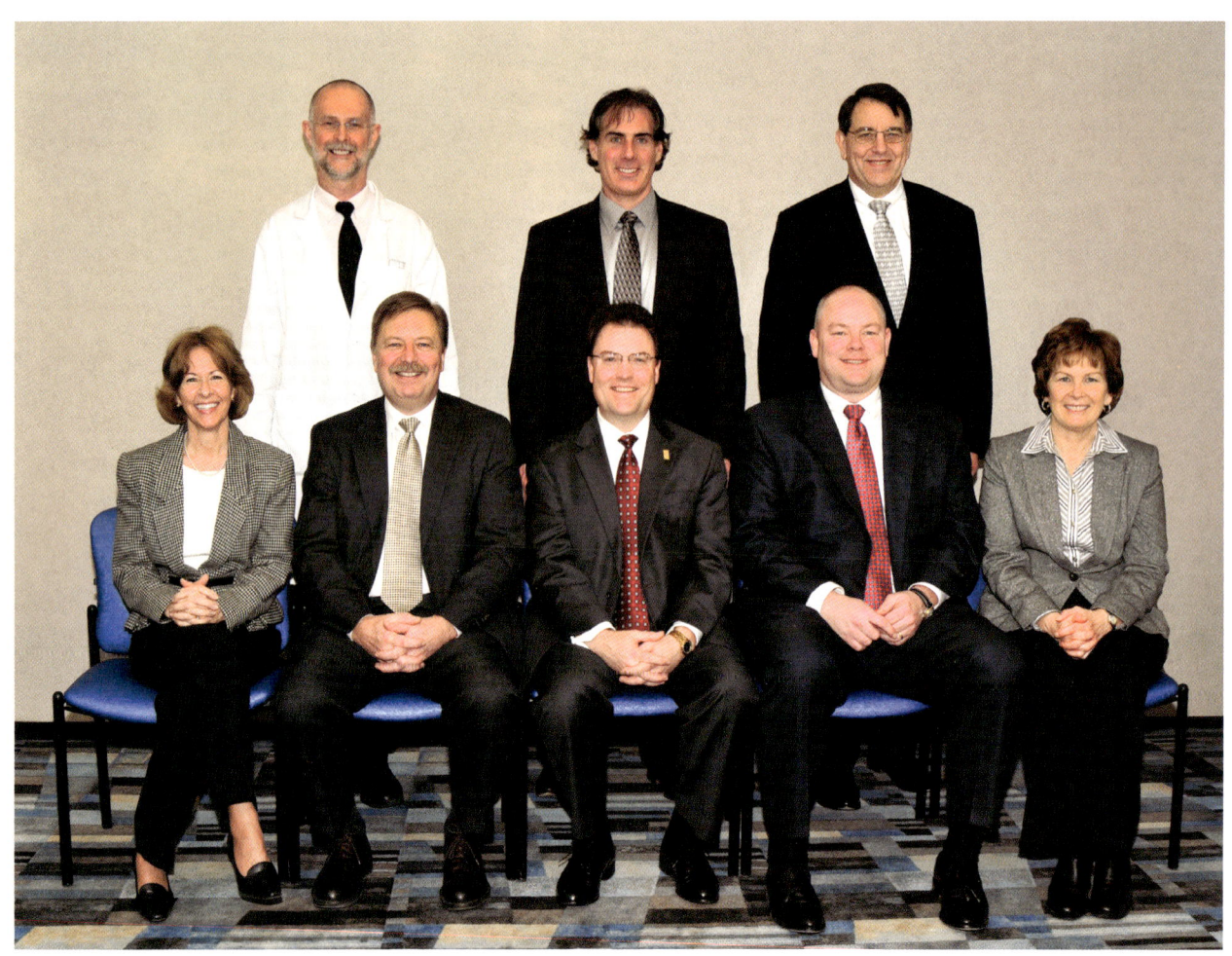

IRMC's board of directors serve on a volunteer basis and represent the best the community has to offer.

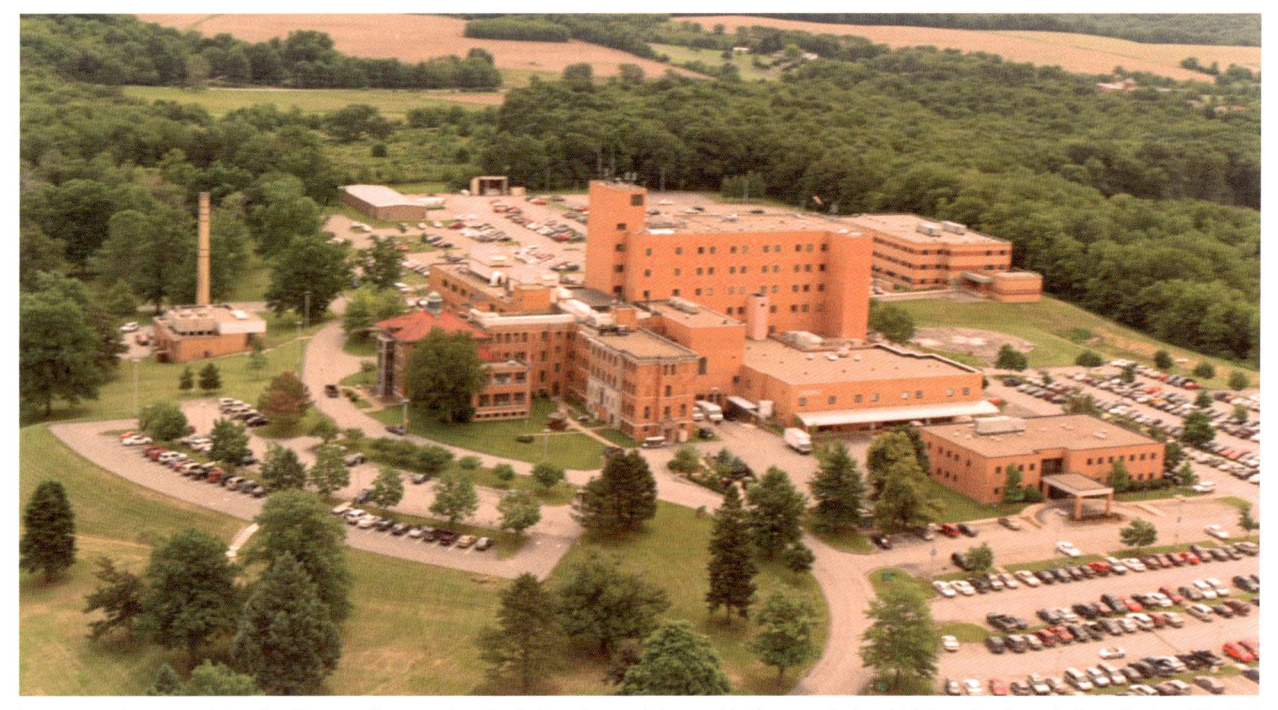

In an area urban enough to offer the amenities people enjoy but rural enough to provide the serenity in which to enjoy them, Indiana Regional Medical Center is key to the area's continued economic development.

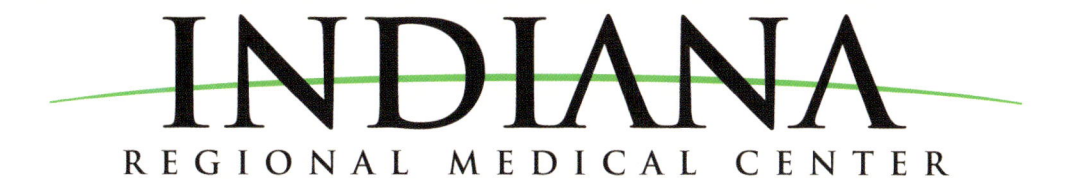

INDIANA
REGIONAL MEDICAL CENTER
SUPPORTING COMMUNITY HEALTH

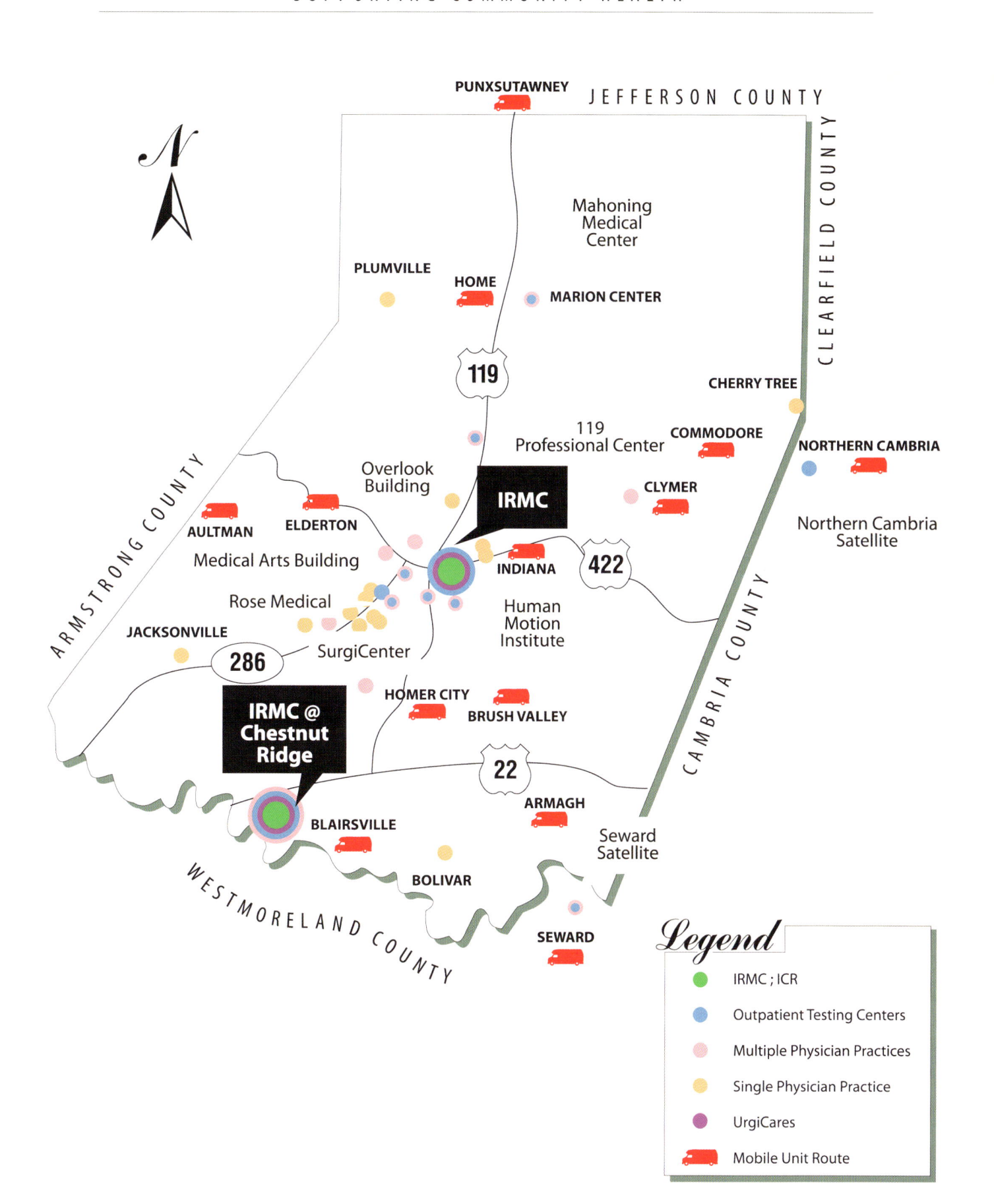

JEFFERSON COUNTY

PUNXSUTAWNEY

Mahoning Medical Center

PLUMVILLE

HOME

MARION CENTER

119

CHERRY TREE

119 Professional Center

COMMODORE

NORTHERN CAMBRIA

Overlook Building

IRMC

CLYMER

Northern Cambria Satellite

AULTMAN

ELDERTON

Medical Arts Building

INDIANA

422

Rose Medical

Human Motion Institute

JACKSONVILLE

286

SurgiCenter

HOMER CITY

BRUSH VALLEY

IRMC @ Chestnut Ridge

22

ARMAGH

BLAIRSVILLE

Seward Satellite

BOLIVAR

SEWARD

ARMSTRONG COUNTY

CLEARFIELD COUNTY

CAMBRIA COUNTY

WESTMORELAND COUNTY

Legend

- 🟢 IRMC ; ICR
- 🔵 Outpatient Testing Centers
- 🩷 Multiple Physician Practices
- 🟡 Single Physician Practice
- 🟣 UrgiCares
- 🚚 Mobile Unit Route

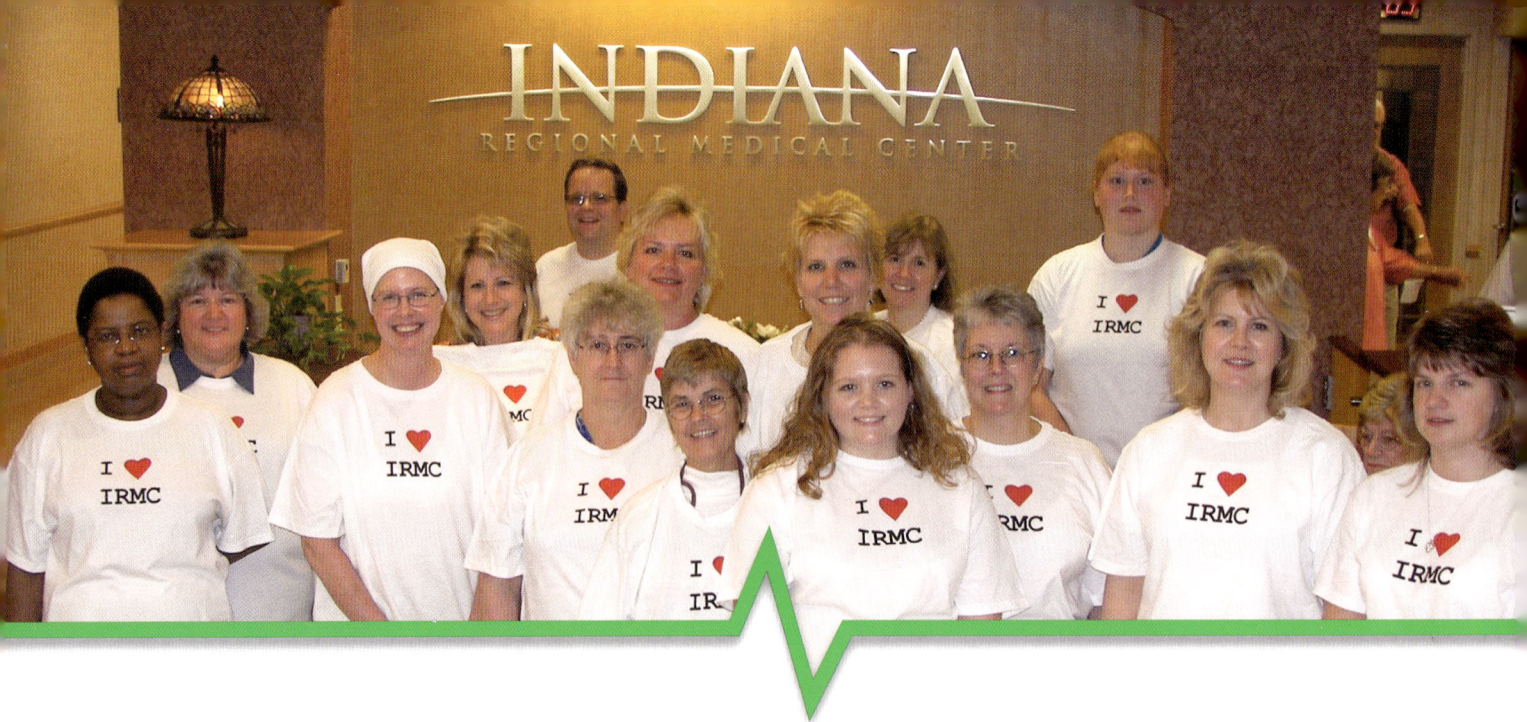

IRMC FAMILY ALBUM

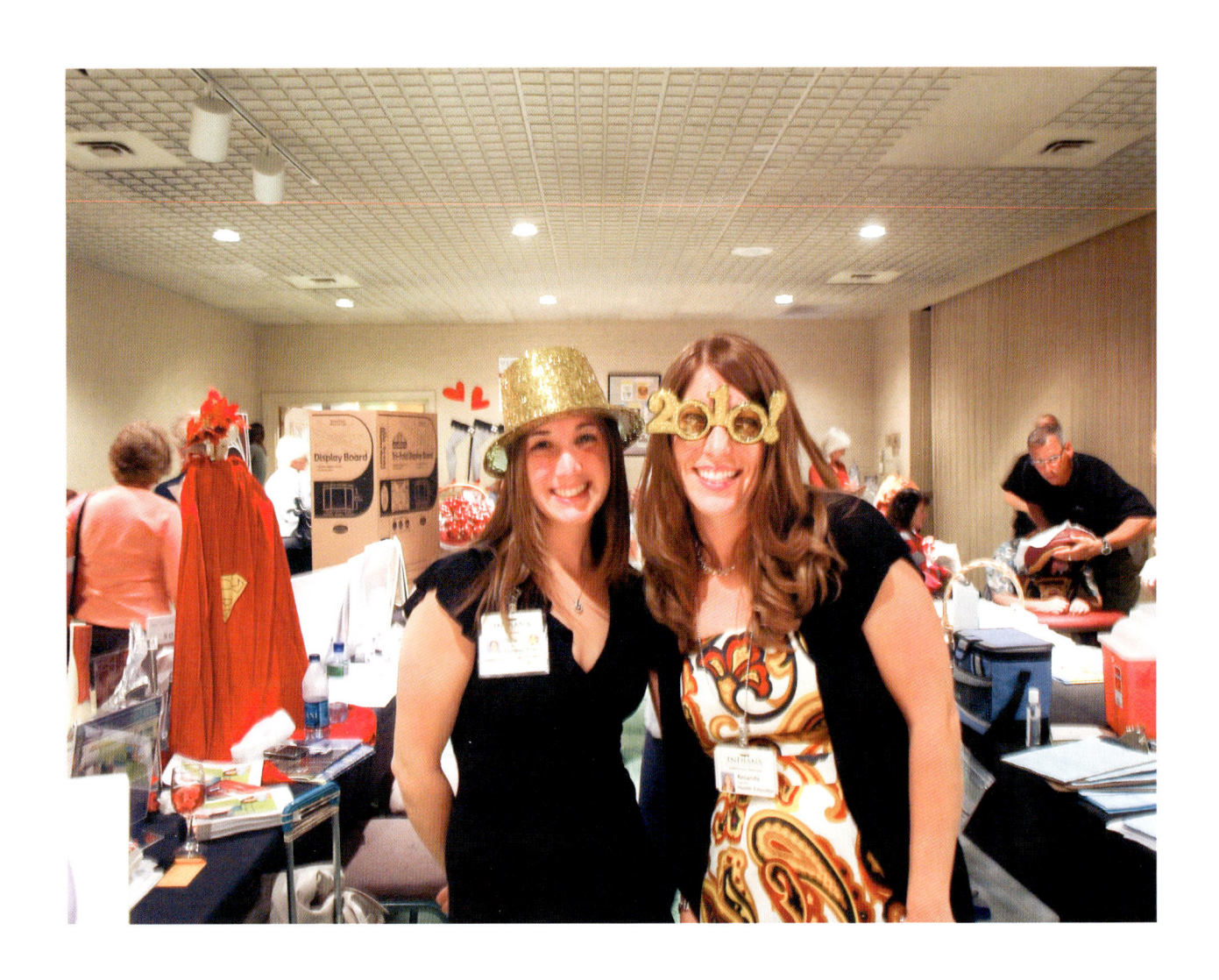

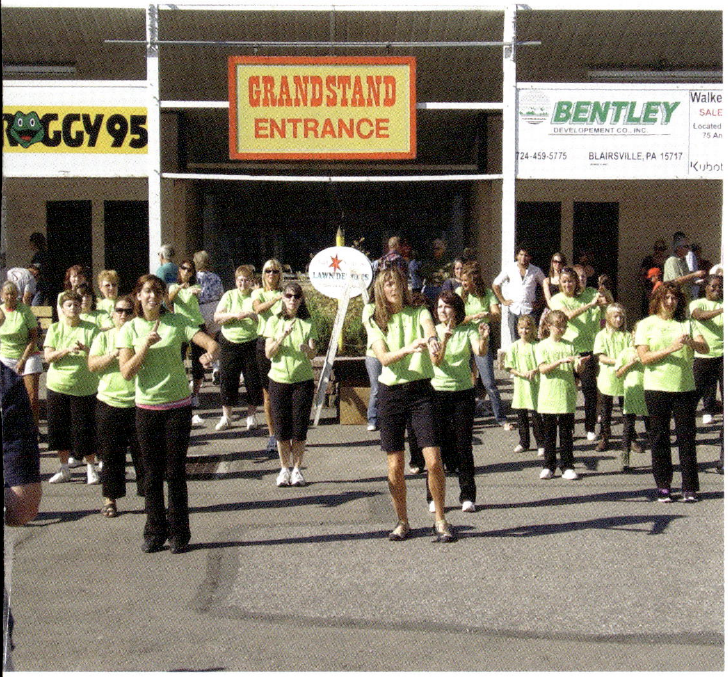
GRANDSTAND
ENTRANCE
BENTLEY
724-459-5775
BLAIRSVILLE, PA 15717

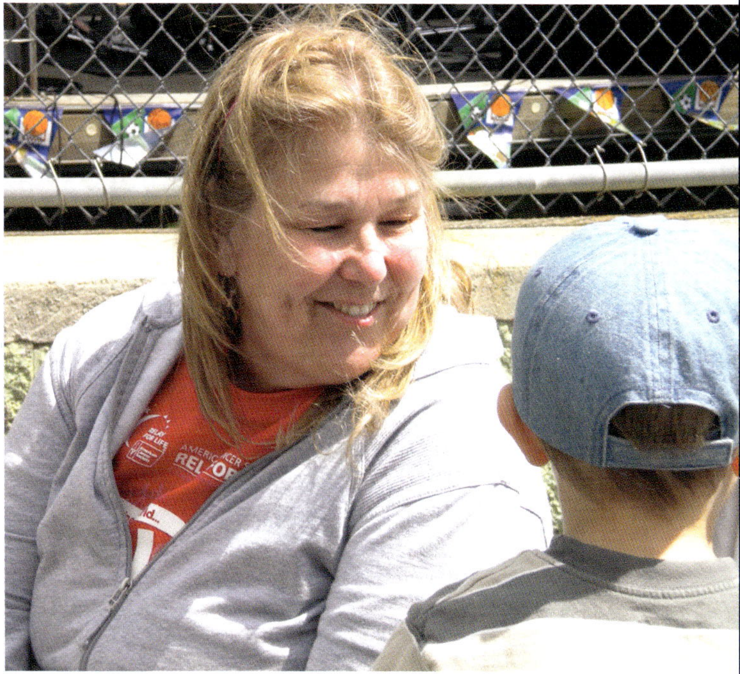

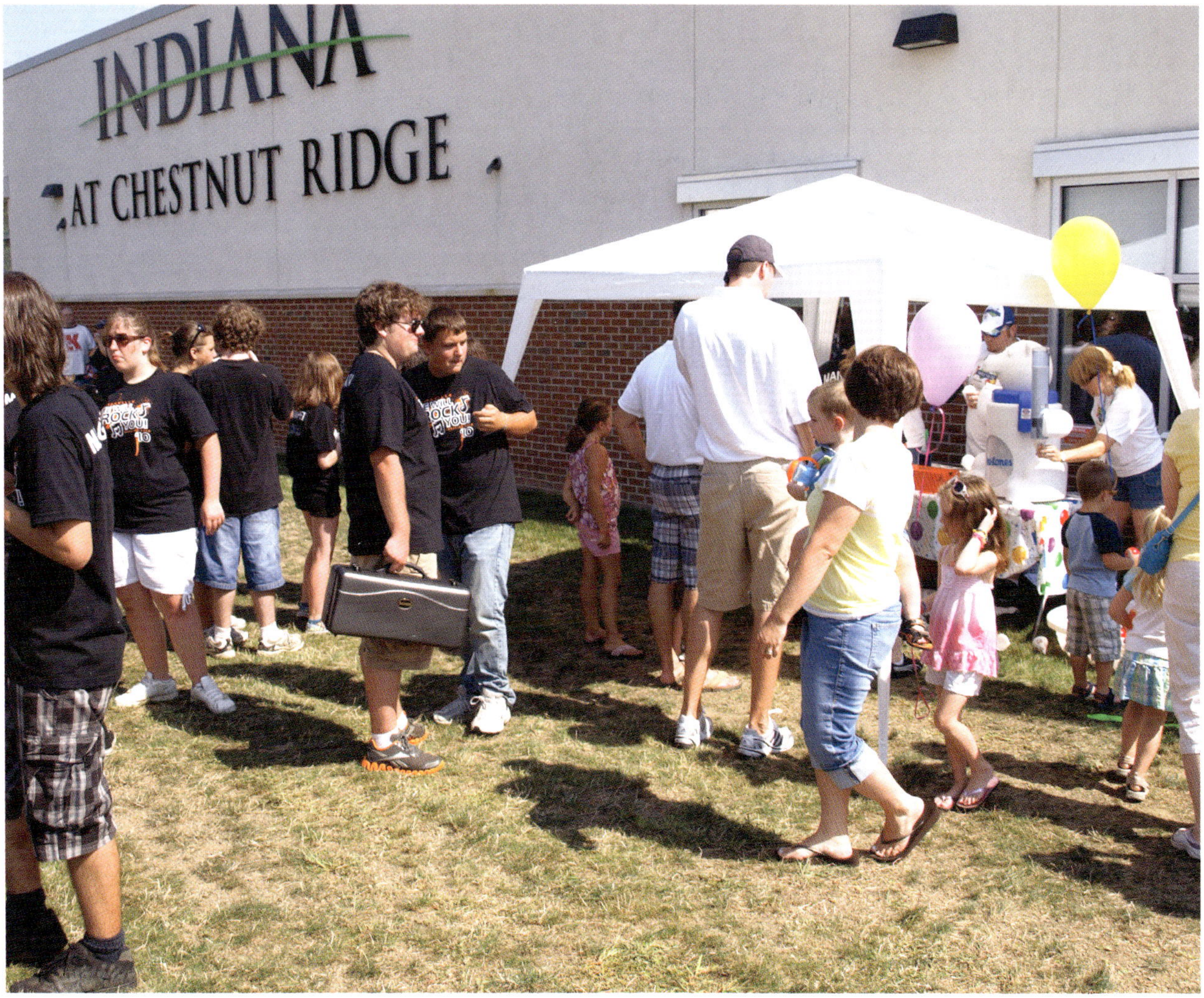
INDIANA
AT CHESTNUT RIDGE

"It is through their efforts that we are able to sustain a winning workplace culture."

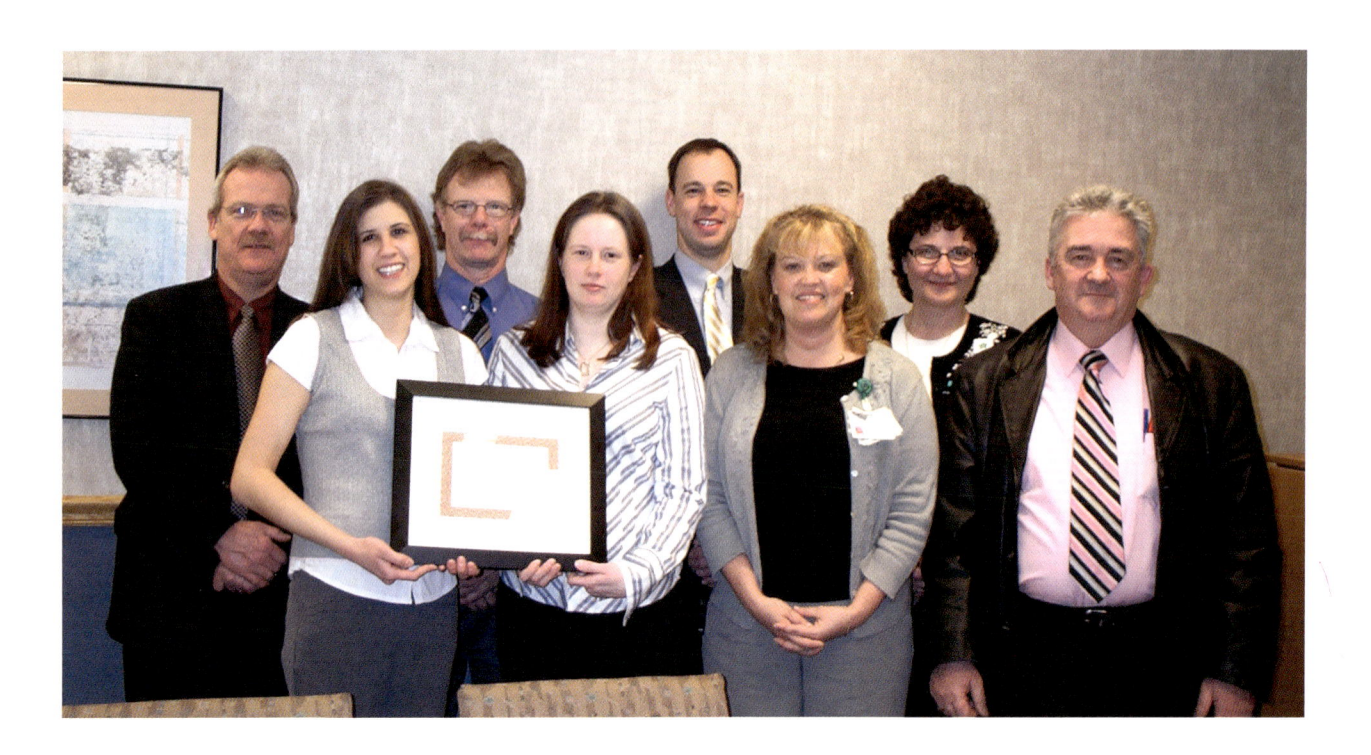

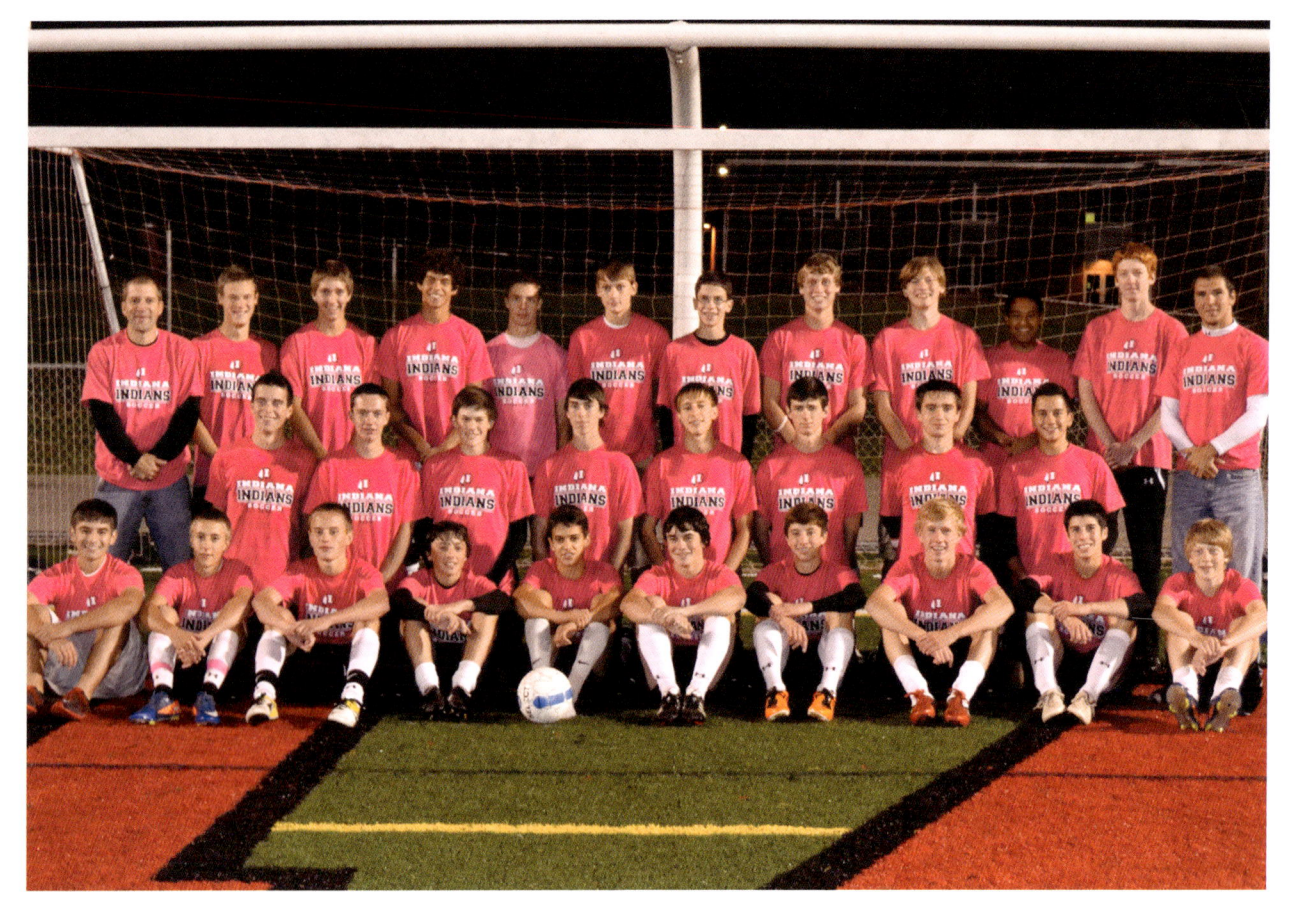

IRMC Family Album — 133

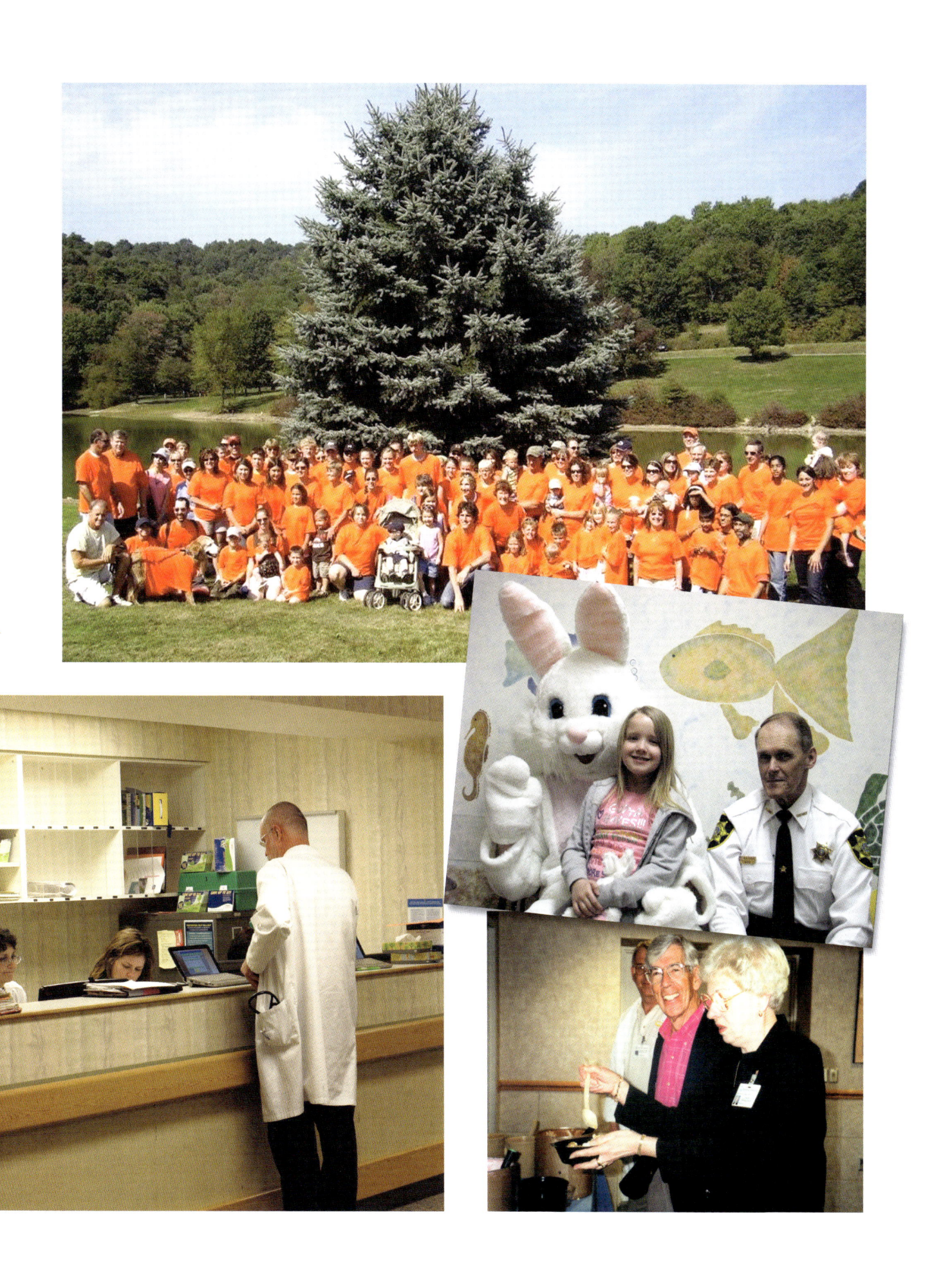

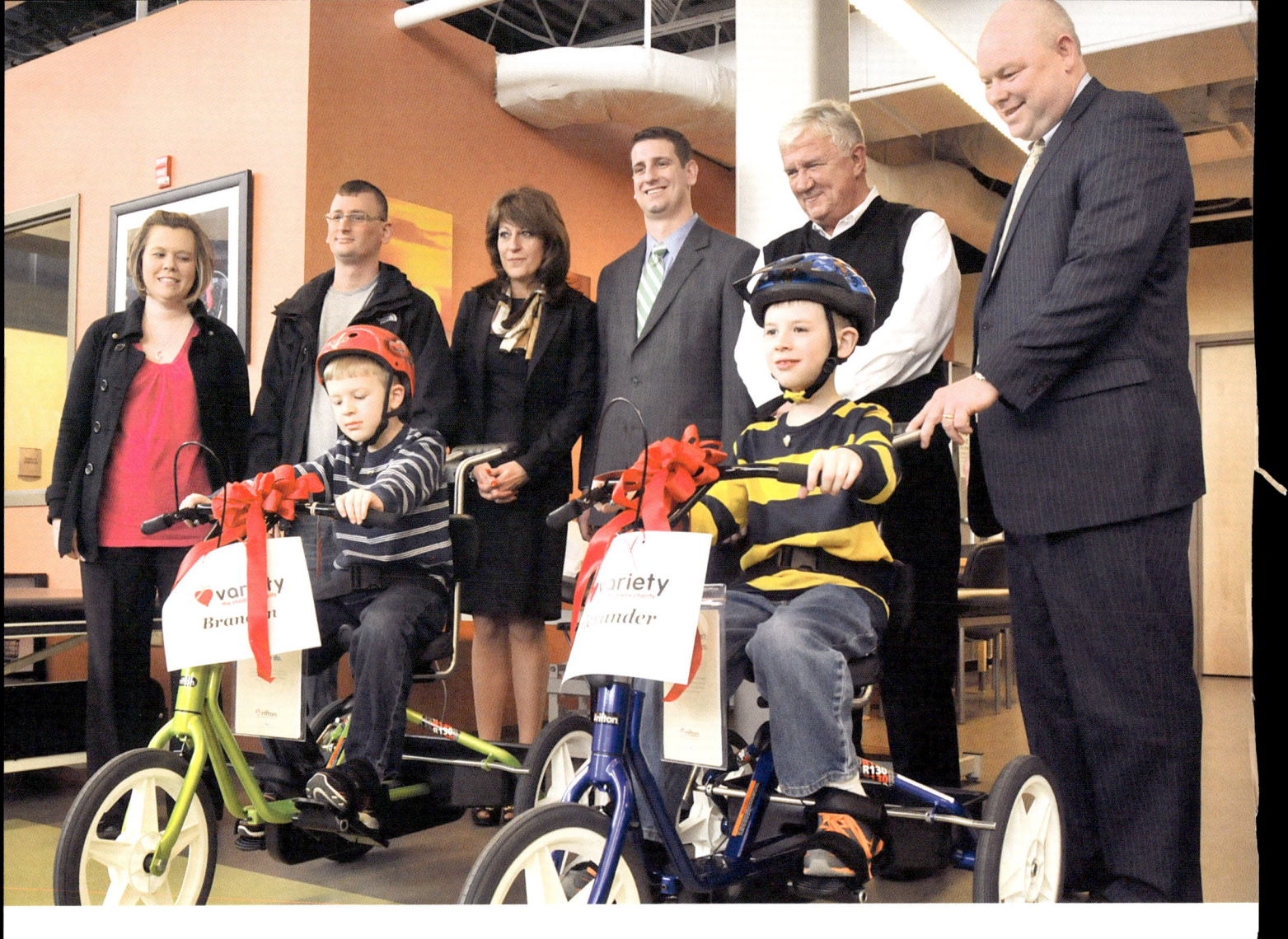

"We've come a long way, but we're going to go a lot further."

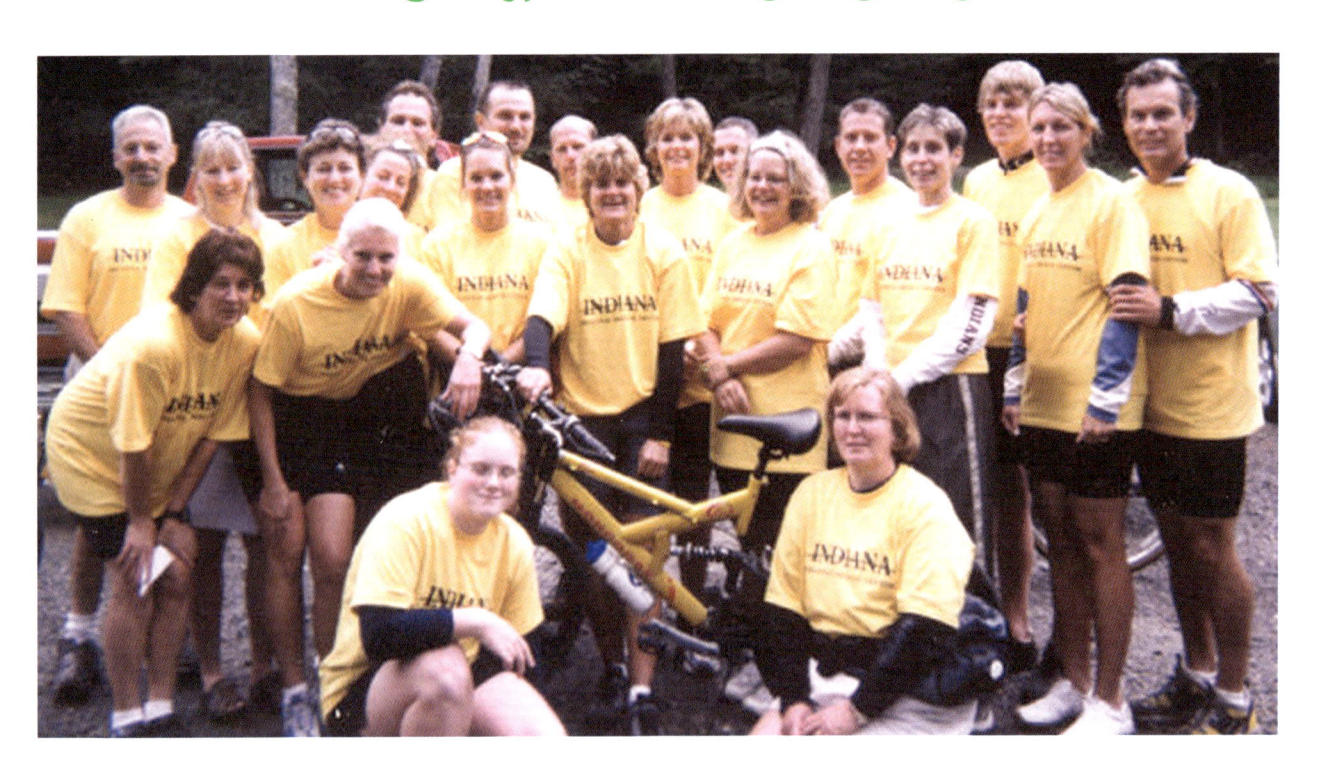

134 — Indiana Regional Medical Center

"I don't know that there is a greater calling on all the planet."

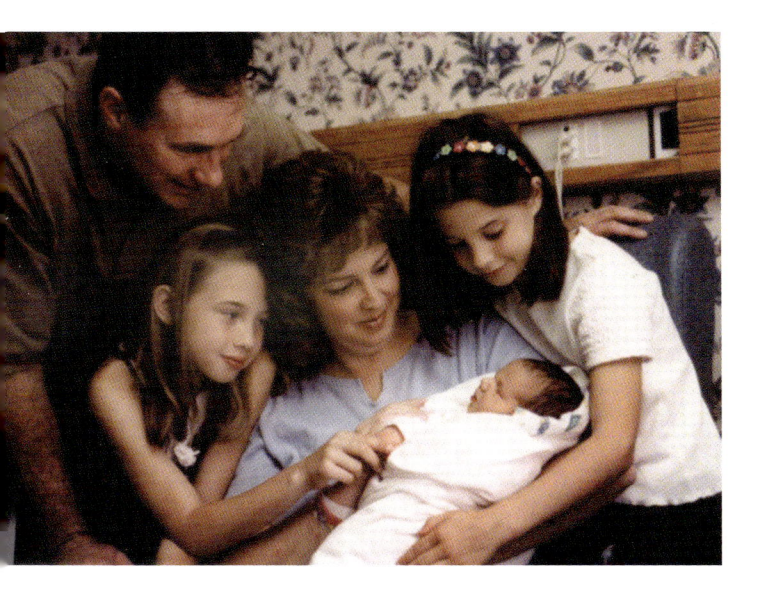

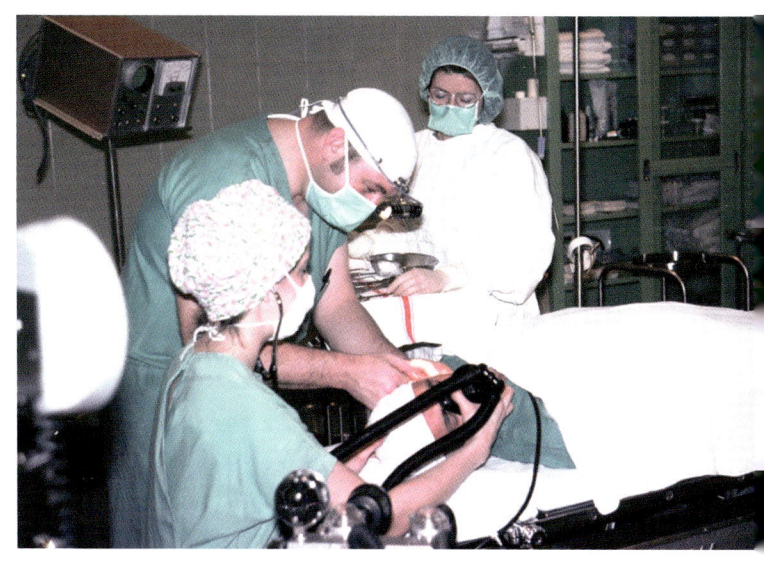

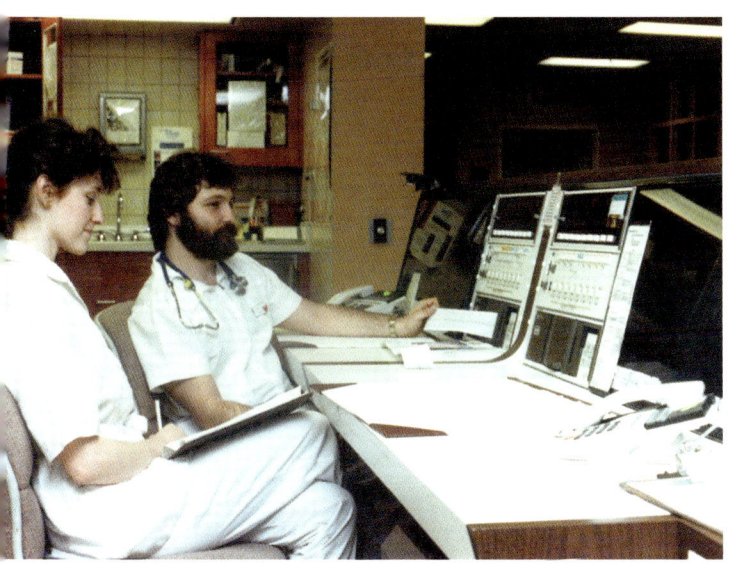

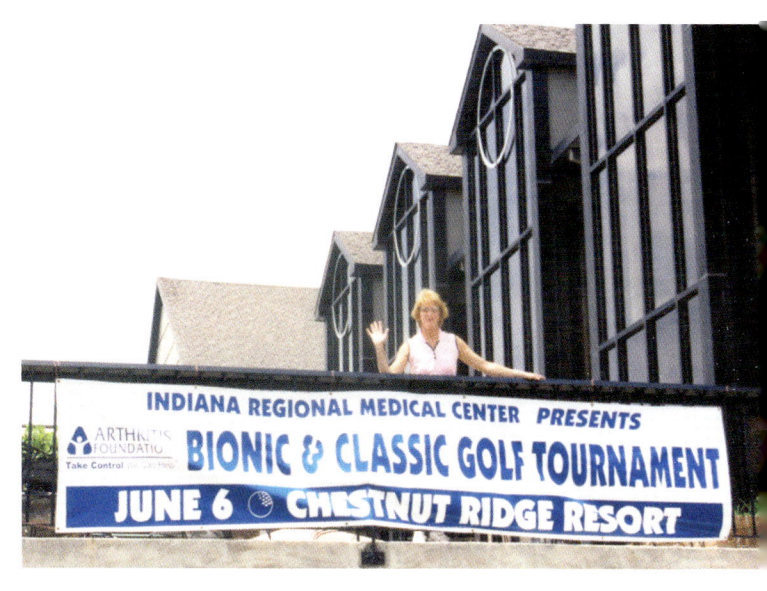

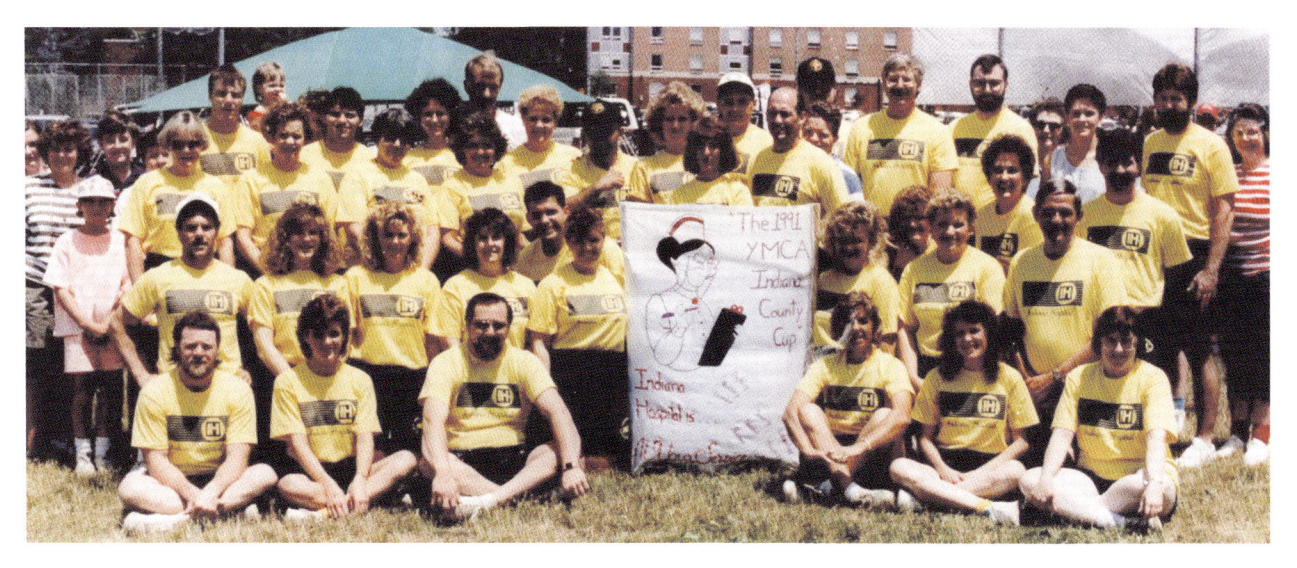

IRMC Family Album — 135

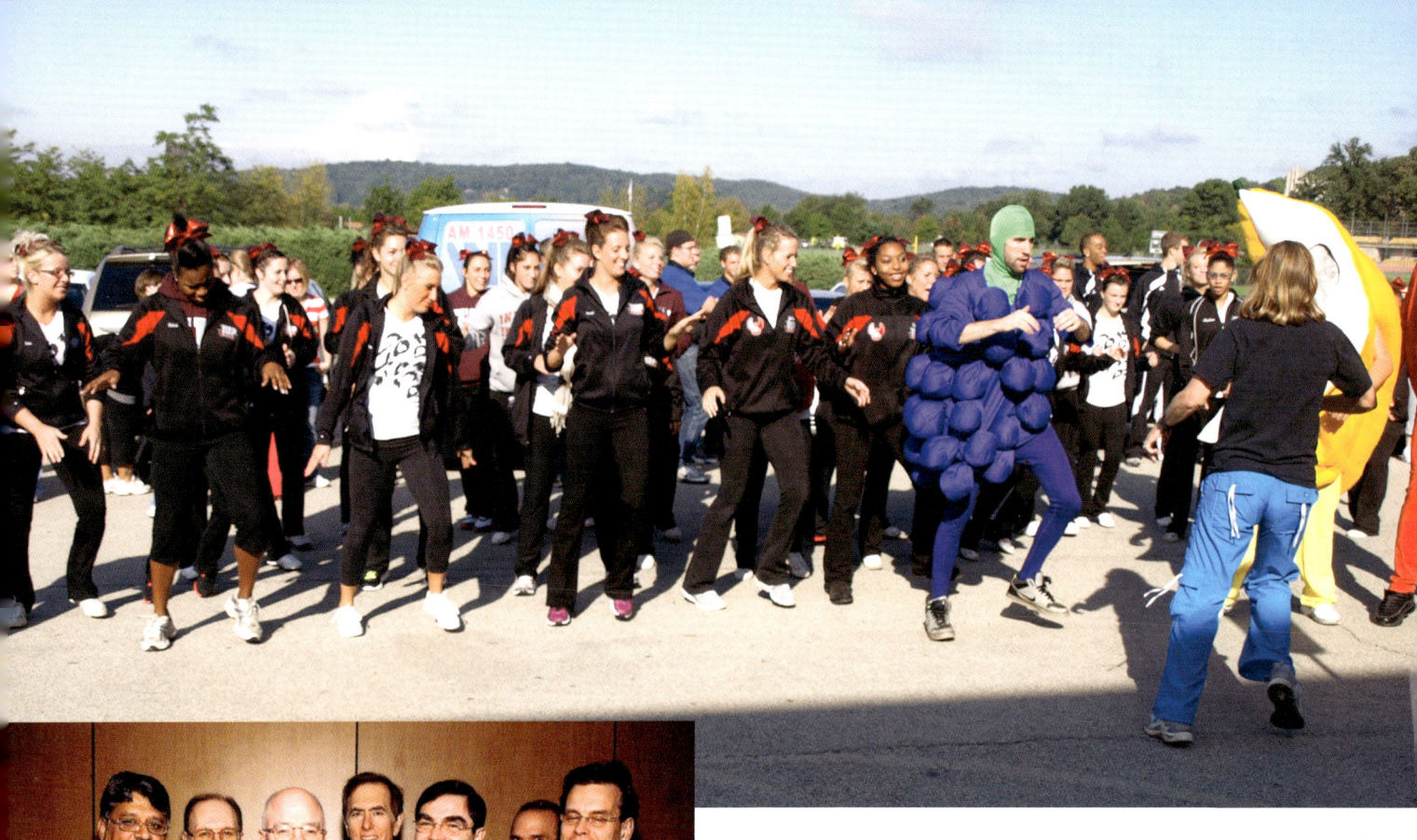

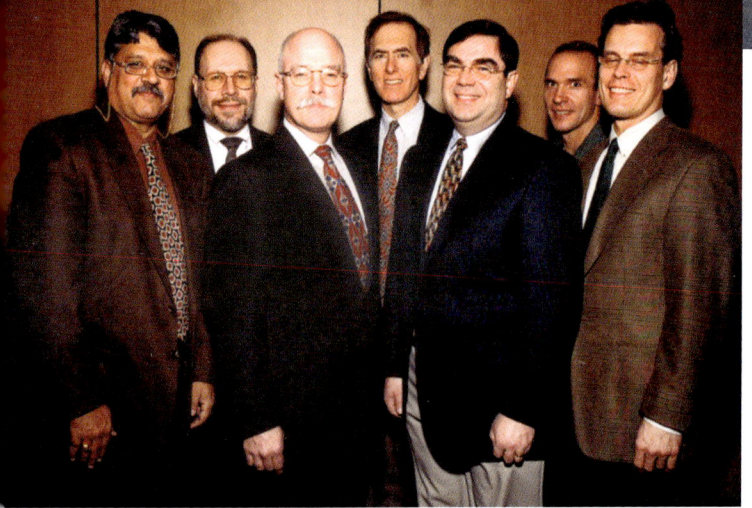

"We're incredibly blessed to have been able to attract and retain an outstanding medical staff."

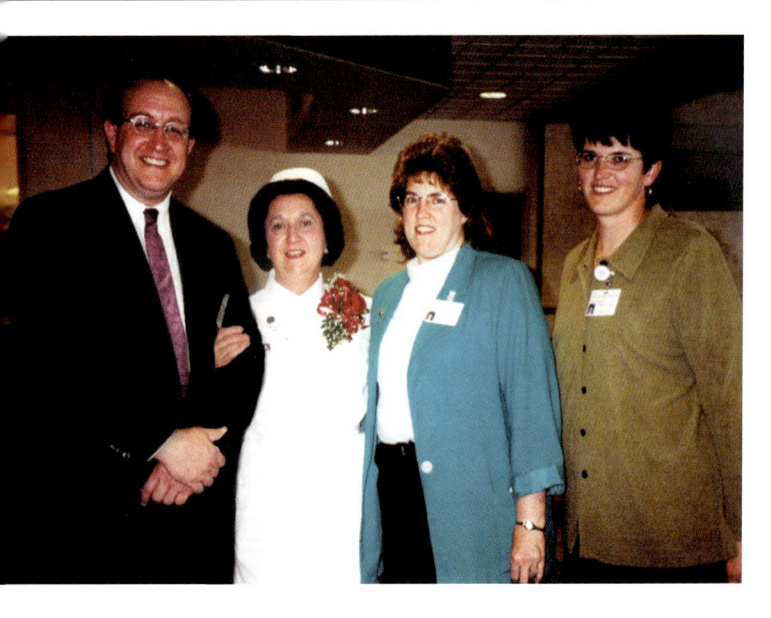

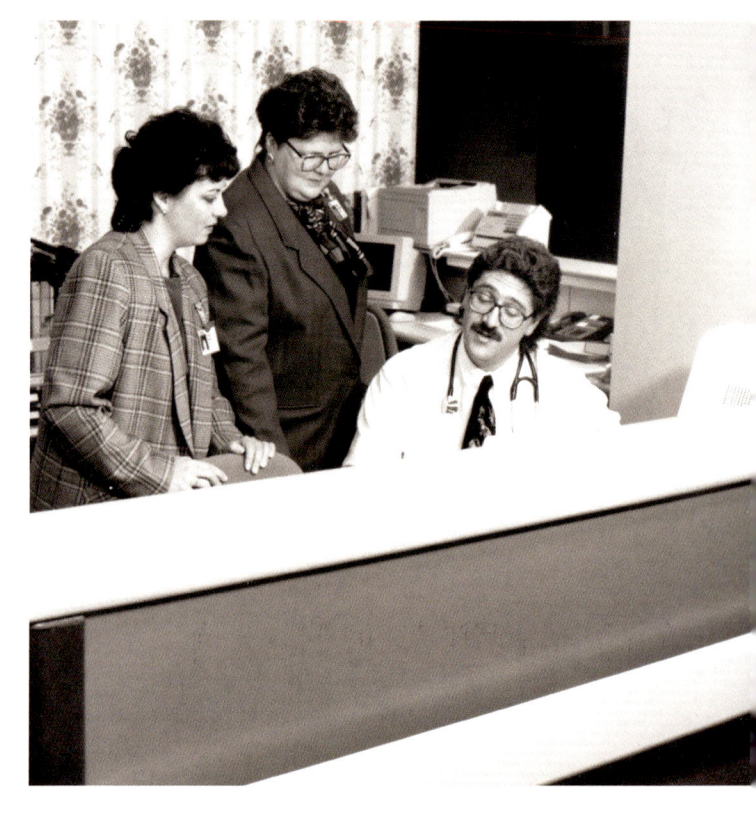

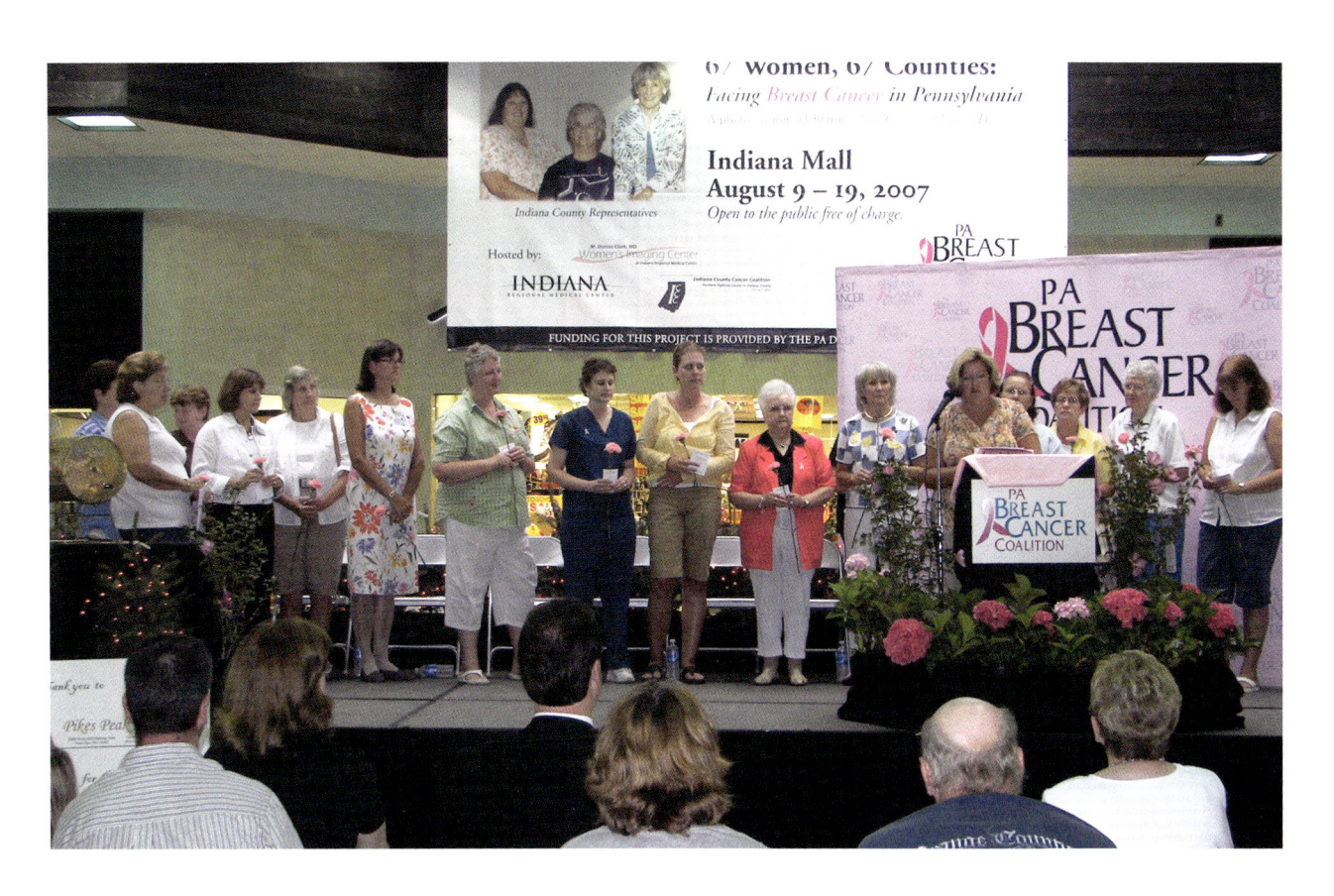

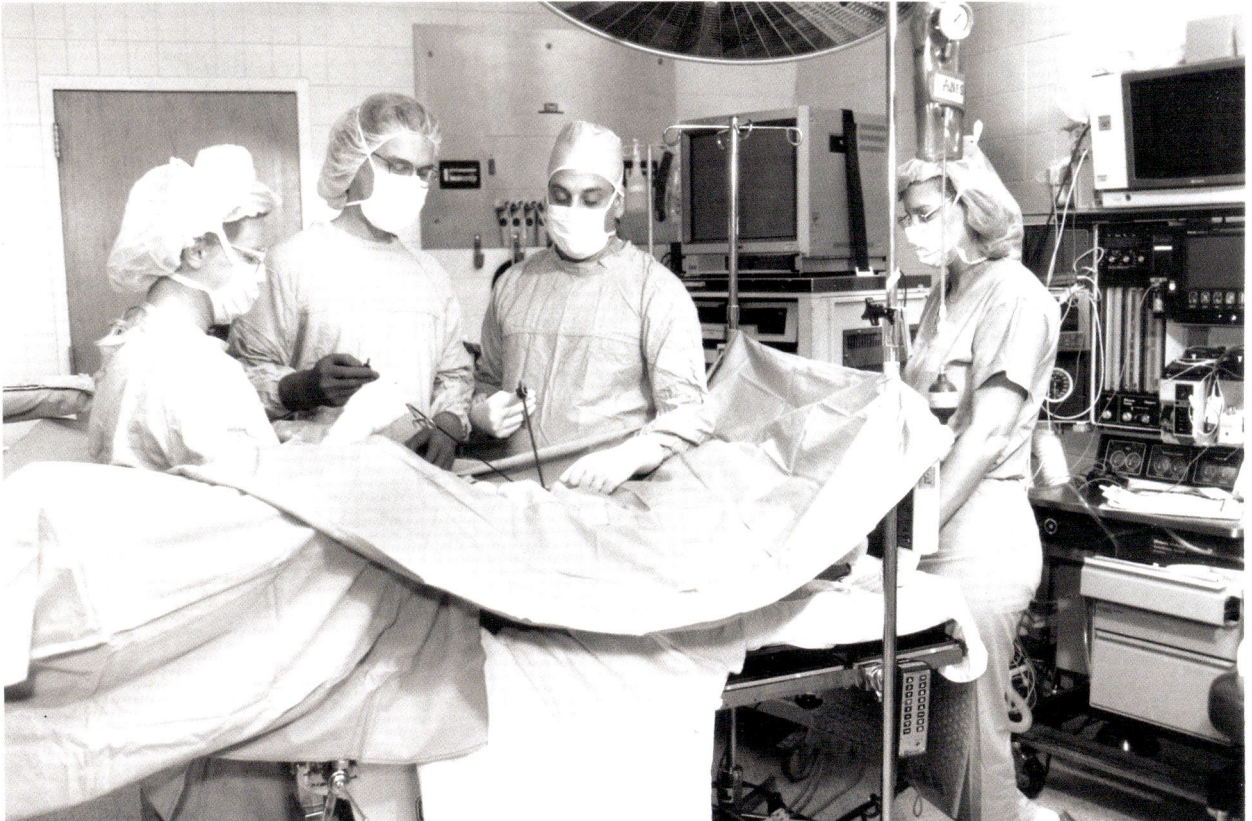

"We've created a culture that believes in itself."

IRMC Family Album — 137

"Our core competency now is our culture of people."

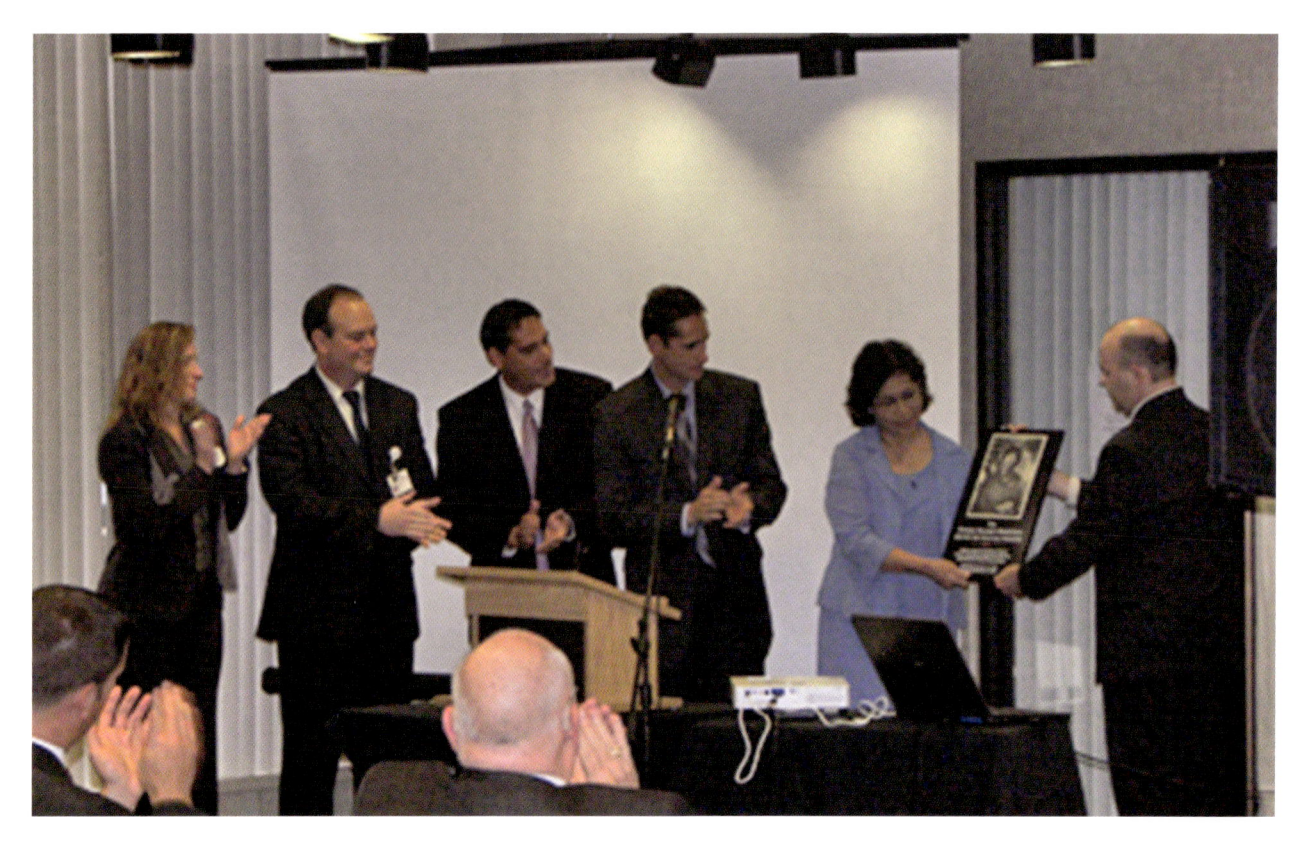

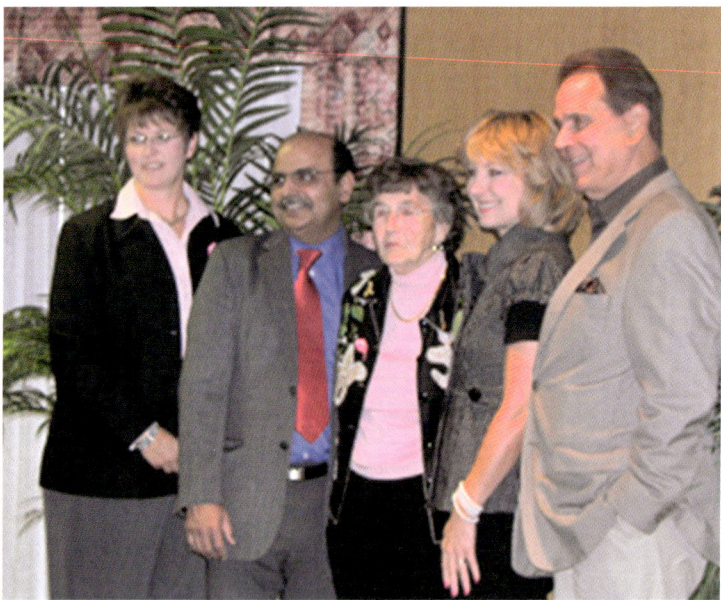

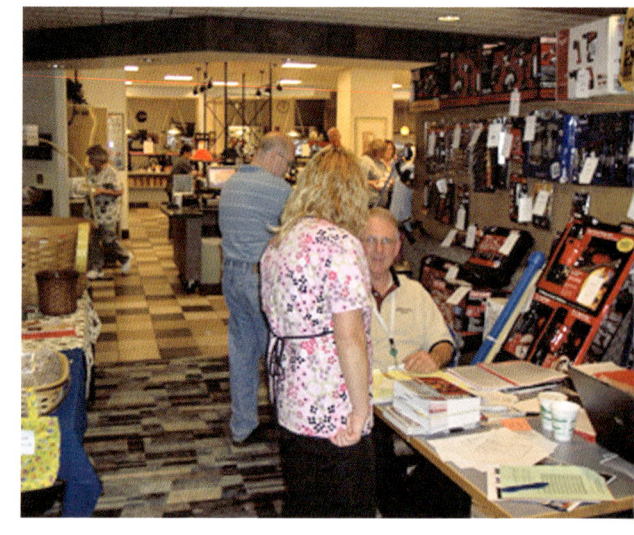

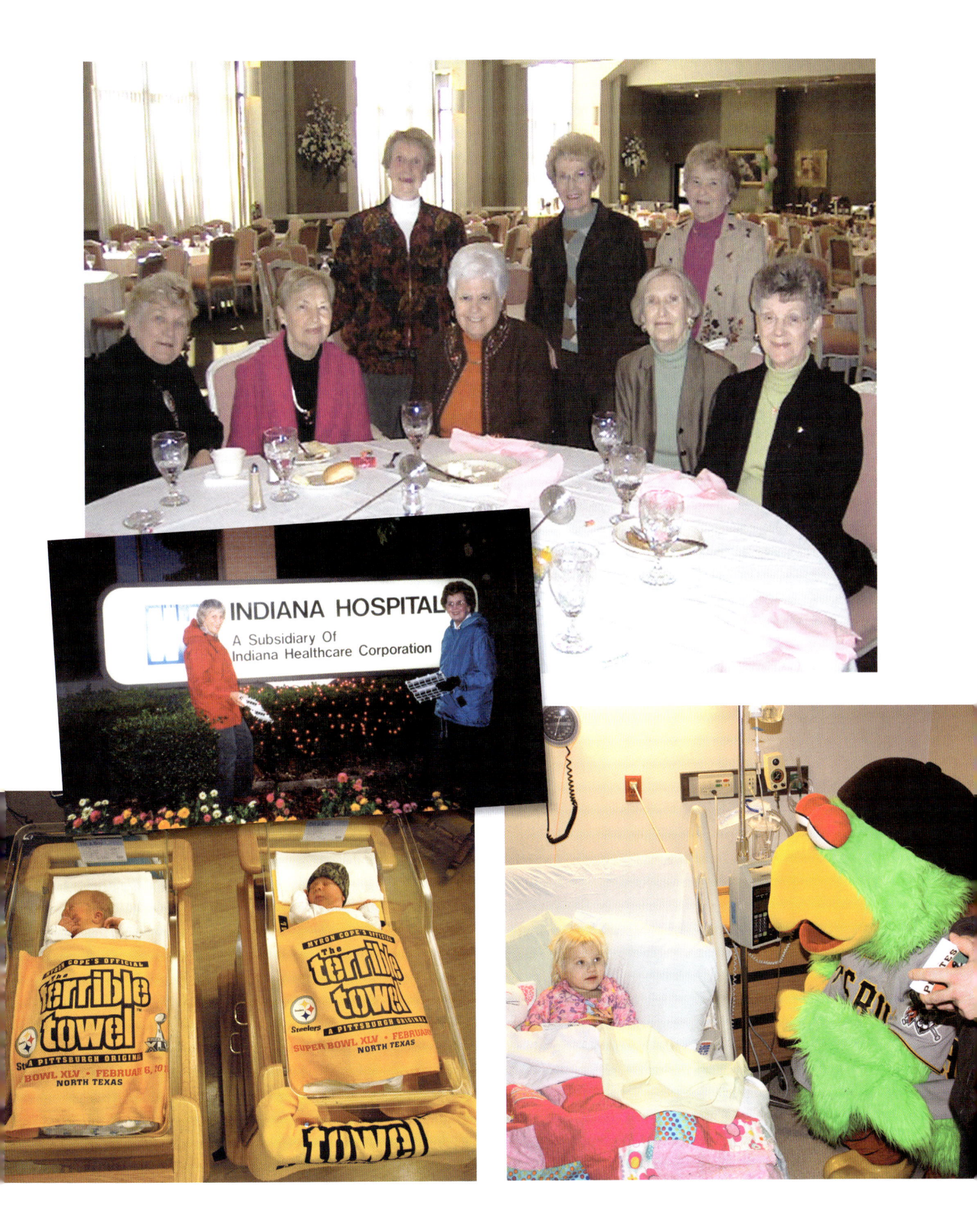

IRMC Family Album —— 139

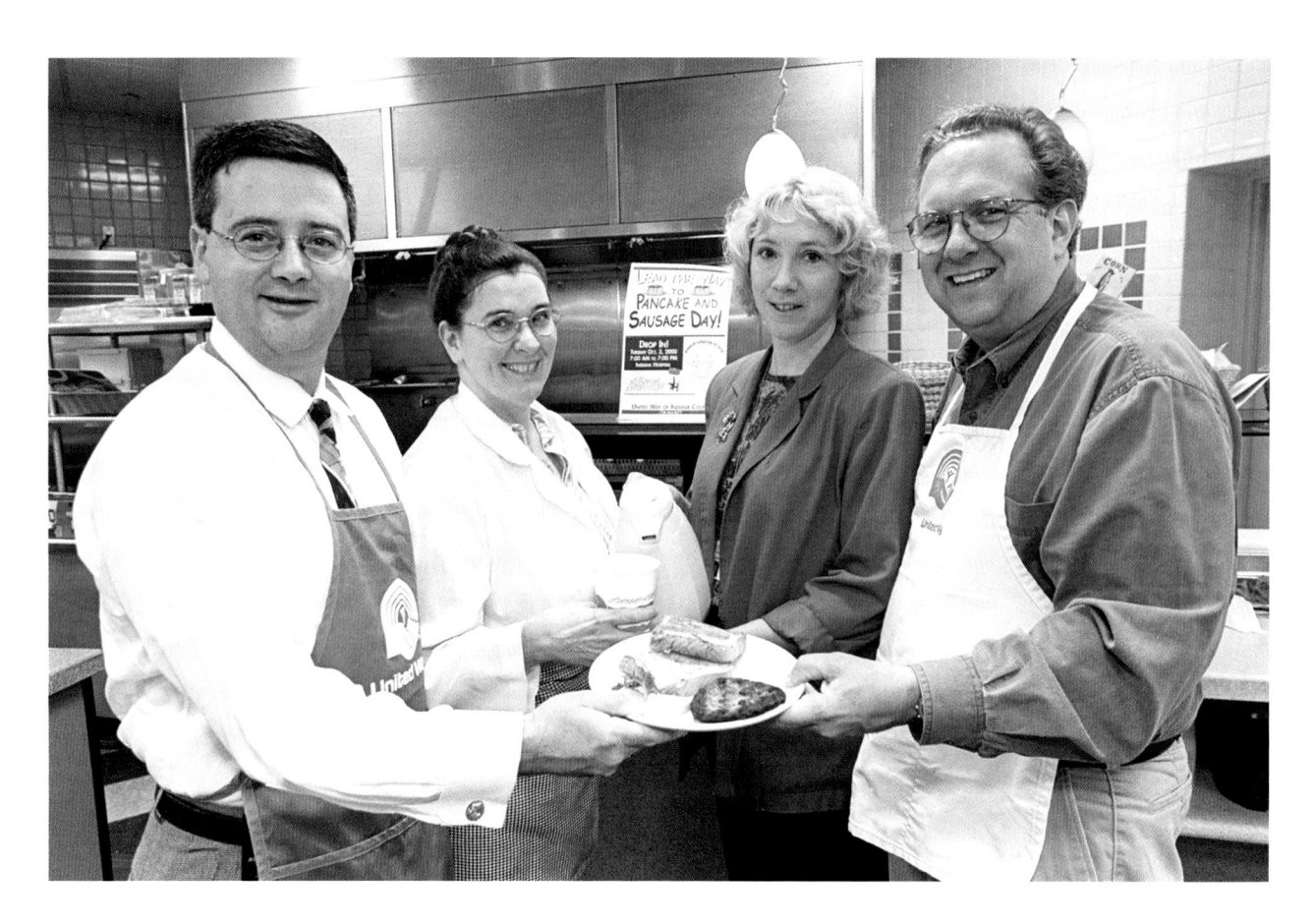

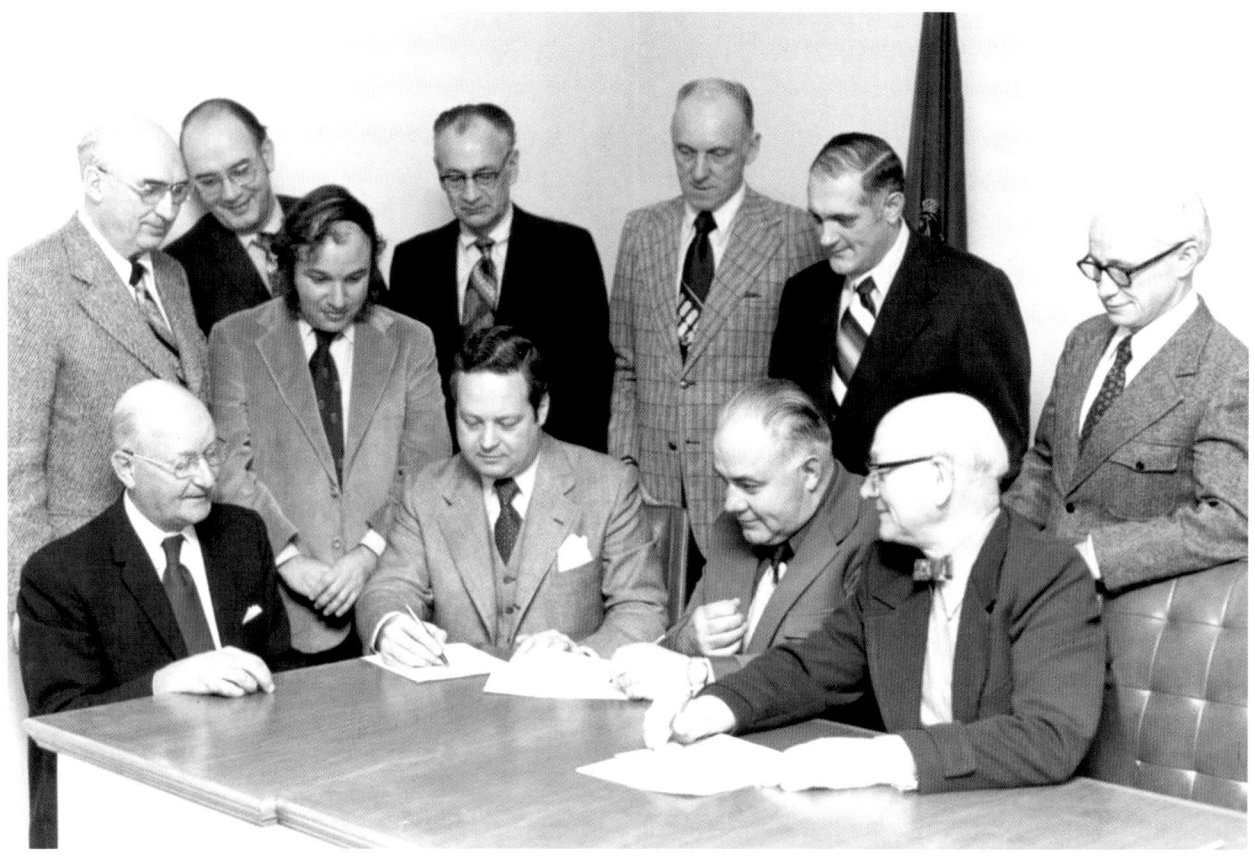

140 — Indiana Regional Medical Center

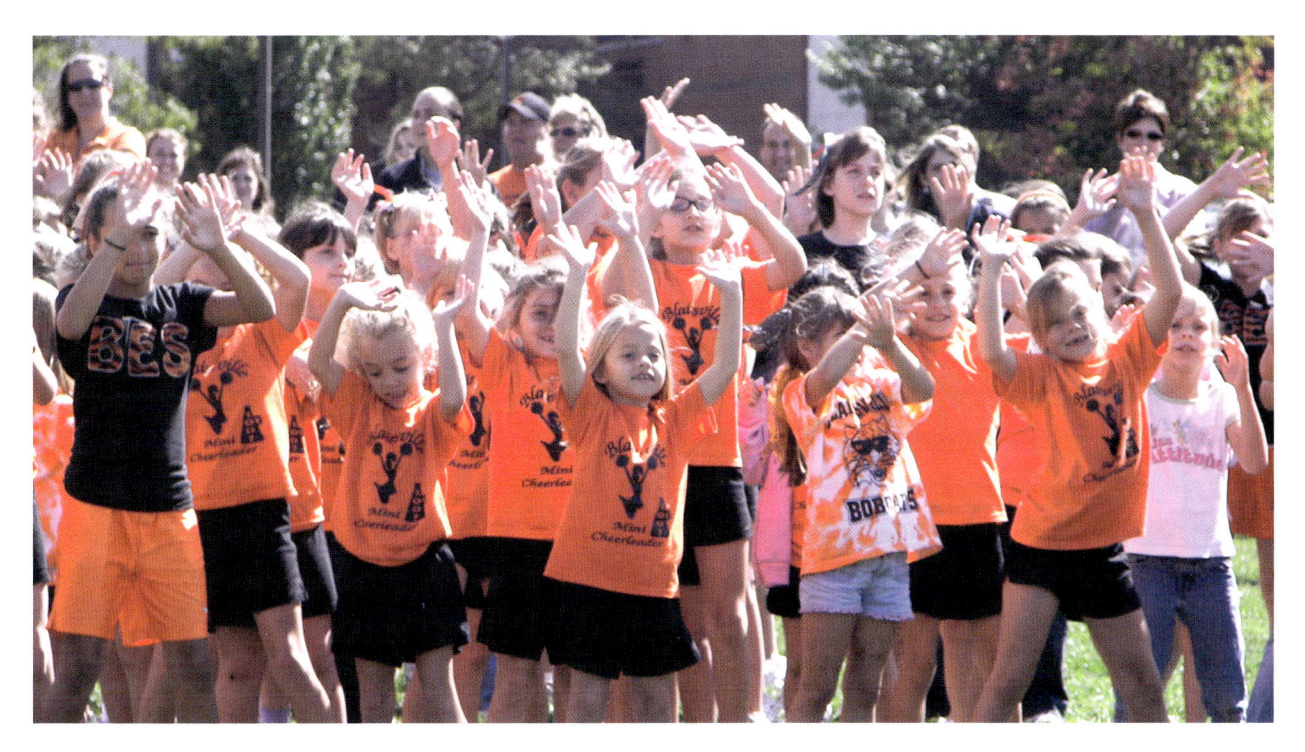

"We've earned the right to remain independent."

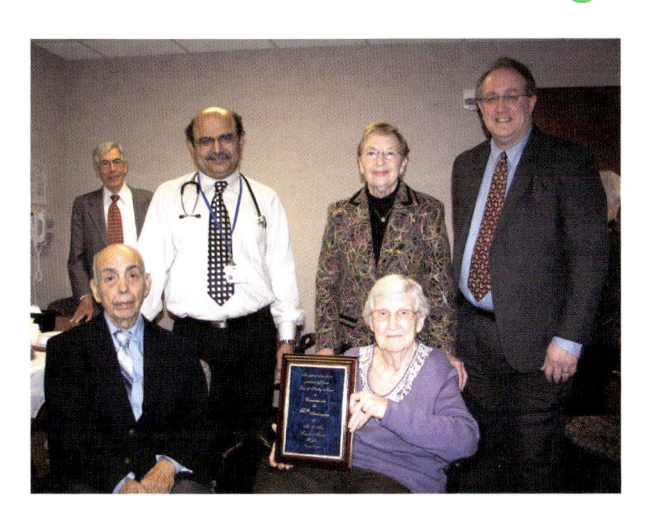

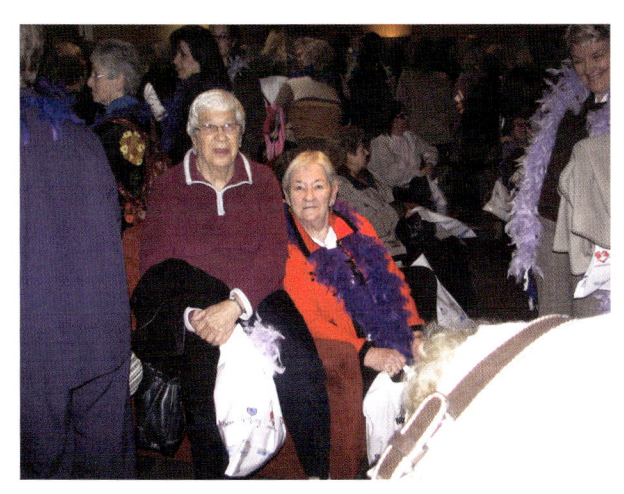

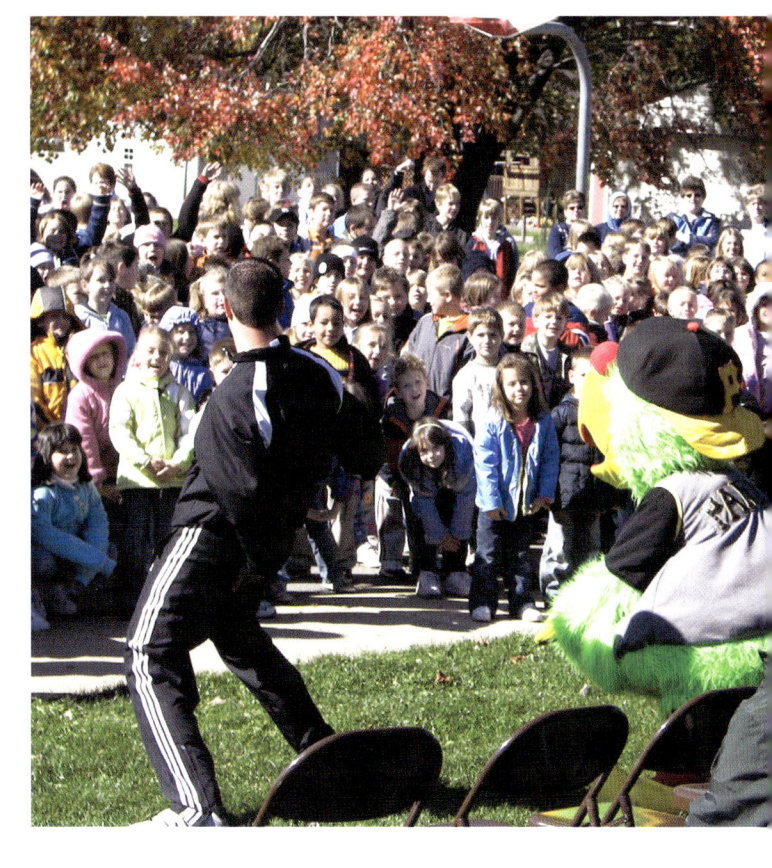

SELECTED REFERENCES

BOOKS

Anderson, William, MD. *A Brief Biographical Sketch of the Medical Profession of Indiana County*

Stephenson, Clarence D. *Indiana County, 175th Anniversary History*, Vols. II and III

NEWSPAPER ARTICLES

"Break Ground Yesterday for Indiana Hospital Addition," *Indiana Evening Gazette*, July 3, 1976

"Cancer center to offer comprehensive care," by Gina DelFavero, *Blairsville Dispatch*, August 29, 2003

"Care and Concern Indiana Hospital's Trademark, *Indiana Evening Gazette*, August 8, 1966

"CEO: Hospital a key to community growth," by Randy Wells, *Indiana Gazette*, October 18, 2005

"Dedication Major Event," *Indiana Evening Gazette*, August 8, 1966

"Doctors paying to practice," by Elaine Jacobs, *Indiana Gazette*, October 26, 2003

"Dream Hospital Open to Public Saturday," *Indiana Evening Gazette*, June 17, 1937

"Faced with Shifting Marketplace, Indiana Hospital Changes Focus," *The Dispatch*, Blairsville, Pa., March 1, 1996

"First Woman Doctor for Indiana County," by Bill Hastings, *Indiana Evening Gazette*, August 31, 1953

"Highlight of Hospital's 35th Anniversary," *Indiana Evening Gazette*, November 1, 1949

"Hospital CEO: Expanded ER should cut wait time," by Randy Wells, *Indiana Gazette*, March 8, 2002

"Hospital eyes more room, more services," by Vicki Ruddock, *Indiana Gazette*, July 10, 1987

"Hospital Gets New Administrator," by Carl Kologie, *Indiana Evening Gazette*, June 11, 1970

"Hospital Plans Call for Expansion, Renovation" *Indiana Evening Gazette*, April 10, 1976

"Hospital's fiscal future uncertain," by Randy Wells, *Indiana Gazette*, October 13, 2003

"Hospitals to get less under Medicare," by Mary Frances Schadl, *Indiana Gazette*, May 23, 1984

"Indiana County Gets a New Hospital," *Indiana Evening Gazette*, October 29, 1914

"Indiana Hospital renovation project ahead of schedule," *Indiana Gazette*, April 12, 1998

"Indiana Hospital to Dedicate Memorial Building on Thursday," *Indiana Evening Gazette*, September 19, 1939

"Indiana Hospital to offer kidney dialysis services," *Indiana Gazette*, August 15, 1988

"Indiana Hospital volunteers provide crucial services," by Randy Wells, *Indiana Gazette*, September 27, 1999

"Indiana Hospital, First Opened in 1914, Protects Health of Countians," *Indiana Gazette*, June 6, 1953

"Indiana Joins in Observance of National Hospital Week," *Indiana Evening Gazette*, May 9, 1970

"Indiana Nursing School Marks Half Century," *Indiana Evening Gazette*, July 27, 1968

"Indiana's Lady Doctor Credits 'Pop' and Principal for Success," by Joe Donnelly, *Indiana Evening Gazette*, September 30, 1953

"IRMC opens Blairsville health center," by Lauren Daley, *Indiana Gazette*, August 28, 2009

"IRMC, Phoenix win nominations," *Indiana Gazette*, September 5, 2010

"Know Your Hospital," *Indiana Evening Gazette*, September 20, 1939

"Laboratory Open House," *Indiana Evening Gazette*, June 11, 1958

"Let Contracts for Buildings," *Indiana Evening Gazette*, August 10, 1938

"Members of Indiana County Medical Society," *Indiana Evening Gazette*, June 29, 1952

"New CEO sees opportunities in challenges facing hospitals," by Randy Wells, *Indiana Gazette*, March 23, 1999

"New Outpatient Services Building Ready for Hospital's Daily Visitors," *The Dispatch,* Blairsville, Pa., March 19, 1992.

An Open Letter to the People of Indiana County, *Indiana Gazette*, May 11, 2002

"Pressure mounting on Indiana Hospital," by Mary Ann Slater, *Indiana Gazette*, October 20, 2000

"Report Made on Hospital," *Indiana Evening Gazette*, May 13, 1958

"Report: IRMC better off financially," by Randy Wells, *Indiana Gazette*, April 29, 2005

"Sandoval resigns top hospital post," *Indiana Gazette*, April 27, 1998

"School of Nursing Ending, Played Key Role," *Indiana Evening Gazette*, December 7, 1976

"16 more doctors added to Indiana Hospital's rolls," *Indiana Gazette*, March 31, 1986

"Staff shortages delay emergency room care," by Helen Noon, *Indiana Gazette*, March 2, 1990

"Substantial Gift for Local Hospital," *The Indiana Progress*, October 1, 1935

"TB Unit Gift Aids Hospital," *Indiana Evening Gazette*, May 3, 1968

"The movement for a Hospital in Indiana," by Clarence Stephenson, *Indiana Gazette*, November 4, 1989

"What the Indiana Hospital Development Fund Means to You," *Indiana Evening Gazette*, May 16, 1975

"Woman's Touch Guides Hospital," *Indiana Evening Gazette,* August 8, 1966

WEBSITES

http://www.digitalhistory.uh.edu/historyonline/childbirth.cfm, Accessed 2/6/13

http://dpsinfo.com/wb/medhistory.html, Accessed 2/6/13

http://www.mcintyrepa.com/Aiselin.htm, Accessed 2/7/13

http://en.wikipedia.org/wiki/History_of_poliomyelitis, Accessed 2/18/13

ABOUT THE AUTHOR

Pat Swinger began writing for The Donning Company Publishers after working with them to publish her hometown's history during its sesquicentennial in 2006. Except for the seventeen years she lived in Kirkwood, during which time she received her degree from Washington University in St. Louis, Pat has lived her entire life in O'Fallon, Missouri. Her passion for the preservation of local histories extends to her work with clients, helping organizations and corporations preserve and tell their own stories.

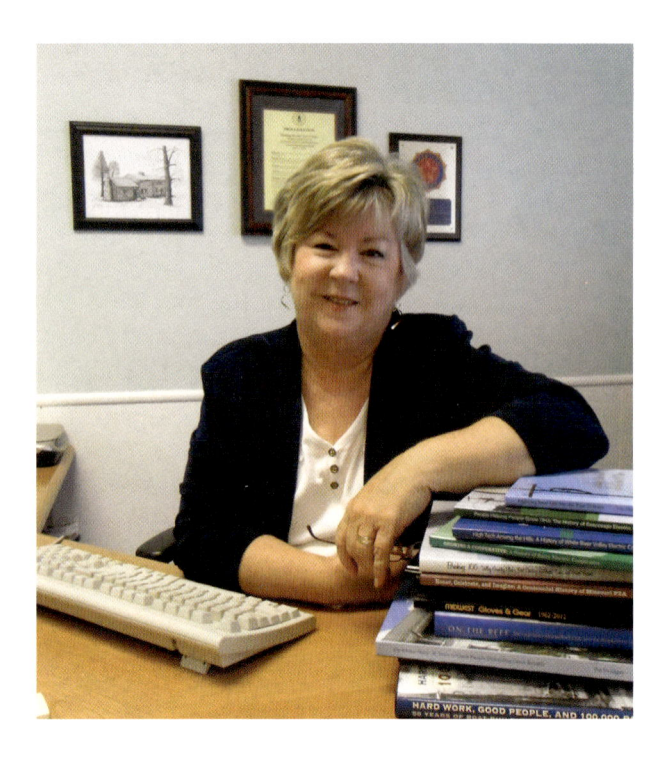

INDIANA
AT CHESTNUT RIDGE

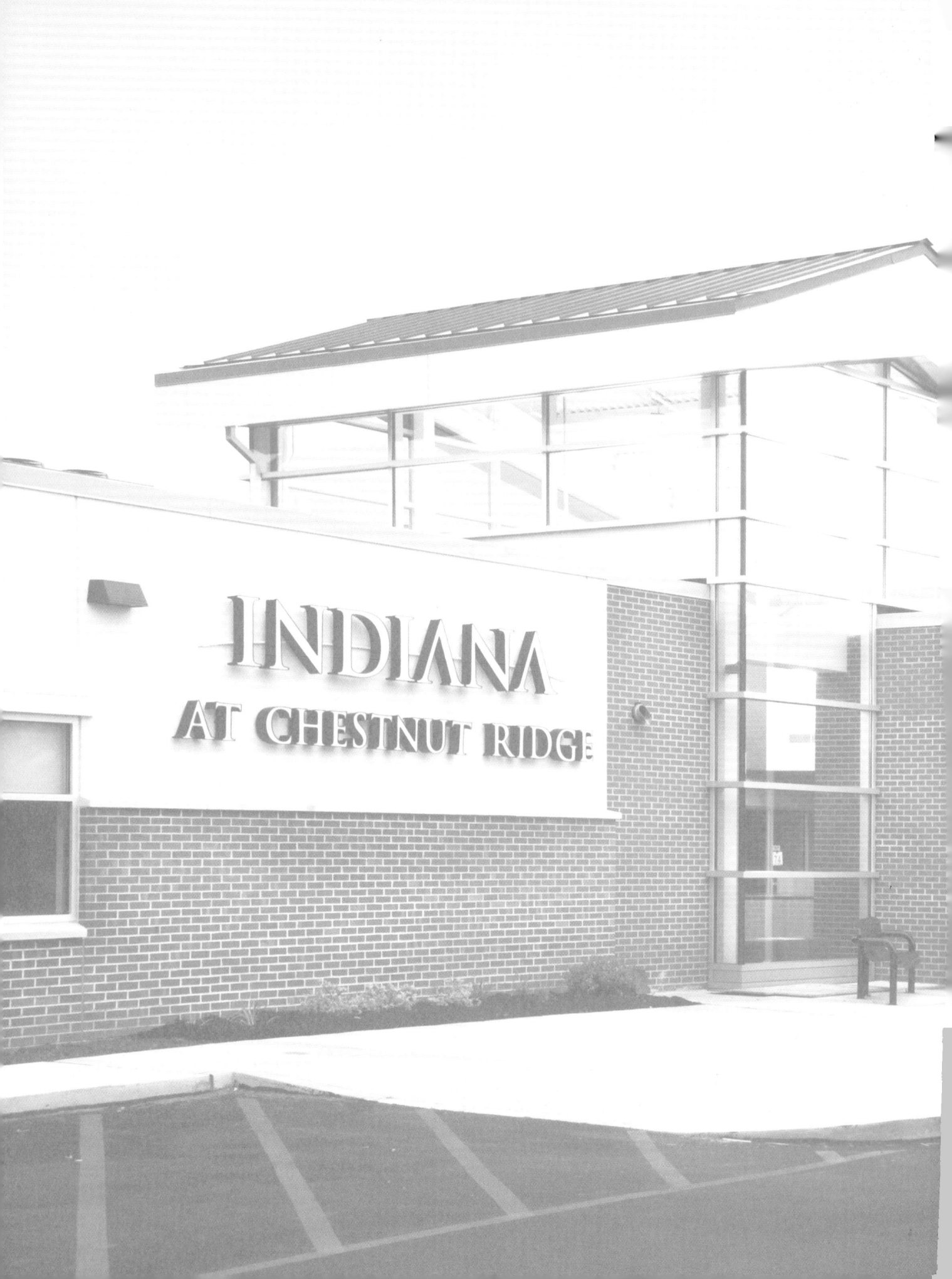